High Altitude Medicine

Jorge Hidalgo • Sabrina Da Re
António Gandra D'Almeida

Editors

High Altitude Medicine

A Case-Based Approach

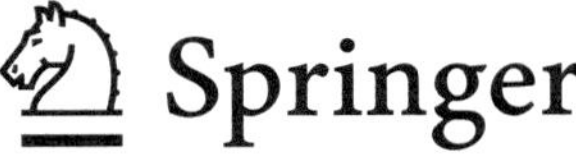

Editors
Jorge Hidalgo
Department of General ICU and
COVID-19 Unit
Belize Helthcare Partners Limited
Belize City, Belize

António Gandra D'Almeida
Department of critical care
Portuguese National Institute of Medical
Emergency
Porto, Portugal

Sabrina Da Re
Department of critical care
Hospital Materno Infantil
La Paz, Bolivia

ISBN 978-3-031-35094-8   ISBN 978-3-031-35092-4   (eBook)
https://doi.org/10.1007/978-3-031-35092-4

This Springer imprint is published by the registered company Springer Nature Switzerland AG
The registered company address is: Gewerbestrasse 11, 6330 Cham, Switzerland

- *Luigi Da Re, Lourdes Gutierrez, and Francesco Da Re for their deep love and understanding.*
- *Salgueiro Casso family.*
- *Health professionals interested in High Altitude pathology.*

Sabrina Da Re

To my parents, my lovely wife Gerhaldine, my daughter Allyson, and my son Benjamin.
—Jorge Hidalgo

I dedicate this book to my family especially to my children. Thank you so much for the love, support, and understanding for all the time that work keeps me away from you.
To Jorge and Geraldine that made this possible.
António Gandra d'Almeida
"The happiest man in the world is the one who knows how to recognize the merits of others and he can rejoice in the good of others as if he were his own."
Johann Wolfgang von Goethe

Foreword

Keen students of high altitude medicine and physiology may recall the exploits of Alexander Kellas on Mt Kamet in 1920. It was in those early years of high altitude exploration that physiology, medicine, and mountains have come together. Since then and over the years giants of high altitude science such as Griff Pugh, Michael Ward, Jim Milledge, John West, and others built the foundations of knowledge we now cherish with the publication of the core text High Altitude Medicine and Physiology in 1989, now in its 6th edition. One could say that a new specialty has been born. In many respects, high altitude medicine is the science of pushing the boundaries. They are boundaries of human endurance—physical and psychological. In 1980, Reinhold Messner conquered Mt Everest without using supplemental oxygen. In 2003, Mr Yūichirō Miura reached the summit of the same mountain aged 80. An American, Jordan Romero succeeded in reaching the summit aged 13. By the age of 15, he became the youngest person to accomplish the prized ascent of Seven Summits. Recently, all 14 eight thousand+ summits have been climbed in marathon succession by Nirmal Purja, who achieved it in under 7 months. From acclimatization, genetic predisposition, endurance training through geriatric and pediatric considerations high altitude medicine is now a vast and growing field. Whilst mountains were and continue to be the domain of professional mountaineers, there is increasing number of people ascending to high altitudes for leisure, taking part in commercial or charity expeditions, as well as heading there for work. It is not surprising that in those austere, remote and physiologically challenging environments, some of them fall ill. Specialists with an interest in mountain medicine are few and resources are not always available in those remote locations. What can be lifesaving is basic knowledge of high altitude medicine. This book, edited by Dr Jorge Hidalgo, aims to introduce concepts from the field in an approachable manner. It is not overbearing with facts and physiology, but at the same time it respects readers' thirst for understanding. The editor's intention has been to use "teaching moments" approach, basing clinical considerations on real cases. This allows to frame the approach to high altitude problems, whilst providing a sketch of the available evidence with regard to treatment. The evidence contours are not exhaustive, but this serves another purpose. Imperfection is an advantage as it fuels growth. A need to revise, reinvent, and re-appraise evidence means that this book has a potential to grow with time becoming a "living text" that adapts to our understanding of high altitude physiology and medicine. Multinational faculty contributing to this book does so with enthusiasm taking a reader on a journey by providing context to each case. I am hopeful that the book will find place not merely in university libraries, but on rough shelves of mountain shelters and remote health posts. Its format lends itself also to becoming an online resource for medics heading into the mountains, as well as those seeking introduction to an amazing medical specialty. Perhaps the knowledge contained within will help to save a life. "Great things are done when men and mountains meet; this is not done by jostling in the street"—remarked William Blake. Perhaps readers will meet with the book and find inspiration within those pages, to delve deeper into the mountains and mountain medicine, and to catch a breath of fresh air—as this is not done simply by jostling in the street.

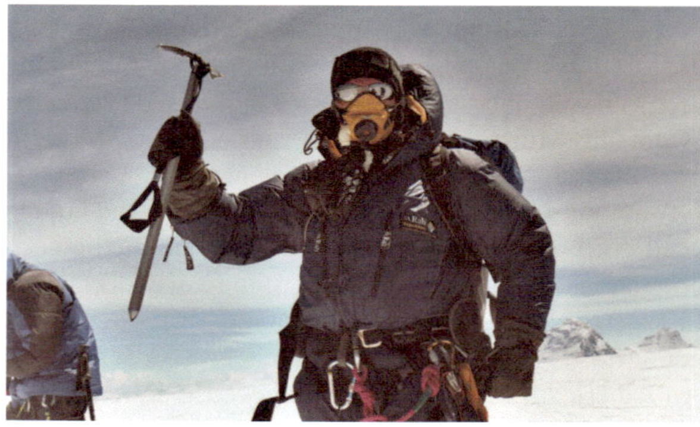

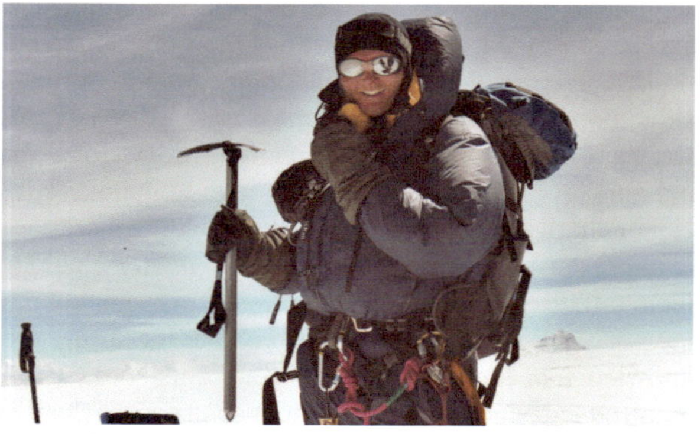

Consultant in Anesthesia and
Intensive Care Medicine
Frimley Health NHS Foundation Trust
Wexham Park Hospital, Slough, UK Piotr Szawarski

Acknowledgments

The preparation of this project *High Altitude Medicine* required the effort of many individuals. We want to thank the authors or collaborators for coming on board on this endeavor, being able to support the pressure of a timeline, taking a moment to satisfy the call for expertise and help, and keeping aside multiple other tasks and, indeed, personal time.

We sincerely appreciate the talent and accomplishments of the Springer professionals, Miranda Finch and in particular, Eugenia Judson, who partnered with us all along and took our manuscript and produced it into this book.

Finally, many thanks to our patients, the ultimate motive of us to be physicians, to whom we must express our gratitude. They trust us with their lives and give us the courage and motive to be consensually learning and actions to make us always keep the utmost attention to details. We welcome all comments, pros, cons, and suggested revisions.

MBBS, MRCPI (Internal Medicine, Dublin),
EDIC, DA (Diploma Anaesthesia, Gold Medal)
Chief Medical Officer and Head Critical Care and
Accident and Emergency
Swami Dayanand Hospital
New Delhi
India

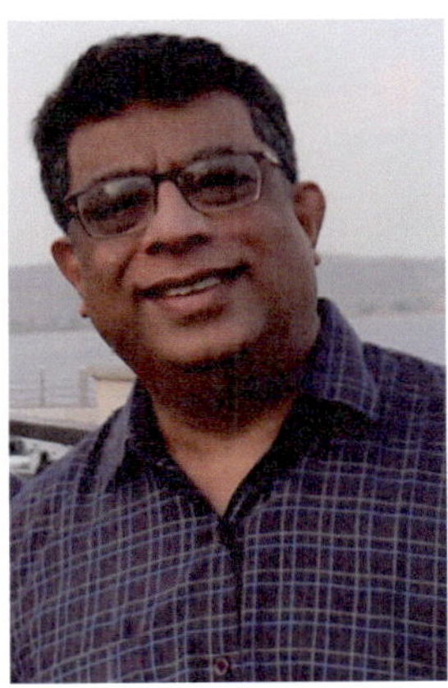

Dr Ranajit Chatterjee

We would like to express our deep gratitude to Professor Ranajit Chatterjee, for his academic contribution, enthusiastic encouragement, and for his useful and constructive recommendations for this project.

Contents

Chapter 1
Introduction to High Altitude Medicine

Jose Alfonso Rubio Mateo-Sidron, Fernando Eiras Abalde, and Jorge Hidalgo

Objectives

Know the pathophysiology of high-altitude diseases (HAI).
Know the clinical presentation of HAI.
Know the preventive measures of HAI.
Know the treatment of HAI.
Know the controversies in HAI.

Case Study

We present the case of a 32-year-old male from Europe (he lives about 2–10 m above sea level). He decided to go on a trip and do mountaineering. He had made several routes throughout his life, but never at such altitude. Its maximum height target was 5790 m. Over the course of 3 days, he progressively climbed, but upon reaching the refuge at 4708 m, he began feeling shortness of breath, fatigue, exhaustion and neurological disorders (improper speech, refusal to eat, incoordination). Nevertheless, he decided continue climbing until his final goal. Due to this progressive clinical deterioration, the team decided to descend to the shelter, where they

J. A. R. Mateo-Sidron
Critical Care Medicine, Hospital Universitario Vithas Arturo Soria, Madrid, Spain

F. E. Abalde (✉)
Intensive Care Unit (ICU), Pontevedra University Hospital Centre, Pontevedra, Spain
e-mail: fernando.eiras.abalde@sergas.com

J. Hidalgo
Critical Care, Belize Healthcare parners, Belize, Belize

J. Hidalgo et al. (eds.), *High Altitude Medicine*,
https://doi.org/10.1007/978-3-031-35092-4_1

began treatment with oxygen. He continued to deteriorate so he was transferred to a hospital.

Upon arrival at the hospital his vital signs were: T^a 35.5 °C HR 110lmp BP 135/85 mmHg FR 36 rpm SatO2 81% with ventimask reservoir. GSC 11/15. Auscultation showed cardiac tachycardia, and pulmonary generalized crackles. In lower limbs, there was mild edema.

Blood test showed: Biochemical: Glucose 113 mg / dl. Urea 34 mg / dl. Creatinine 0.7 mg / dl. Na 145 mEq / L. K 4.2 mEq / L. Arterial blood gas: pH 7.41 pCo2 40 mmHg pO2 51 mmHg SatO2 81% HCO3 26. Hemogram: Hb 13.9 g / dl. Platelets 85 × 109 / L. Leukocytes 7 × 109 / L. Coagulation: Normal. ECG: Sinus tachycardia. Normal QTc. Normal PR. Chest X-ray: bilateral diffuse interstitial infiltrates. Echocardiogram at bedside: No relevant alterations.

Treatment with dexamethasone and broad-spectrum antibiotics were started. Cultures were carried out.

At 24 h of admission, he persisted with progressive clinical deterioration, with worsening on the Glasgow to 7/15 and greater respiratory compromise in terms of mechanics, saturation, and hypoxia; therefore, it was decided to analogous sedation and relaxation, orotracheal intubation and connection to invasive mechanical ventilation. Throughout the days, the patient developed progressive neurological and respiratory improvement, which allowed extubating 5 days after admission to the ICU. Being discharged after 7 days.

Discussion of the Case

In our case, a patient without comorbidity who lives in an area of low altitude with respect to sea level, decides to undertake an ascent to more than 2500–3000 m. In addition, he does not carry out prophylactic measures prior to the ascent.

Based on the beginning of symptoms a few days after starting the ascent. Thorough clinical history, physical examination, and complementary tests, we can make differential diagnoses. The diagnostic hypothesis is: High altitude illness (HAI) which includes Acute Mountain sickness (AMS), High altitude cerebral edema (HACE) and High altitude pulmonary edema (HAPE).

On the one hand, the patient had some respiratory symptoms: cough, dyspnoea which progresses to cyanosis, tachypnoea, orthopnoea, and symptoms compatible with pulmonary edema. X-ray and laboratory tests were not suggestive of infectious disease, and echocardiography showed preserved LVEF.

HAPE is a non-cardiogenic pulmonary edema. Irregular pulmonary vasoconstriction, excessive perfusion in some areas, increased pulmonary capillary pressure and finally failure due to capillary "stress" occurs. Also, endothelial dysfunction due to hypoxia.

On the other hand, there were neurological symptoms: alterations in the level of consciousness, confusion, and ataxia of gait, progressing to further deterioration of the Glasgow.

HACE is produced by alteration of brain autoregulation in the presence of hypoxic cerebral vasodilation and permeability of the blood-brain barrier; all contribute to brain edema.

After starting treatment with corticosteroids and connection to mechanical ventilation, significant clinical improvement began.

Pathogeny

HAI encompasses the syndromes that can occur after an initial ascent to a high altitude, generally>2000-2500 m, or with a new ascent while at a high altitude. HAI includes: AMS, HACE, and HAPE [1].

The main mechanism that triggers these pathologies is hypobaric hypoxia (Hp). Hypoxia is defined as the reduction in the partial pressure of oxygen (PaO2) at the cellular level. This is the main causal agent of height-related diseases [2–4]. As the barometric pressure drops, so does the available oxygen. At high altitudes, especially when tissue oxygen demands are high, the marked reduction in pressure gradient and available oxygen can cause tissue hypoxia. There are other factors that influence barometric pressure, with little influence at low altitudes, but greater at high altitudes such as temperature and latitude [2].

The physiological compensation mechanisms for this Hp are acute or chronic:

Acute compensation mechanisms are divided into two stages (acclimatization and adaptation). The acclimatization stage runs from the ascent until about the fifth day. (a) Acute respiratory adaptation (hyperventilation) is the most immediate response. The hypoxic ventilatory response (HVR) is produced by the stimulation of peripheral chemoreceptors, producing an increase in minute ventilation. Increased ventilation increases alveolar pO2, reduces alveolar pCO2, increases pH. On the other hand, central chemoreceptors in the brain medulla respond to alkalosis in the cerebrospinal fluid (CSF) by inhibiting ventilation, so that the complete hypoxic ventilatory response is attenuated. (b) Acute circulatory adaptation (tachycardia). There is an increase in heart rate and cardiac output, increasing the supply of cellular oxygen. The other acute stage is Adaptation, which is established after the fifth day and produces an increase in haematocrit and improves the capacity to transport oxygen [2, 5–8].

Regarding chronic mechanisms, three are fundamentally three: (a) Erythrocytosis, defined as the increase in the number of red blood cells, which improves the O2 transport, causing an increase in blood viscosity. Increase in the synthesis of erythropoietin (EPO) by the kidney, stimulating the production of red blood cells in the bone marrow, the synthesis of 2,3-Diphosphoglycerate (2,3-DPG) is increased, producing a shift of the haemoglobin dissociation curve to the right. (b) Pulmonary vasoconstriction. HVR causes increased pulmonary vascular resistance, increased pulmonary arterial pressure, all with the aim of maintaining constant blood flow. Secondarily, the right ventricle hypertrophies when it must pump against a higher pressure. Cardiac output is initially elevated, with subsequent normalization. (c) At the tissue level, hypoxia-inducible factor 1 (HIF-1) is elevated, stimulates vascular endothelial growth factor (VEGF), which stimulates angiogenesis and nitric oxide synthesis. All this produces greater blood flow, greater supply of oxygen to the tissues, improvements in oxidative metabolism and the exchange of tissue gases [2, 6–9].

In the development of AMS and HACE, it is considered a continuum of the same disease by many authors, the mildest forms being AMS and the most serious being HACE. The event that initiates AMS is excessive cerebral vasodilation in response to hypoxemia [2, 3, 5]. There is also mild astrocytic inflammation caused by a redistribution of fluid from the extracellular to the intracellular space without evidence of cerebral edema. All of this can trigger the activation of the trigeminal vascular system, causing headaches and nausea [10, 11]. If it continues to evolve, it will develop HACE. Edema formation occurs in HACE (the relationship between cerebral edema and AMS is less clear), initially cytotoxic (intracellular) edema, later extravascular ionic edema, evolving to vasogenic edema with protein extravasation and, finally, loss of integrity of the BBB with extravasation of red blood cells and microbleeds [12]. Brain edema will cause increased intracranial pressure (ICP), which if not stopped could cause brain herniation and finally evolve to death [13].

HAPE is initiated by an increase in pulmonary arterial pressure, by an initial cascade of physiological responses that seek to compensate the hypoxia but which over time become harmful [5, 7]. This elevated pulmonary pressure, associated with unevenly perfused areas; by regional phenomena of uneven vasoconstriction; they result in a failure of the integrity of the alveolar-capillary barrier and an irregular pulmonary edema throughout the lung. This process continues with the breakdown of the alveolar-capillary barrier, producing leakage into the alveolar space of liquid, proteins and cells. This extravascular fluid in the alveolar spaces will make gas exchange difficult. If this is perpetuated, it will produce alveolar haemorrhage. There is a probable genetic component in the development of HAPE, not yet well studied, due to the interpersonal variability of the response to exposure in height [2, 5, 14].

Clinic

As we discussed earlier, most experts consider AMS and HACE to be different stages of severity of the same process [7, 15].

AMS Clinic

The onset of symptoms is highly variable. It can start very early, 1–2 h after the ascent, although it usually takes 6–12 h or up to 24 h. On the other hand, symptoms usually resolve within a day or two, if there is no further ascent.

Symptoms can be mild or very disabling. Among them mainly are headache, fatigue, light-headedness, anorexia, nausea, vomiting, and sleep disorders [16].

HACE Clinic

What characterizes and makes HACE different from the rest of the pathologies of the HAI spectrum are the neurological symptoms and signs; these include altered level of consciousness, irritability, confusion, drowsiness, stupor, coma, gait disturbance. Ataxia is one of the most characteristic symptoms; they also tend to have tandem gait involvement and much less frequent finger-nose involvement [10, 11, 15].

The appearance of general neurological signs should make us think about the probable evolution from AMS to HACE. This transition may be progressively or abruptly.

HAPE Clinic

Initial symptoms usually appear 2–4 days after the ascent, although sometimes it occurs earlier. It occurs more often at night or after strenuous exertion. Development after a week at the same altitude is very rare.

The most frequent symptoms of HAPE at the beginning are non-productive cough and dyspnoea on exertion. This progresses to dyspnoea at rest or with minimal effort, productive cough (pink, frothy sputum, or frank blood). All of this associated with tachycardia, tachypnoea, tirage, or low-grade fever. Crackles are frequent. The highlight of this pathology is the great dissociation between the patient's great hypoxemia and clinically finding a better patient than expected for this hypoxemia [4, 5].

The association between AMS / HACE and HAPE is frequent, especially as we increase in height [17].

One of the problems that are established to identify this pathology is that the symptoms are frequently confused with an infection of the upper respiratory tract or dyspnoea secondary to altitude or exhaustion.

There are another series of diseases related to altitude that we include in this section, as they are not specific to altitude, although they usually appear in these conditions.

Acute hypoxia. High altitude pharyngitis and bronchitis. Headache at high altitude. High altitude syncope. Organic brain syndrome. Peripheral edema. Periodic sleep breathing. Ultraviolet keratitis. High altitude retinopathy. Hypothermia and frostbite. Deterioration at high altitude. Pulmonary edema. Monge's disease, chronic mountain polycythaemia. High-altitude pulmonary hypertension. Pregnancy problems: pre-eclampsia, hypertension, and low-birth-weight babies. T cell dysfunction [18–20].

Diagnosis

AMS Diagnosis

AMS is diagnosed clinically in those patient who, having recently ascended high altitudes (generally more than 2000 m), initiates typical symptoms referred to in the section (CLINIC SECTION) [21].

Diagnosis is made by physical examination, vital signs, laboratory values, and SpO2 oxygen saturation.

If the symptoms appear more than 2 days after reaching the altitude, there is absence of headache, and there is not an improvement after administration of supplemental oxygen, this should make us consider an alternative diagnosis.

Radiographic or laboratory tests are not warranted unless the diagnosis is unclear [21–23].

There are diagnostic support scoring systems such as the Lake Louise AMS score (Table) [23]. Which is the most widely used standardized method today. There are another series of interesting tools such as Screening for acute mountain sickness.

HACE Diagnosis

The diagnosis is clinical, we must suspect it in a patient who makes an ascent in height and initiates neurological symptoms and signs (CLINICAL SECTION). The complementary tests are only useful to exclude other diagnoses, except brain magnetic resonance imaging (MRI).

In laboratory tests, an increase in the white series stands out. There is usually hypoxemia, respiratory alkalosis, and low saturation in pulse oximetry. CSF biochemistry will be normal, with increased opening pressure. The chest radiograph may reveal pulmonary edema or be normal. Brain computed tomography (CT) may show brain edema and signal attenuation [21, 23, 24].

Finally, in MRI, it is the most useful test, the characteristic pattern of magnetic resonance is observed, consisting mainly of involvement of the corpus callosum - preferably in the splenium (SCC). In FLAIR sequence, a lesion is marked in SCC, confirmed by DWI, with increased values in the apparent diffusion coefficient (ADC), which indicates a greater diffusion of the water compatible with vasogenic edema. The MRI can remain altered for days or weeks, highlighting that hemosiderin deposits could remain for years. There is no correlation between MRI severity and subsequent clinical outcome [25, 26].

2018 Lake Louise acute mountain sickness score

Headache		
	0 points	None at all
	1 points	A mild headach
	2 points	Moderate headache
	3 points	Severe headache, incapacitating
Gastrointestinal symptoms		
	0 points	Good appetite
	1 points	Poor appetite or nausea
	2 points	Moderate nausea or vomiting
	3 points	Severe nausea and vomiting, incapacitating
Fatigue and/or weakness		
	0 points	Not tired or weak
	1 points	Mild fatigue/weakness
	2 points	Moderate fatigue/weakness
	3 points	Severe fatigue/weakness, incapacitating
Dizziness/light-headedness		
	0 points	No dizziness/light-headedness
	1 points	Mild dizziness/light-headedness
	2 points	Moderate dizziness/light-headedness
	3 points	Severe dizziness/light-headedness, incapacitating
AMS clinical functional score		
Overall, if you had AMS symptoms, how did they affect your activities?		
	0 points	Not at all
	1 points	Symptoms present, but did not force any change in activity or itinerary
	2 points	My symptoms forced me to stop the ascent or to go down on my own power
	3 points	Had to be evacuated to a lower altitude

HAPE Diagnosis

It develops in those patients who, after an ascent, start the respiratory symptoms previously referred to (CLINIC SECTION). The diagnosis, as in the other pathologies related to the height, is based on the history and the physical examination.

Outstanding findings on examination include tachycardia, tachypnoea, tracing, low-grade fever, and lung crackles. The oxygen saturation by pulse oximetry is significantly decreased below that expected for altitude. Laboratory tests are not specific for diagnosis. The white series, brain natriuretic peptide (BNP), troponin may be elevated. [27, 28].

Chest X-ray may be helpful with chest X-ray. In it, bilateral alveolar infiltrates - very rare unilateral involvement - are usually observed, patchy predominantly in the right central hemithorax - not always -, which increase in size and converge with the progression of the disease [21, 28–30].

Chest computed tomography (CT) usually shows patchy lobular ground glass and consolidation opacities, reflecting a heterogeneous alveolar filling.

Echocardiography reveals an increase in pulmonary artery pressure and, occasionally, a dysfunction of the right heart. Lung ultrasound detects an increase in extravascular lung water consisting of B lines [31].

Differential Diagnosis (DD)

AMS DD

The AMS generates doubts at the time of diagnosis, since it has a heterogeneous clinic that can be confused with exhaustion or a viral clinic, like influenza, asthenia, generalized fatigue, myalgia, headache, exhaustion. On other occasions it is confused with dehydration - thirst, weakness, headache, and nausea- (the latter with a good response to fluid replacement) [4, 32, 33].

HACE DD

Hypothermia and taking medications can cause neurological alterations, so we must keep them in mind when establishing the diagnosis of HACE. When a focal neurological affectation is present (hemiparesis, speech alteration or a visual deficit) it should make us consider an alternative diagnosis (ischemic stroke, haemorrhage). There is an extensive list of pathologies with which to perform the differential diagnosis.

Ingestion of toxins, carbon monoxide toxicity, anxiety, brain neoplasms, Diabetic ketoacidosis, hypoglycaemia, hyponatremia, hypothermia, brain abscess, infection, Guillain-Barré syndrome, intracranial haemorrhage, ischemic stroke, transient ischemic attack, migraine, dehydration, King's syndrome [15, 32, 33].

HAPE DD

The main DD of HAPE is infectious. To differentiate it from pulmonary infectious pathology, we can help ourselves with the little clinical expressiveness of the picture in relation to the great hypoxemia and radiological affectation that the patient presents; as well as a good response to the supplementary oxygen therapy administered and the decrease in height. On the other hand, infectious pathology usually lasts longer. Pneumonia, although it can coexist with HAPE, is rare.

DD includes viral upper respiratory infection, pneumonia, bronchospasm, asthma, acute decompensated heart failure, exercise-associated hyponatremia, myocardial infarction, pulmonary embolism and pneumothorax [1, 5, 28, 33]

Treatment

AMS and HACE Treatment

Decrease in height is the best measure for AMS and HACE treatment. It is necessary in cases of progression of AMS, severe disease or HACE. The resolution of symptoms is variable for everyone, but usually improves after the descent from 300 to 1000 m [1].

Administered supplemental oxygen improves AMS symptoms and may serve as an alternative to descent or when symptoms are severe. Its use is necessary in cases of severe AMS progression or HACE [1, 35].

Portable hyperbaric chambers are effective in treating severe AMS or HACE. Symptoms improve significantly, but they usually reappear within 12 h. Its use should not delay the descent [1, 34, 35].

Acetazolamide treatment accelerates acclimatization to high altitudes. Only one study has examined it for the treatment of AMS, most use it in prevention. The dose studied was 250 mg every 12 h (72), although the usual dose is 125–250 mg twice a day (up to 750 mg a day) [1, 34, 36].

Dexamethasone is effective in improving symptoms, but it does not facilitate acclimatization. It should be used in moderate / severe AMS or HACE as soon as it is available. There are few studies, but extensive experience with its use in this pathology. The recommended dose is an 8 mg dose followed by 4 mg every 6 h until symptoms resolve. It can be used alone or in combination with acetazolamide [1, 34, 36].

As in all patients, we must assess ABCDE. Monitor the HACE patient for the probability of a low level of consciousness and the need for airway isolation. In addition, it is vitally important to monitor hypotension that may have repercussions in a probable cerebral ischemia due to alteration of cerebral autoregulation. On the other hand, once in a hospital centre, monitor intracranial pressure (ICP) to initiate general measures to control intracranial hypertension, if necessary, to avoid secondary brain damage.

HAPE Treatment

Although some treatments are the same for HAPE as for AMS / HACE, there are some differences, due to the pathophysiological difference of the disease.

The descent is indicated, when possible or when oxygen therapy treatment does not improve symptoms. It is also important to reduce physical activity to a minimum, as well as increasing the temperature [1, 34].

Supplemental oxygen is the vital part in the treatment of HAPE. When available, it should be given to achieve an SpO2 goal of>90% to relieve symptoms. Decreases hypoxemia, reduces pulmonary artery pressure, reverses capillary leak, and improves symptoms [1, 34].

The use of portable hyperbaric chambers should not delay descent in situations where descent is feasible. It can be combined, if available with oxygen therapy, pharmacotherapy. There are no systematic studies, but if it is collected in the literature. In the hospital environment, being at a lower altitude and having high-flow oxygen therapy; the use of hyperbaric therapy is usually not necessary [1, 34].

There is no systematic evidence that CPAP or EPAP improves patient outcomes compared to oxygen alone or in conjunction with medications [1, 37].

Nifedipine works by reducing pulmonary vascular resistance and pulmonary arterial pressure. Its usefulness is based on a single study, and it is proposed that it can be used as an adjuvant therapy when there is no oxygen available or portable hyperbaric chamber, or when the descent is difficult. Prospective study proposed little utility. Recommended dosages vary, but a common regimen is to administer 30 mg (slow-release formulation) every 12 h [1, 34, 38].

There is little evidence of the use of beta-agonists in HAPE. Although they could be useful [1].

The use of PDE-5 phosphodiesterase inhibitors: Sildenafil and tadalafil produce pulmonary vasodilation and decrease the pressure of the pulmonary artery. No systematic study has evaluated it, but physiologically it seems that they may be useful. Its use is considered as a therapy when there is no available oxygen or portable hyperbaric chamber, or when the descent is difficult and nifedipine is not available. Avoid combined use of nifedipine and sildenafil or tadalafil should be avoided due to risk of hypotension [1, 39].

Regarding the use of dexamethasone, there is discrepancy among the experts. A priori it could be useful (prevention of HAPE, reduction of lung inflammation). No study has established whether it is effective. There is no recommendation in this regard. If may be useful when coexisting with AMS / HACE [1, 40].

Prevention

Within prevention, it is important to carry out a physical examination, as well as a clinical interview before the ascent; so we can predict those people with a higher risk of developing disease at altitude.

Those people who have been to a high altitude before, knowing the behaviour that they have previously had, will serve as a predictor of behaviour when they are exposed to that same height. We have the biggest problem in those people who have never been exposed to heights; for this, there is a model to identify people at risk of suffering a serious altitude illness, although this model is currently being questioned [22, 41].

AMS/HACE Preventive

Gradual ascent is a very useful measure in preventing disease. A gradual ascent is recommended, planning the ascent speed, and above all, even more importantly the overnight altitude [1, 34].

Acetazolamide should be taken prophylactically, in people at moderate or high risk of AMS with high-altitude ascent. Facilitates acclimatization. The recommended prophylaxis dose for adults is 125 mg every 12 h (up to 750 mg daily) [1, 34].

Dexamethasone does not facilitate acclimatization. There is a benefit in preventing AMS. Doses are 2 mg every 6 h or 4 mg every 12 h (Consider even 4 mg every 6 h in very high-risk situations). It can be used as an alternative to acetazolamide for adult travellers at moderate or high risk of AMS [1, 34].

Acetazolamide and dexamethasone should be started the day before the ascent, but still have beneficial effects if started on the day of the ascent.

Ibuprofen can be used for the prevention of AMS in people who do not want to take other preventive medication.

The use of paracetamol or budesonide inhaled is not recommended [1].

When possible, ascent in stages and pre-acclimatization can be considered as a method of prevention of AMS. In literature it is not studied at all. It seems, is that spending 6–7 days at a moderate altitude (2200–3000 m) before proceeding to a higher altitude reduces the risk of AMS [1, 34].

Hypoxic tents can be helpful in facilitating acclimatization and prevention of AMS, provided sufficiently long exposures are taken regularly.

Products derived from coca or Gingko biloba, reduced AMS in some trials, but in others. No recommendation can be made [1, 42].

Other methods without evidence: antioxidants, iron, dietary nitrates, leukotriene receptor blockers, phosphodiesterase inhibitors, salicylic acid, spironolactone, and sumatriptan, "forced"or "excessive" hydration [1].

HAPE Preventive

Some of the prophylactic methods are the same for AMS / HACE as for HAPE, important differences in pathophysiology establish small changes.

A gradual ascent is the main method of preventing HAPE. Although it is true that no studies have evaluated it prospectively, there is a clear relationship between the rate of ascent and the incidence of diseases [1, 34, 39].

Nifedipine is recommended for the prevention of HAPE in people susceptible to HAPE. The recommended dose is 30 mg prolonged-release every 12 h. It should start the day before the ascent and continue until the descent begins or 4–7 days have passed at the highest elevation [1, 34, 39].

Tadalafil can be used for the prevention of HAPE in known susceptible individuals who are not candidates for nifedipine [1, 34, 39].

Dexamethasone can be used to prevent HAPE in known susceptible individuals who are not candidates for nifedipine and tadalafil [1, 34, 39].

Acetazolamide accelerates acclimatization and should be effective in prevention. If that could be recommended for prevention in people with a history of HAPE [1, 34, 39].

Salmeterol is not recommended for HAPE Prevention [1, 34].

Pre-acclimatization and staggered ascent: No studies have examined this in HAPE. But it seems clear that it would be recommended [1, 34].

Question Discussion

We have already discussed many of the controversies throughout the topic, and we will leave many others behind; but I would like to emphasize the following.

Is there increased cerebral blood flow in patients with AMS?

Hypoxemia produced by AMS may involve increased cerebral blood flow (CBF). The CBS is not clear that there are differences between those with and without AMS. There are controversial results, possibly due to changes in the diameter of the middle cerebral artery (CBS remained unchanged); changes in internal carotid artery diameter were not correlated with high altitude headache [36, 43].

What is the dose of acetazolamide in prophylaxis?

Acetazolamide is important in the prophylaxis of AMS. There is much debate about the appropriate dose. Most studies suggest that 125 mg twice a day is sufficient, but higher doses may be necessary in too rapid ascents and / or ascents to very high final altitudes [1, 36, 44].

Is the use of intermittent hypobaric or normobaric hypoxic exposures useful prior to ascent?

Studies have reported conflicting results regarding intermittent hypobaric or normobaric hypoxic exposures, with some studies showing benefit and others showing no clear effect [45, 46].

Key Points
- Early identification of diseases associated with altitude is important. Especially HACE and HAPE.
- The evaluation of patients prior to the ascent and the implementation of prevention measures play an important role in this type of pathology.
- The most important prevention is gradual ascent, acetazolamide and sometimes dexamethasone or nifedipine.
- Hyperbaric hypoxia is the main trigger mechanism, understanding the pathophysiology allows us to understand how to address it.
- Once the disease is established, administering supplemental oxygen, lowering the height, hyperbaric chambers, and sometimes dexametamethasone are vital for the patient.

References

1. McIntosh SE, Freer L, Grissom CK, Auerbach PS, Rodway GW, Cochran A, et al. Wilderness medical society clinical practice guidelines for the prevention and treatment of frostbite: 2019 update. Wilderness Environ Med. 2019 Dec;30(4S):S19–32.
2. West JB. American College of Physicians, American Physiological Society. The physiologic basis of high-altitude diseases. Ann Intern Med. 2004;141(10):789–800.
3. Anholm JD, Foster GP. Con: hypoxic pulmonary vasoconstriction is not a limiting factor of exercise at high altitude. High Alt Med Biol. 2011;12(4):313–7.
4. Hackett PH, Roach RC. High-altitude illness. N Engl J Med. 2001;345(2):107–14.
5. Gallagher SA, Hackett PH. High-altitude illness. Emerg Med Clin North Am. 2004;22(2):329–55. viii
6. Tinoco-Solórzano A, Nieto Estrada VH, Vélez-Páez JL, Molano Franco D, Viruez SA, Villacorta-Córdova F, Avila Hilari A, Cahuaya Choque CA. Medicina intensiva en la altitud. revisión de alcance. Revista de Medicina Intensiva y Cuidados Críticos. 2020;13(4):218–25.
7. Schoene RB. Illnesses at high altitude. Chest. 2008 Aug;134(2):402–16.
8. Monge C, Leon-Velarde F, Rivera M, Palacios J. Altura: Conocimientos Basicos: Realizacion: Unidad De Diagnostico De Tolerancia A La Altura (Udta) I Hipoxia (médica) I Edema. Inst Investig Altura UPCH. 2000;1(1):1–11.
9. West JB. Physiological effects of chronic hypoxia. N Engl J Med. 2017;376(20):1965–71.
10. Sanchez del Rio M, Moskowitz MA. High altitude headache. Lessons from headaches at sea level. Adv Exp Med Biol. 1999;474:145–53.
11. Wilson MH, Newman S, Imray CH. The cerebral effects of ascent to high altitudes. Lancet Neurol. 2009;8(2):175–91.
12. Meier D, Collet T-H, Locatelli I, Cornuz J, Kayser B, Simel DL, et al. Does this patient have Acute Mountain sickness?: the rational clinical examination systematic review. JAMA. 2017;318(18):1810–9.

13. Dickinson J, Heath D, Gosney J, Williams D. Altitude-related deaths in seven trekkers in the Himalayas. Thorax. 1983;38(9):646–56.
14. MacInnis MJ, Wang P, Koehle MS, Rupert JL. The genetics of altitude tolerance: the evidence for inherited susceptibility to acute mountain sickness. J Occup Environ Med. 2011;53(2):159–68.
15. Basnyat B, Murdoch DR. High-altitude illness. Lancet Lond Engl. 2003;361(9373):1967–74.
16. Bezruchka S. High altitude medicine. Med Clin North Am. 1992;76(6):1481–97.
17. Hultgren HN, Honigman B, Theis K, Nicholas D. High-altitude pulmonary edema at a ski resort. West J Med. 1996;164(3):222–7.
18. Paralikar SJ, Paralikar JH. High-altitude medicine. Indian J Occup Environ Med. 2010;14(1):6–12.
19. Zafren K, Honigman B. High-altitude medicine. Emerg Med Clin North Am. 1997;15(1):191–222.
20. Alexander JK. Coronary problems associated with altitude and air travel. Cardiol Clin. 1995;13(2):271–8.
21. Luks AM, Swenson ER, Bärtsch P. Acute high-altitude sickness. Eur Respir Rev Off J Eur Respir Soc. 2017;26(143):160096.
22. Richalet J-P, Larmignat P, Poitrine E, Letournel M, Canouï-Poitrine F. Physiological risk factors for severe high-altitude illness: a prospective cohort study. Am J Respir Crit Care Med. 2012;185(2):192–8.
23. Roach RC, Hackett PH, Oelz O, Bärtsch P, Luks AM, MacInnis MJ, et al. The 2018 Lake Louise Acute Mountain sickness score. High Alt Med Biol. 2018;19(1):4–6.
24. Stokum JA, Gerzanich V, Simard JM. Molecular pathophysiology of cerebral edema. J Cereb Blood Flow Metab Off J Int Soc Cereb Blood Flow Metab. 2016;36(3):513–38.
25. Bailey DM, Bärtsch P, Knauth M, Baumgartner RW. Emerging concepts in acute mountain sickness and high-altitude cerebral edema: from the molecular to the morphological. Cell Mol Life Sci CMLS. 2009;66(22):3583–94.
26. Hackett PH, Yarnell PR, Weiland DA, Reynard KB. Acute and evolving MRI of High-altitude cerebral edema: microbleeds, edema, and pathophysiology. AJNR Am J Neuroradiol. 2019;40(3):464–9.
27. Jones BE, Stokes S, McKenzie S, Nilles E, Stoddard GJ. Management of high altitude pulmonary edema in the Himalaya: a review of 56 cases presenting at Pheriche medical aid post (4240 m). Wilderness Environ Med. 2013;24(1):32–6.
28. Swenson ER, Bärtsch P. High-altitude pulmonary edema. Compr Physiol. 2012;2(4):2753–73.
29. Vock P, Brutsche MH, Nanzer A, Bärtsch P. Variable radiomorphologic data of high altitude pulmonary edema. Features from 60 patients. Chest. 1991;100(5):1306–11.
30. Fiorenzano G, Dottorini M. Unilateral High-altitude pulmonary edema. Ann Am Thorac Soc. 2017;14(9):1492–3.
31. Ma D, Bao H, Zhang H, Shi H, Li C, Li W, et al. Application of lung ultrasound examination in severe high altitude pulmonary edema. Zhonghua Wei Zhong Bing Ji Jiu Yi Xue. 2017;29(9):815–20.
32. Hackett PH, Roach RC. High altitude cerebral edema. High Alt Med Biol. 2004;5(2):136–46.
33. Rodway GW, Hoffman LA, Sanders MH. High-altitude-related disorders--Part I: Pathophysiology, differential diagnosis, and treatment. Heart Lung J Crit Care. 2003 Dec;32(6):353–9.
34. Bärtsch P, Swenson ER. Clinical practice: acute high-altitude illnesses. N Engl J Med. 2013;368(24):2294–302.
35. Bärtsch P, Merki B, Hofstetter D, Maggiorini M, Kayser B, Oelz O. Treatment of acute mountain sickness by simulated descent: a randomised controlled trial. BMJ. 1993;306(6885):1098–101.
36. Bartsch P, Bailey DM, Berger MM, Knauth M, Baumgartner RW. Acute mountain sickness: controversies and advances. High Alt Med Biol. 2004;5(2):110–24.
37. Johnson PL, Johnson CC, Poudyal P, Regmi N, Walmsley MA, Basnyat B. Continuous positive airway pressure treatment for Acute Mountain sickness at 4240 m in the Nepal Himalaya. High Alt Med Biol. 2013;14(3):230–3.

38. Oelz O, Maggiorini M, Ritter M, Waber U, Jenni R, Vock P, et al. Nifedipine for high altitude pulmonary oedema. Lancet Lond Engl. 1989;2(8674):1241–4.
39. Fagenholz PJ, Gutman JA, Murray AF, Harris NS. Treatment of high altitude pulmonary edema at 4240 m in Nepal. High Alt Med Biol. 2007;8(2):139–46.
40. Mairbäurl H, Baloglu E. Con: corticosteroids are useful in the management of HAPE. High Alt Med Biol. 2015;16(3):190–2.
41. Canouï-Poitrine F, Veerabudun K, Larmignat P, Letournel M, Bastuji-Garin S, Richalet J-P. Risk prediction score for severe high altitude illness: a cohort study. PLoS One. 2014;9(7):e100642.
42. Seupaul RA, Welch JL, Malka ST, Emmett TW. Pharmacologic prophylaxis for acute mountain sickness: a systematic shortcut review. Ann Emerg Med. 2012;59(4):307–317.e1.
43. Wilson MH, Edsell MEG, Davagnanam I, Hirani SP, Martin DS, Levett DZH, et al. Cerebral artery dilatation maintains cerebral oxygenation at extreme altitude and in acute hypoxia--an ultrasound and MRI study. J Cereb Blood Flow Metab Off J Int Soc Cereb Blood Flow Metab. 2011;31(10):2019–29.
44. Dumont L, Mardirosoff C, Tramèr MR. Efficacy and harm of pharmacological prevention of acute mountain sickness: quantitative systematic review. BMJ. 2000;321(7256):267–72.
45. Schommer K, Wiesegart N, Menold E, Haas U, Lahr K, Buhl H, et al. Training in normobaric hypoxia and its effects on acute mountain sickness after rapid ascent to 4559 m. High Alt Med Biol. 2010;11(1):19–25.
46. Beidleman BA, Muza SR, Fulco CS, Cymerman A, Ditzler D, Stulz D, et al. Intermittent altitude exposures reduce acute mountain sickness at 4300 m. Clin Sci Lond Engl 1979. 2004;106(3):321–8.

Chapter 2
History of High Altitude Medicine

Ahsina Jahan Lopa, Ranajit Chatterjee, and Sharmili Sinha

HAPE

Introduction

Human race has always been eager for the quest to reveal the unknown, to reach unimaginable destinations, to explore the depth of the deepest ocean or to climb and conquer the inaccessible mountain peaks. The thirst of climbing the snow-capped mountains, in extreme cold and thin air, lead to numerous ailments. Many fell ill and lost their lives, haunted by the wrath of nature. Slowly but steadily however, mankind started getting acquainted with these unusual ailments. As the number of expeditions increased, a new science developed- high altitude medicine. In modern times, millions of people, many of them amateurs, rush for pure recreation and adventurism. This chapter aims at going to the depth of this interesting development which took place over centuries.

A. J. Lopa (✉)
ICU and Emergency Department, Shahabuddin Medical College Hospital, Dhaka, Bangladesh

R. Chatterjee
Anesthesiology and Critical Care, Swami Dayanand Hospital, Delhi, New Delhi, India

S. Sinha
Critical Care Medicine, Apollo Hospital, Bhubaneswar, Odisha, India

© The Author(s), under exclusive license to Springer Nature Switzerland AG 2023
J. Hidalgo et al. (eds.), *High Altitude Medicine*,
https://doi.org/10.1007/978-3-031-35092-4_2

History of High-Altitude Medicine

That high altitude can have deleterious effects on the body has long been recognized. Perhaps the first reference to illness associated with altitude was recorded nearly 2000 years ago by Tseen Hanshoo, who described the "Great and Little Headache" mountains on the journey along the Silk Road [1]. A description of a monk foaming at the mouth during the ascent of a mountain pass in AD 403 is believed to have been a form of high-altitude sickness [2].

Soroche and Puna

Breathlessness due to lack of oxygen at high altitudes was misinterpreted though ages . In the sixteenth century, there is a popular belief that the air of the mountain is poisonous known as the "Sickness of the Andes" or "Soroche". In certain parts of Peru and Bolivia this was also called "Puna". People of Europe never experienced this phenomenon until thy started exploring the heights of Mt. Blanc in eighteenth century.

Ballooning and High Altitude

Beginning with the eighteenth century, ballooning has continually achieved higher altitudes. From Charles's 3000-metre (10,000-foot) ascent in 1783 to U.S. Army Air Corps Capt. Hawthorne C. Gray's fatal ascent to 12,950 metres (42,470 feet) in 1927, the maximum altitude was only limited by the pilot's need for oxygen. Paul Bert was the first person to clearly state that the deleterious effects of high altitude were caused by the low partial pressure of oxygen (PO2), and later research was accelerated by high-altitude stations and expeditions to high altitude [3].

Exploring the Everest

Harsh weather conditions had spoilt many near successful events and lot of lives had been lost in those great heights. Also, the rumours of unseen but ferocious and ghostly creatures had also been circulated amongst travellers. On June 8 1924, George Mallory and Andrew Ivrine was observed within 600 ft. from the peak by fellow photographer and climber Noel Odell. But they were swept away by an enormous storm. Mallory's body was recovered after 75 years in 1999. Surprisingly, he was remarkably intact. History was created when Sir Edmund Hillary and Tenzing Norge conquered the highest peak on earth, the invincible mount Everest in 1953. In 1960, Charles Houston, an Aspen internist, described noncardiogenic pulmonary edema i.e. high-altitude pulmonary edema (HAPE), in a healthy 21-year-old cross-country skier.[4] More "firsts" followed, over the next three decades. Junko Tabei, a Japanese teacher, climbed the peak in 1975. The first solo ascent by Reinhold Messner was an incredible feat as the first traverse (up one side of the mountain and down the other) and the first descent on skis.

Conquering the Height Without Oxygen

But all of these climbers had relied on bottled oxygen to achieve their high-altitude feats. Could Mt. Everest be conquered without it? As early as the 1920s, mountain climbers debated the pros and cons of artificial aids. One, George Leigh Mallory, argued "that the climber does best to rely on his natural abilities, which warn him whether he is overstepping the bounds of his strength. With artificial aids, he exposes himself to the possibility of sudden collapse if the apparatus fails." In 1920, the British physiologist Alexander M. Kellas predicted that "Mount Everest could be ascended by a man of excellent physical and mental constitution in first-rate training, without adventitious aids if the difficulties are not too great. "The philosophy that nothing should come between a climber and his mountain continued to have adherents 50 years later. In 1960–1961, Sir Edmund Hillary concluded that oxygen levels at the summit of Mt. Everest were only enough to support a body at rest—and that the oxygen demands of a climber in motion would certainly be too great. But nothing seems to be impossible for mankind. Sometime between 1 and 2 in the afternoon on May 8, 1978, Reinhold Messner and Peter Habeler achieved what was believed to be impossible—the first ascent of Mt. Everest without oxygen. Messner described his feeling: "In my state of spiritual abstraction, I no longer belong to myself and to my eyesight. I am nothing more than a single narrow gasping lung, floating over the mists and summits. The feat of these two gentlemen (termed by many fellow climbers as lunatics) puzzled the whole medical community and forced them to rethink about the unexplored areas of human physiology. The large number of Indian troops stationed in the Himalayas provided further description of HAPE in otherwise healthy young men.5 In 1991, a group of experts met to define criteria for the diagnosis of illnesses associated with high altitude. These are known as Lake Louis Criteria.

The "Great and the Little Headache"

The history of scaling heights started 2000 years ago by travellers travelling through the silk route from China to India. One of the principle difficulties they faced was headache. Tseen Hansoo described this headache while writing his experience traveling the silk route [5]. He named the area "Great Headache Mountain" and "Little Headache Mountain." Modern evidence that headache occurs frequently at high altitude comes from studies of people living in the South American Andes and from soldiers of the Indian Army who moved frequently between sea level and altitudes up to 6000 meters in the Himalayas [6].

Headache is a common symptom in almost half of the thousands of people who Ski, trek or climb, at heights over 3000 meters (9900 feet). Mexico City is at a height of 2240 m from sea level. The Mexico city Olympics of 1968 witnessed migraine headache occurring more frequently amongst athletes and specterors than Olympics held at lower altitudes.

Headache may be a prominent symptom in people with chronic exposure to high altitude. A door-to-door population-based epidemiological study of the prevalence of migraine and headache in a sample of 3246 people older than 15 years of age was carried out in Cuzco, a high-altitude town in the Peruvian Andes, located at 3380 m. Among the 3246 screened people, there were 172 cases of migraine and 930 cases of headache, yielding a crude 1-year prevalence of 5.3% for migraine (2.3% among men and 7.8% among women) and 28.7% for headache (17.5% among men and 38.2% among women). The prevalence of headache was higher at high altitudes than at sea level [7].The incidence of High altitude headache is directly proportional to age because the lungs' efficiency in supplying oxygen to the body declines with age in all individuals, oxygen levels in the blood may decrease even further with advancing age in those who reside at high altitudes. Since migraine occurs more commonly when the blood level of oxygen falls, this might explain why headaches seem to increase with age in those who live at higher altitudes.

We now recognize that nearly one in four people who ascend to 2600 m (8500 feet) above sea level develop symptoms referred to as acute mountain sickness (AMS). Headache is the most prominent symptom of AMS and may be accompanied by other symptoms including Sleep disturbances, Loss of appetite, Nausea, Dizziness, Vomiting,Fatigue and Weakness.

The most important variables affecting the incidence of AMS according to studies include an individual's birthplace, acclimatization in the week before the travel, the rate of change in altitude and days of rest while ascending. Rest days were most potent protective variable.

How Can You Identify with Acute Mountain Sickness Headache?

Mountaineers slowly started learning the symptoms and signs of AMS headache. This unique headache is usually intense, throbbing and is either generalized or in the forehead. It develops within 6 h to 4 days of arrival at high altitude and can last for up to 5 days. The headache often worsens with exertion, coughing, straining or lying flat. Facial flushing, eye redness and sensitivity to light may accompany headache. The headache does not appear to be the result of low blood oxygen (hypoxia) alone because the attack often doesn't begin for hours to days after thriving at the higher altitude. Furthermore, oxygen therapy does not usually relieve the headache. Fortunately, these headaches generally go away after descent to sea level, although in unusual instances the headache may persist for several days to months. The underlying cause of the headache remains unknown. Swelling of blood vessels has been considered as a potential cause, but not confirmed with experimental studies. Some experts feel that the brain swells with increased pressure within the headache, but no direct evidence exists for this explanation either.

In addition to these medications, there are several tricks to avoiding or limiting the discomfort of adjusting to high altitude for those who are susceptible, mountaineers started learning as to how to tackle headache by simply by avoiding dehydration, gradual ascent with adequate rest. Medicines developed gradually over years and headache now can easily be managed. The whole process of learning took decades.

Conclusion

In this way, slowly but steadily, mankind started to explore the unknown, scaled the greatest heights, learnt the skills to conquer it even without supplemental oxygen, won over severe headache and acclimatised with this most adverse of environments. I salute those unsung heroes whose sacrifice today gives us the courage to write such a book.

References

1. West JB, Alexander M. Kellas and the physiological challenge of Mt. Everest. J Appl Physiol. 1987;63:3–11.
2. Rennie D. The great breathlessness mountains. JAMA. 1986;256:81–2.
3. West JB, et al. Early history of high altitude physiology. Ann N Y Acad Sci. 2016;1365(1):33–42.
4. Houston CS. Acute pulmonary edema of high altitude. N Engl J Med. 1960;263:478–80.
5. Singh I, Kapila CC, Khanna PK, Nanada RB, Rao BD. High-altitude pulmonary edema. Lancet. 1965;191:229–34.
6. Krieger BP, de la Hoz RE. Altitude-related pulmonary disorders. Crit Care Clin. 1999;15:265–80.
7. Jaillard AS, Mazetti P, Kala E. Prevalence of migraine and headache in a high-altitude town of Peru: a population-based study. Headache. 1997;37(2):95–101. https://doi.org/10.1046/j.1526-46 10.1997.3702095.x.

Chapter 3
Genetics in High Altitude Medicine

Prithwis Bhattacharyya, Prakash Deb, and Debasis Pradhan

Case Scenario

A team of four young people who are inhabitants of low altitude areas of Indian subcontinent went for an expedition in one of the mountain peaks in Nepal with an altitude of ~7000 m. The team had an expert High altitude climbing Sherpa along with porters who are inhabitants of high-altitude Himalayan ranges. On reaching an altitude of 4700 m some of the team mates started having headache, nausea and breathlessness. They had tachycardia, low SpO2 (~78–84%) detected in pulse oximeter. They were given supplemental oxygen and symptoms improved. To the surprise of the teammates, one member in their group had climbed to the destination even without a single episode of discomfort or any complain comparable with the sherpa and the potters.

Q. *What could be the probable reason of this medical condition in the group member? What are the other complications possible in high altitude climbers? Why was the group member or the Sherpa resilient to the high-altitude changes?*

A: The symptoms are suggestive of Acute Mountain Sickness, which develops due to low barometric pressure of oxygen in high altitude leading to some physiological changes in an attempt to increase oxygen delivery to the vital organs. High

P. Bhattacharyya (✉)
Department of Critical Care Medicine, Trauma and Emergency Medicine, Pacific Medical College, Udaipur, Rajasthan, India

P. Deb
Department of Anaesthesiology, Critical care and Pain medicine, AIIMS, Guwahati, Assam, India

D. Pradhan
Anaesthesia, NHS Derby and Burton, Derby, UK

J. Hidalgo et al. (eds.), *High Altitude Medicine*,
https://doi.org/10.1007/978-3-031-35092-4_3

altitude illness may be in the form of High-altitude loss of appetite, headache, pulmonary hypertension, pulmonary edema or cerebral edema etc.

There are phenotypic differences in the individuals residing at high altitude like Sherpas with that of low altitude dwellers. These changes help adapt them not only to the low oxygen conditions but also to the extreme physical excursion. There are advantages of natural selection to this group of people and is still ongoing. Genes responsible for the adaptative changes have been studied and are distinct even in different high-altitude inhabitants. Even with same types of physical built or rate of ascent or time for acclimatization, susceptibility to high altitude sickness is also different among low altitude dwellers which may be due to variants in genetic loci.

Introduction

Human physiology experiences diverse adaptive changes in high altitude in response to low atmospheric oxygen. Some of the changes are acute occurring in people living at the sea level reaching to high altitude, while others are consistent with high altitude inhabitants. Some of the conditions are common and easily reversible with descend, increasing inspired fraction of oxygen or barometric pressure as in passenger aircraft. Complications like High altitude pulmonary edema and High-altitude cerebral edema are life threatening and requires immediate recognition and treatment. The ability to tolerate hypoxia and the susceptibility to high altitude illnesses are different amongst the natives of different high-altitude locations. Extensive researches in this field found many phenotypic differences in high altitude Tibetans, Andeans, Chinese and Ethiopian population and a potential link with genetic changes has been described. Some populations have been exposed to the chances of natural selection and the process is ongoing leading to different levels of tolerance and adaptative changes in hypoxic conditions.

Role of Genetics in High Altitude Adaptation

Acute mountain sickness occurs in low landers due to sudden ascent to high altitude (≥ 2500 m) and is attributed to the less barometric pressure of oxygen in alveoli and blood. To sustain vital function in spite of less availability of oxygen, there is requirement of higher oxygen delivery and need to increase basal metabolic rate in this population which manifests itself through different signs and symptoms. For high altitude dwellers, the maximum oxygen consumption rate or aerobic capacity is comparable with the people living at sea level and is higher than the low altitude people who climbed to high altitude level. High landers have adapted well to low level of hemoglobin to maintain oxygenation even during heavy physical excursion. Prevalence of High-altitude headache and

Acute Mountain sickness in low landers reaching high altitude compared to high altitude inhabitants show an advantage of natural selection in population who settled there thousands of years ago, which is evident on recent genomic studies.

People migrated to high altitude locations from their places of origin under various survival challenges. Over thousands of years of inhabitation have given them the privilege of natural selection to settle with a lower basal metabolic rate, higher aerobic capacity and other hematological and cardiorespiratory adjustments. The evolutionary steps are however distinct among different groups of people residing in high altitude locations in different parts of the globe.

For example, Tibetans have higher resting minute ventilation and hypoxic ventilatory response compared to Andean high landers. These are dominant adaptive changes seen in low landers exposed acutely to high altitude in an attempt to increase oxygen delivery and increase dramatically to a high level acutely and settle down to a lower range over days and months. The change in adaptive features among different groups of high-altitude residents are not uniform which raised the possibility of distinct genetic factors. Beall C M described in details about other phenotypic differences between Tibetans and Andeans and pointed towards different evolutionary routes towards the adaptive changes in the high-altitude conditions necessitating the identification of responsible genes and their connection to the adaptive behavior in these high-altitude dwellers. Both Andeans and Tibetans have adapted well to high altitudes; However, there are phenotypic differences and the tolerance to mountain sickness along with evidence of genetic deviations. Chronic mountain sickness developing in highlanders is a result of multiple phenotypic changes happening secondary to the attempts of adjustment to low oxygen level. Most of the features are neurological like headache, dyspnea, somnolence, depression, tiredness. Palpitation etc. and are attributed to the polycythemia and higher blood viscosity. The prevalence of mountain sickness is higher in Andean highlander of south America (10–15%) compared to Tibetans due to higher erythropoietin secretion in response to lower atmospheric oxygen. These individuals are susceptible to the development of stroke, ischemic heart disease at an early age. Excessive erythropoiesis leads to pulmonary hypertension and predispose them to right ventricular failure [1, 2, 3]. The hypoxia is the basis of these symptoms in high altitude as evidenced by reversal of the conditions on descending or by phlebotomy. The lesser incidence of pulmonary hypertension in Tibetan may also be due to higher production of Nitric oxide and a less profound hypoxic pulmonary response compared to low landers and other high landers.

Hypoxia Inducible Factor Pathway

To understand the variability of the predisposition between low and high landers and also amongst different high-altitude populations we will explore the available researches and evidences on the pathways leading from hypoxia exposure to outcome and their link to different genes. Dr. Gregg L Semenza identified the Hypoxia inducing factor, a transcriptional factor which acts as master switch by sensing oxygen in body. They transfer the genetic information from a DNA sequence to mRNA. In response to hypoxia there is an increase in the concentration of HIF α which binds to HIF β to affect the release of hypoxia response elements (HRE). These transcription factors have control over the genes that mediate multiple physiological responses happening in the high-altitude residents at low oxygen concentration and these are:

- Regulation of genes involved in erythropoiesis
- VEGF induced by HIF has been linked to the pro-angiogenetic activity.
- Regulation of mitochondrial function and energy utilization
- Control of Nitric oxide metabolism genes, controlling pulmonary vasodilatation and pulmonary artery hypertension
- Regulating genes for anaerobic metabolism
- Carotid body chemosensory response [4]

Genes Identified in High Altitude Adaptations

Advancement in technologies of genomic studies like candidate gene sequencing, SNP genotyping arrays, whole exome sequencing, microarray etc. has helped make a remarkable progress in High Altitude Medicine by identifying the possible areas of interest in whole genome. Genome wide Association studies can be applied to find correlation between a specific Genotype and adaptive phenotype in different high-altitude dwellers [5]. Multiple genes have been identified in the last few years of extensive research in the field of genetic adaptation of high-altitude inhabitants and some of them are:

Peroxisome proliferator activated receptor alpha (PPARA), Endothelial PAS domain protein – 1 (EPAS 1), Egl-9 family hypoxia inducible factor 1 (EGLN1), hypoxia inducible factor 1 alpha subunit (HIF 1A), hypoxia inducible factor 1 alpha subunit inhibitor (HIF1AN), Nuclear factor erythroid 2-like 2 (NFE2L2), Protein Kinase AMP Activated catalytic subunit alpha 1 (PRKAA1), Acidic Nuclear Phosphoprotein 32 Family Member D (ANP32D), SUMO specific peptidase 1 (SENP1), Aryl Hydrocarbon Receptor Nuclear Translocator 2 (ARNT 2), Thyroid Hormone Receptor Beta (THRB), Histidine rich glycoprotein (HRG), cytochrome p450 family 1 (CYP1B1), Vascular Endothelial Growth factor A (VEGFA) etc.

The genetic variation in the populations of different high-altitude regions have been described long back and the need for extensive research had also been felt. Numerous studies have been conducted in the last two decades and have led to the identification of numerous genetic variants, mutation and their phenotypic outcomes in both high-altitude populations and the low altitude susceptible.

EPAS1 (Endothelial PAS domain protein 1) located on chromosome 2 encodes for HIF2 α which is responsible for various hypoxic responses in high altitude as described earlier. Genetic variants in EPAS1 have been linked to the downregulation of erythropoietin under hypoxic conditions in Sherpas, a Tibetan ancestry known for their capacity to tolerate high altitude. Single nucleotide polymorphisms (SNPs) occurring in EPAS1 gene has been implicated in adaptation to the high altitude and reduced incidence of mountain sickness in Tibetan population [6]. Similarly, polymorphisms in EPAS1 gene have been described in Chinese Han population which make them less susceptible to high altitude headache. It is clear that presence of an adaptive allele i.e. a particular genotype makes a population suffer less than another [7].

SNP of rs6756667 EPAS1 gene has been linked to lowering the risk of high-altitude appetite loss though the mechanism of it is not well established. PPARA gene located in chromosome 22 is responsible for the higher risk of high-altitude appetite loss in Chinese Han population and exerts its action through the PPAR alpha, a transcription factor responsible for regulating genes involved with glucose and lipid metabolism. Increased Insulin release secondary to gluconeogenesis stimulated by PPAR alpha in response to hypoxia leads to elevated risk of appetite loss [8]. Variants of EPAS1 and VEGFA genes may make individuals susceptible to the development of acute mountain sickness, which may be used to screen the at-risk population before reaching high altitude. EGLN1 decrease hydroxylation of HIF 1 alpha during hypoxia. EGLN1 mutation has been linked to the erythropoiesis.

Placental circulation, fetal growth and pregnancy outcome is influenced by hypoxic conditions. However, the high-altitude Tibetans and Andeans have many phenotypic adaptations and changes leading to better fetal weight and outcomes compared to Chinese and European counterparts, changes been linked to the SNP of PRKAA1 locus which is otherwise associated with diseases like WPW syndrome and myotonia. Unlike Tibetan population, where EGLN1, EPAS1 SNP is linked with hemoglobin concentration, Ethiopian high landers have demonstrated two genes, ARNT2 and THRB which are linked to the hemoglobin concentration via HIF pathway during adaptation to hypoxia [9]. Mutation in BHLHE41 gene reduce sleep quota and adapting to the consequences of less sleep. The same gene has also been found to have interaction with hypoxia adaptation in Ethiopian highlanders [9].

In a study conducted on Chinese Han soldiers, Allele T in one single Nucleotide Polymorphism, rs2070699 of EDN1 gene has been found to correlate with occurrence of acute mountain sickness. So, EDN1 gene polymorphism may be a predicted genetic factor in acute mountain sickness. This was associated with increased tryptophan and serotonin level in TT/TG genotype in SNP rs2070699.

ANP32D, SENP1 genes have been identified in Andean high landers and their downregulation has been implicated in the adaptability in hypoxic conditions [10].

Similarly, ACE gene polymorphism has been linked to the higher oxygen saturation in peruvian Quechua high landers though there are conflicting data regarding higher presence of the same in sea level residents also [11]. Carriers of three gene variants MTMR4, TMOD3, VCAM1 have been found to be protective in those Highlander Kyrgyz who are known to be protected from high altitude pulmonary hypertension. A specific haplotype located at HIF 2 alpha (EPAS1) gene have been found in high altitude pulmonary hypertension susceptible individuals [12]. High altitude pulmonary edema susceptible mountaineers also had two mutations in gene HRG and CYP1B1. Dysregulation at these two loci leads to increased tendency of vascular permeability leading to edema.

Conclusion

The role of genetics in high-altitude acclimatisation and disorders is well known and there has been ongoing research in this domain over last two decades, thanks to the availability of advanced genomic study tools. One important aspect of genomic study in High altitude medicine is the possible therapeutic application as some of the most commonly implicated genes like EPAS1, EGLN1 can be targeted by pharmacological agents [13]. This can be considered as potential therapeutic intervention in mountain sickness, pulmonary vascular disease and other vascular events. Some individuals who are at high risk of developing the high attitude illness can be screened prior. Understanding genetic basis of many adaptive changes may allow the scientists to explore newer pathways and links to phenotypes, the same may also have implications even in disorders distinct from High Altitude illness.

References

1. Monge CC, Arregui A, Leon-Velarde F. Pathophysiology and epidemiology of chronic mountain sickness. Int J Sports Med. 1992;13(Suppl 1):S79–81.
2. Penaloza D, Arias-Stella J. The heart and pulmonary circulation at high altitudes: healthy highlanders and chronic mountain sickness. Circulation. 2007;115:1132–46.
3. Penaloza D, Sime F. Chronic cor pulmonale due to loss of altitude acclimatization (chronic mountain sickness). Am J Med. 1971;50:728–43.
4. Prabhakar NR, Semenza GL. Regulation of carotid body oxygen sensing by hypoxia-inducible factors. Pflugers Arch. 2016;468:71–5.
5. Eichstaedt CA, Benjamin N, Grünig E. Genetics of pulmonary hypertension and high-altitude pulmonary edema. J Appl Physiol. 2020;128:1432–8. https://doi.org/10.1152/japplphysiol.00113.2020. Epub 2020
6. Beall CM, Cavalleri GL, Deng L, et al. Natural selection on EPAS1 (HIF2alpha) associated with low hemoglobin concentration in Tibetan highlanders. Proc Natl Acad Sci U S A. 2010;107:11459–64.
7. Shen Y, Zhang J, Yang J, et al. Association of *EPAS1* and *PPARA* gene polymorphisms with high-altitude headache in Chinese Han population. Biomed Res Int. 2020;2020:1593068. https://doi.org/10.1155/2020/1593068.
8. Pan W, Liu C, Zhang J, et al. Polymorphisms in PPARA and EPAS1 genes and high-altitude appetite loss in Chinese young men. Front Physiol. 2019;10:59. https://doi.org/10.3389/fphys.2019.00059.
9. Molinaro L, Pagani L. Human evolutionary history of eastern Africa. Curr Opin Genet Dev. 2018;53:134–9.

10. Zhou D, Udpa N, Ronen R, et al. Whole-genome sequencing uncovers the genetic basis of chronic mountain sickness in Andean highlanders. Am J Hum Genet. 2013;93:452–62.
11. Bigham AW, Kiyamu M, Leon-Velarde F, et al. Angiotensin-converting enzyme genotype and arterial oxygen saturation at high altitude in Peruvian Quechua. High Alt Med Biol. 2008;9:167–78.
12. Scheinfeldt LB, Soi S, Thompson S, et al. Genetic adaptation to high altitude in the Ethiopian highlands. Genome Biol. 2012;13:R1.
13. Ronen R, Zhou D, Bafna V, et al. The genetic basis of chronic mountain sickness. Physiology (Bethesda). 2014;29:403–12.

Chapter 4
High Altitude Medicine, Its Relevance and Classification According to Meters

Jorge Enrique Sinclair De Frías, Jorge Sinclair Avila,
Sabrina Da Re Gutierrez, and Jorge Hidalgo

Introduction

Millions of visitors travel to high altitude recreation areas in the United States, central and south Asia, Africa, and South America each year. In addition, millions of individuals worldwide live in large cities above 2500 m (8 200 ft) such as El Alto (4150 m) and La Paz (3640 m) in Bolivia, Quito (2850 m) in Ecuador, and Bogotá (2620 m) in Colombia.

Travelling to high altitude exposes the human body to a variety of stresses: extremely low temperatures, high velocity winds, low humidity, high intensity solar radiation, and reduced atmospheric pressure. Moreover, the state of sub-optimal O_2 availability in tissues and organs leads to deficiencies in biological processes [1].

J. E. Sinclair De Frías (✉)
Department of Physiology, University of Panama, Panama City, Panama

J. Sinclair Avila
Critical Care Department, Hospital Punta Pacífica, Panama City, Panama

S. Da Re Gutierrez
Department of Intensive Care Medicine, Materno Infantil Hospital, La Paz, Bolivia

J. Hidalgo
Department of Critical Care, Belize Healthcare Parners, Belize City, Belize

Physiological changes during ascent will depend on factors such as degree of change in elevation, degree of hypoxia, rate of ascent, level of acclimatization, exercise intensity, previous history of severe high-altitude illness, genetics, and age [2].

Incidence and severity of altitude illness are directly related to elevation and rapidity of ascent. Lowlander visitors who rapidly travel to high altitude are at greater risk of developing acute altitude illness as a rapid ascent does not allow an adequate acclimatization. Acute illness includes acute mountain sickness (AMS), high-altitude pulmonary edema (HAPE), and high-altitude cerebral edema (HACE); being HAPE the leading cause of death from altitude illness. HAPE incidence varies from 0.01% to 2% in most studies [3]. HACE is less common than AMS, however it carries a worse prognosis if not quickly recognized and treated. HACE and HAPE are more common with a longer duration of visit and higher sleeping altitude. On the other hand, highlanders or permanent residents do not suffer from acute altitude illness; however, they can be affected by chronical conditions such as chronic mountain disease and high-altitude pulmonary hypertension.

Clinicians working in or near mountainous areas must be familiarize with the presentation and management of high-altitude illness. In addition, all health care providers are frequently consulted with questions of prevention and treatment of high-altitude medical problems; therefore, a better understanding of physiologic and deleterious effects of high altitude is essential.

Definition [3, 4]

High Altitude: 1500 m to 3500 m (4 921 ft. to 11,483 ft)
Lower partial pressure of inspired oxygen (P_{IO2}) results in a decreased exercise performance, increased ventilation with lowering of arterial partial pressure of carbon dioxide (Pa_{CO2}), and minor impairment of arterial oxygen transport with an arterial oxygen saturation (Sa_{O2}) of at least 90%, but with significant impairment of arterial oxygen partial pressure (Pa_{O2}). Some predisposed individuals may desaturate to less than 90% at altitudes as low as 2500 m (8 202 ft). Acute high-altitude illness is common in this range of altitude, while severe altitude illness is rare.

Very High Altitude: 3500 m to 5500 m (11 483 ft. to 18,045 ft)
Maximum Sa_{O2} falls below 90% with a $Pa_{O2} < 60$ mm Hg. Extreme hypoxemia may occur during exercise, sleep, and HAPE. Likelihood of altitude illness is high, and the risk of severe acute high-altitude illness is important.

Extreme Altitude: Higher Than 5500 m (18 045 ft)
Marked hypoxemia, hypocapnia, and alkalosis. Acclimatization can't compensate progressive deterioration of physiologic functions; therefore, no permanent resident can live above 5500 m. When ascending to this altitude, a period of acclimatization is needed; abrupt ascent without supplemental oxygen will result in severe altitude illness.

Environment Considerations

Deleterious effects of altitude are primarily caused by hypobaric hypoxia. P_{IO2} is equal to the fractional concentration of oxygen times the barometric pressure minus the water vapor pressure of the body.

$$P_{IO2} = 0.2093 \left(P_B - 47\,\mathrm{mm\,Hg} \right)$$

where 0.2093 is the fractional concentration, P_B is the barometric pressure, and 47 mm Hg is the water pressure at 37 C. The fractional concentration of oxygen remains constant at any altitude; therefore, reduced P_{IO2} is determined solely by the fall in P_B which decreases in a logarithmic manner as altitude increases. Moreover, water pressure is unaltered by altitude. Consequently, it reduces the P_{IO2} at altitude more than at sea level. Understanding this is important, as acute altitude illness results mainly from this state of acute oxygen insufficiency.

At sea level, the P_B is of 760 mm Hg. At 5800 m, P_B is one half that of sea level; while on the summit of Mt. Everest (8848 m [29,029 ft]), the P_B and P_{IO2} are about one-third of sea level values. Rapid ascent to this summit will result in loss of conscious and death, however a gradual ascent will reduce symptoms and associated mortality [5].

Although altitude is the main determinant of P_B and its resulting physiologic stress, other factors can contribute to a reduction in P_B such as latitude and environmental factors (season, weather, and temperature) [6]. The earth and its atmospheric envelope are slightly flat at poles and bulging at the equator; thus, the pressure at a given altitude at the equator tends to be higher than at distances from the equator [7]. Season of the year also affects the atmospheric envelope. During summer, the sun's rays heat the air more, creating a higher column and thus increasing the pressure. During winter, P_B is lower compared to summer, making relative altitudes physiologically higher.

As altitude increases, temperature decreases and the effect of cold adds to the effect of hypoxia in provoking cold relating injuries and HAPE [8]. Reduced atmospheric protection from ultraviolet radiation increases the risks of sunburn, skin cancer, and snowblindness. Sunlight reflection in glaciers can cause radiation of heat in the absence of wind, leading to heat exhaustion which is often unrecognized in cold environment. Moreover, in extreme altitudes, water can only be obtained by melting down snow or ice. In addition, water loss through lungs and skin is increased. All these factors can lead to dehydration.

References

1. Purkayastha SS, Ray US, Arora BS, Chhabra PC, Thakur L, Bandopadhyay P, Selvamurthy W. Acclimatization at high altitude in gradual and acute induction. J Appl Physiol (1985). 1995;79(2):487–92. https://doi.org/10.1152/jappl.1995.79.2.487.

2. Richalet JP, Larmignat P, Poitrine E, Letournel M, Canouï-Poitrine F. Physiological risk factors for severe high-altitude illness: a prospective cohort study. Am J Respir Crit Care Med. 2012;185(2):192–8. https://doi.org/10.1164/rccm.201108-1396OC. Epub 2011 Oct 27
3. Roach RC, Lawley JS, Hackett PH. High altitude physiology. In: Auerbach PS, editor. Wilderness medicine. 7th ed. Philadelphia: Mosby/Elsevier; 2017. p. 2–8.
4. Paralikar SJ, Paralikar JH. High-altitude medicine. Indian J Occup Environ Med. 2010;14(1):6–12. https://doi.org/10.4103/0019-5278.64608. PMID: 20808661; PMCID: PMC2923424
5. Clarke C. Acute Mountain sickness: medical problems associated with acute and subacute exposure to hypobaric hypoxia. Postgrad Med J. 2006;82(973):748–53. https://doi.org/10.1136/pgmj.2006.047662. PMID: 17099095; PMCID: PMC2660503
6. West JB, Lahiri S, Maret KH, Peters RM Jr, Pizzo CJ. Barometric pressures at extreme altitudes on Mt. Everest: physiological significance. J Appl Physiol Respir Environ Exerc Physiol. 1983;54(5):1188–94. https://doi.org/10.1152/jappl.1983.54.5.1188.
7. Balke B, Nagle FJ, Daniels J. Altitude and maximum performance in work and sports activity. JAMA. 1965;194(6):646–9.
8. Reeves JT, Wagner J, Zafren K, et al. Seasonal variation in barometric pressure and temperature in Summit County: effect on altitude illness. In: Sutton JR, Houston CS, Coates G, editors. Hypoxia and molecular medicine. Bulrington, VT: Queen City Press; 1993.

Chapter 5
Physiology of High-Altitude Illness

Jorge Sinclair Avila, Sabrina Da Re Gutierrez, Lorenzo Olivero, and Jorge Enrique Sinclair De Frías

Case Presentation

A 30-year-old previously healthy man has decided to jump into a hiking expedition at the highest point of Panama, the Baru Volcano (~3400 m/11000 ft.). He takes no medication and does not use tobacco, alcohol, or illicit drugs. The man is in excellent physical condition and passes the preliminary physical examination before starting to climb. The ascending route used to be 8 h long to reach the top of the volcano. However, after 7 h, he experiences fatigue and unfocused thinking while climbing. He begins to note that his friends are also fatigued and have increased their respiratory rate. He got a pulse oximeter which revealed a heart rate of 111/min and 91% oxygen saturation. They decided to camp near the top of the volcano. On the second night, they experienced increasing urinary frequency despite not increasing liquid intake. With time, they gradually begin to feel better.

Question—What is the explanation for his presentation?

Answer—Hypobaric Hypoxia—This patient presents transient fatigue, tachycardia, tachypnea, and enhanced diuresis with a subsequent return to an asymptomatic state. This presentation is highly suggestive of a **high-altitude physiologic response.** The low partial pressure of oxygen at high altitudes triggers a series of adaptive mechanisms in response to hypoxia.

J. Sinclair Avila (✉)
Critical Care Department, Hospital Punta Pacífica, Panama City, Panama

S. D. R. Gutierrez
Department of Intensive Care Medicine, Materno Infantil Hospital, La Paz, Bolivia

L. Olivero
Department of Medicine, University of Panama, Panama City, Panama

J. E. Sinclair De Frías
Department of Physiology, University of Panama, Panama City, Panama

J. Hidalgo et al. (eds.), *High Altitude Medicine*, https://doi.org/10.1007/978-3-031-35092-4_5

35

Early while ascending, the activation of the sympathetic system and the peripheral chemoreceptors increase heart rate and minute ventilation in an attempt to improve the delivery of oxygen to the tissues. The resulting tachypnea leads to respiratory alkalosis. In addition, increasing glycolysis within the erythrocyte promotes the synthesis of 2,3- BPG leading to a right shift of the oxygen hemoglobin dissociation curve. This right shift reduces the affinity of hemoglobin for O2, which means that O2 is released more readily to the tissues.

Later changes in the patient's organism include increased red blood cell count mediated by erythropoietin (EPO) release, normalization of arterial pH through bicarbonate excretion (renal compensation in response to respiratory alkalosis), and vascular changes such as increased pulmonary arterial pressure and cerebral blood flow to compensate for reduced arterial oxygen content. Inadequate adaptation will result in high altitude-related diseases, such as acute mountain sickness, pulmonary edema, and cerebral edema.

Principles of Hypobaric Hypoxia and Its Physiology

Overview

Oxygen is one of the essential atoms for the survival and proper function of tissue cells in the human body. It plays a critical role in the electron transport chain leading to energy production [1]. Air is a mixture of gases, in which the percentage of oxygen (O_2) remains approximately around 21%, even at high altitude [2].

Atmospheric pressure, also known as barometric pressure, is caused by the air's weight above the measuring point. It directly correlates with the partial pressure of oxygen (pO_2); a lower atmospheric pressure results in a lower pO2. This phenomenon is explained by gravitational force, which tries to attract objects to the earth's center. As mentioned, the air mass will be the determinant in calculating the atmospheric pressure. This can be explained by Newton's second law of motion, where Force (F) = mass x acceleration. The atmospheric pressure represents the F, and it can be calculated by multiplying the weight of air (mass) x 9.8 m/s^2 (gravitational acceleration of earth); therefore, the greater the weight of air, the greater the pressure. This explains why there is higher atmospheric pressure at sea level (760 mmHg), with higher air mass above, compared to lower atmospheric pressures over sea levels. Lower atmospheric pressures will result in lower partial pressure of inspired oxygen (FiO2); therefore, FiO2 presents a negative linear correlation with altitude.

This decrease in atmospheric pressure is the primary cause of the hypoxia problems in high-altitude physiology because as the atmospheric pressure decreases, the oxygen partial pressure (Po_2) decreases proportionately. This makes it difficult for oxygen to diffuse into the pulmonary capillaries, depriving of O_2 the peripheral tissue cells.

Investigators have been interested in clarifying how some populations can live at such high altitude and their mechanisms of adaptation [3]. Although, now we know that people living at high altitudes have been adapting their bodies and generationally evolving, including genetic changes, to bear with the low oxygen pressure [4]. These adaptations, which take the place of a chronic exposition to low inspired oxygen pressure, differ from "acclimatization," a group of changes (early and late) in people who usually are not exposed to these oxygen levels (lowlanders). For example, people ascending to high altitudes for pleasure, work, and athletic competition, including skiing, trekking, and mountaineering, are prone to be acutely exposed to these low levels of oxygen and experience the changes we will discuss now.

Acclimatization

Acclimatization is a normal compensatory process that occurs in response to the low level of oxygen at high altitudes and occurs in different organ systems during the first hours to days. The physiologic changes typically become significant at elevations >2500 m (8202 ft).

Respiratory Changes

Decreased PiO2 at high altitudes triggers various mechanisms in the respiratory system. Insufficient acclimatization of the respiratory system results in high altitude sickness, which will be reviewed in the following chapters.

During normal conditions, the primary respiratory stimulus for regulating ventilation is the partial pressure of carbon dioxide ($PaCO_2$). Since the partial pressure of oxygen (PO_2) ranges typically between 60-100 mmHg and remains almost constant with the variation of tidal volume. Levels less than 60 mmHg become an essential stimulus to the peripheral chemoreceptors [5]; these receptors sense changes in PCO_2, PO_2, and pH and are located in the aortic arch and the bifurcation of the carotids (carotid bodies) and send stimulus to the respiratory center located in the reticular formation of the medulla oblongata and pons via CN X and CN IX.

The dorsal respiratory group (DRG) of the respiratory center in the medulla controls the inspiration, whereas the ventral respiratory group controls the expiration. In the respiration cycle, inspiration is an active process. However, the expiration, which usually is a passive process, can become active when we need more robust work of breathing like our patient. These nuclei increase the frequency of action potentials to the respiratory muscles via phrenic and intercostal nerves, increasing the respiratory rate and amplitude, resulting in increased minute ventilation [6]; this response is termed hypoxic ventilatory response [7, 8].

While this integrative response occurs initially and helps increase the alveolar ventilation and PO_2 for a while in our patient, this comes at the expense of increased CO_2 removal and respiratory alkalosis, blunting both central and peripheral respiratory chemoreceptor activation limiting subsequent ventilatory drive and creating a ceiling for the ventilatory response.

The peripheral chemoreceptors are sensitive to changes in PCO_2, PO_2, and pH. In contrast, central chemoreceptors located in the medulla are highly sensitive to changes in pH (H^+) and communicate directly with the DRG [6].

With the help of the carbonic anhydrase, CO_2 combines with water (H_2O) and produces HCO_3^- and H^+; however, the blood-brain barrier is relatively impermeable to H^+ and HCO_3^-. Contrarily, CO_2 can cross the blood-brain barrier and is converted in the cerebrospinal fluid to H^+ and HCO_3^- decreasing the pH. But in our hyperventilating patient, low PCO_2 means low H^+ concentration and a higher pH. This will inhibit central and peripheral chemoreceptors and offset the increase in ventilation rate.

This integrative response is not influenced by athletic training but by external factors, like alcohol and sedative/hypnotics. Instead, respiratory stimulants (e.g., progesterone) and sympathomimetics (e.g., coca, caffeine) increase this response [9]. Within several days the renal response will become helpful in balancing the respiratory alkalosis from the resulted hypoxic ventilatory response.

Renal Changes

The kidney is crucial in facilitating acclimatization and helping prevent mountain sicknesses. Nearly 100% of HCO3 is reabsorbed during normal conditions in the proximal tubules. HCO_3^- is polar and poorly soluble in lipids to cross membranes. Thus, it needs to be combined with secreted H^+ to form CO_2 and H_2O catalyzed by the brush border carbonic anhydrase to be reabsorbed. CO_2 and H_2O cross the lumen membrane and then are converted back to HCO_3^- and H^+ inside the cell catalyzed by the intracellular carbonic anhydrase. Therefore, HCO_3^- is reabsorbed in the basolateral membrane either by cotransport with Na^+ or antiport with Cl^- [6] (Fig. 5.1).

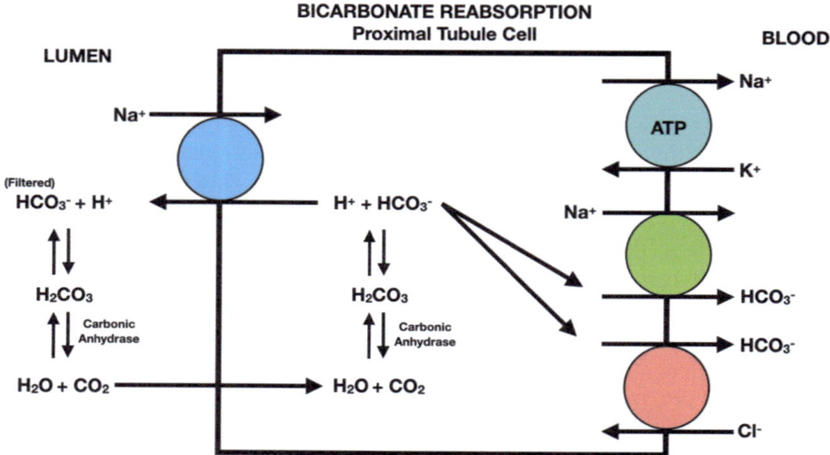

Fig. 5.1 Bicarbonate reabsorbption

Bicarbonate reabsorption depends primarily on the glomerular filtration rate and plasma concentration of HCO_3^-; therefore, when plasma levels of HCO_3^- are greater than 40 mEq/L, the reabsorption mechanism becomes saturated; hence any filtered HCO_3^- that cannot be reabsorbed will be excreted.

Besides the filtered load, two other mechanisms are essential for regulating the reabsorption of HCO_3^-: extracellular fluid volume and PCO_2. For example, volume depletion activates the renin-angiotensin-aldosterone system to promote isotonic volume reabsorption; HCO_3^- is one of the reabsorbed components along with water and other ions involved in the restoration of the volume status; this is called contraction alkalosis.

On the other hand, the effect of CO_2 on the reabsorption of HCO_3^- is not completed understood, but it is thought that higher levels of CO_2 inside the proximal tubular cell will be available to generate H^+ that can be secreted to promote HCO_3^- reabsorption. Conversely, less CO2 is available to generate H+ for secretion in respiratory alkalosis, which means less HCO_3^- that can be reabsorbed [10].

Following the hypoxic ventilatory response, the kidney initiates the compensation:

HCO_3^- excretion increases, and the pH decreases toward normal especially in the cerebrospinal fluid, as well as in the brain tissues and fluids surrounding cells in the respiratory center, thus increasing the respiratory stimulatory activity of the center and the offsetting effects will be reduced, allowing ventilation to increase again as the alkalosis is reduced. Thus, within 2–3 days new steady-state in the acid-base status is established [11, 12].

The respiratory alkalosis that occurs in high altitudes can be treated with carbonic anhydrase inhibitors (e.g., acetazolamide). These drugs increase HCO_3^- excretion, creating a mild compensatory metabolic acidosis that facilitates acclimatization.

Cardiovascular Changes

Systemic changes - increasing sympathetic activity as the patient is going higher in altitude transiently increases cardiac output, blood pressure, heart rate, and venous tone [13]. However, later the kidneys enhance diuresis from HCO3- diuresis; therefore, the heart rate will be elevated still but with a low stroke volume due to decreased plasma volume [14].

Pulmonary Vasoconstriction - Hypoxic pulmonary vasoconstriction (HPV) is an intrinsic homeostatic mechanism of the pulmonary vasculature.

Intrapulmonary arteries constrict in response to alveolar hypoxia, diverting blood to better-oxygenated lung segments, thereby optimizing ventilation/perfusion matching and systemic oxygen delivery; this is called the Euler-Liljestrand reflex mechanism. In contrast, hypoxia in other organs causes vasodilation to increase perfusion. The low ambient partial pressure of inspired oxygen (PiO_2) at high altitude causes global HPV throughout the lungs, leading to **increased pulmonary arterial pressure**, and finally causes pulmonary hypertension (PH) [15].

Exaggerated or heterogeneous HPV contributes to high-altitude pulmonary edema. Besides that, it is traduced in high right ventricle post-load and can develop in right ventricle failure and cor pulmonale, which will be discussed separately in this book.

Increased cerebral blood flow - Cerebral perfusion autoregulation is determined by the mean arterial pressure, intracranial pressure, temperature, and local metabolites. It is predominantly modulated by pCO_2; increased levels of pCO_2 (low pH) promote vasodilation and increase cerebral blood flow to remove excess CO_2. Whereas decreased pCO_2 causes vasoconstriction and decreases cerebral blood flow. The pO_2 modulates cerebral perfusion only in severe hypoxic conditions ($pO_2 < 50$ mmHg), vasodilating the cerebral vasculature in response to hypoxia. In our hyperventilating patient, hypocapnia attenuates hypoxic vasodilation. However, the net change in response to hypoxia is an increase in cerebral blood flow [16].

Hematologic Changes

Increased levels of 2,3 BPG - Initially, increased pH from respiratory alkalosis due to hyperventilation shifts the O2-hemoglobin dissociation curve to the left, resulting in increased binding of oxygen to hemoglobin and less oxygen delivery to the tissues. After a few hours, increased glycolysis rises 2,3-diphosphoglycerate levels, shifting the curve back to the right. The pro of this right-shifted curve is that it improves oxygen delivery by facilitating oxygen unloading to the tissues. However, the con is that it is more challenging to load oxygen to hemoglobin in the lungs during the gas exchange [6].

Increased red blood cell production - Ascent to high altitude increases red blood cell concentration (polycythemia). This is achieved by releasing hypoxia-inducible factors (HIFs), thereby inducing cell-type-specific gene expression changes that result in increased erythropoietin (EPO) production in the kidney hemoglobin concentration. As we know, the transportation of oxygen within the blood is mainly bound to hemoglobin (98%); an increase in hemoglobin concentration means that the O_2-carrying capacity is increased, which increases the total O_2 content of blood in spite of arterial pO_2 being decreased. Polycythemia is advantageous in O_2 transport to the tissues, but it is disadvantageous in blood viscosity, which could increase resistance to blood flow.

The following table summarizes the essential features of acclimatization to high altitude (Tables 5.1 and 5.2).

Table 5.1 Correlation between altitude with barometric pressure and PO_2 in the air

Altitude (m/ft)	Barometric Pressure (mmHg)	PO_2 in the air (mmHg)
0	760	149
1000/3281	679	132
2000/6062	604	117
3000/9842	537	103
4000/13123	475	90
5000/16404	420	78
8848/29029[a]	253	43

[a]Mount Everest's altitude

Table 5.2 Acclimatization to high altitude

Parameter	Early changes	Late changes
pCO2	Decreased	Decreased
pO2	Decreased	Decreased
Arterial pH	Decreased	Normal (renal compensation)
Hemoglobin (Hb)	Normal	Increased
Arterial O2 content	Decreased	Normal

Evidence Contour

how the physiological responses performed during high altitude acclimatization were still conflicting, as many factors could influence the physiological processes, such as altitude, rate of ascent, nutrition, supplements, physical status, psychical status, and exercise.

Rate of Ascent

Although data are lacking regarding the rate of ascent preventing high altitude illness, consensus and guidelines recommend an ascent rate of 300–500 m/day above 2500–3000 m, with a day of rest every 3–4 days. Slow rate protocols of ascent in many studies have been shown to prevent acute mountain sickness (AMS) and other high-altitude illnesses, but not all the studies include data regarding physiologic responses consistent with acclimatization [17–20].

Preaclimatization

This measure has become more popular nowadays. Several equipment and protocols simulating low oxygen pressures, like intermittent exposure hypoxic chambers, have become available, however lack of randomized control studies using this strategy and comparing physiologic parameters in acclimatization makes this strategy remains with a low level of evidence [21–25].

Alcohol, Sedative/Hypnotics, and Acclimatization

Respiratory depressors like alcohol, sedative, hypnotics, and some recreational drugs are well known to blunt respiratory response, although limited data involving these molecules in high altitudes are available.

However, the current recommendation is to avoid respiratory depressors, especially in the first 2 days of ascending [26, 27].

Diet and Altitude

several exercise programs (e.g., altitude training for cyclists and endurance athletes) include dietary recommendations within their guidelines. Diets seeking a quicker response to hypoxic factors and a more vigorous increase of EPO have become the subject of some new studies. Although more evidence is needed regarding nutritional demands in acute exposure to high altitude; the dramatic increase in the rate of energy expenditure in low oxygen pressure settings compared to normoxia claims to assure sufficient dietary macronutrients, especially dietary carbohydrates (CHO) to replace muscle glycogen stress during ascending [28, 29].

Iron, antioxidants, and other supplements initially showed promising results [30, 31], but recent data have shown no benefit or mixed results [32, 33].

Exercise

Exercise in the early hours of altitude exposure results in a marked increase in the severity and incidence of high altitude illnesses increasing oxygen consumption and fluid retention [34]. Mild pulmonary hypertension at rest can be markedly increased by vigorous exercise, with pulmonary pressure reaching near-systemic levels, especially in people with a history of high-altitude pulmonary edema (HAPE).

On the other hand, sedentary climbers are prone to achieving slow acclimatization and are at risk of high-altitude illness. Therefore, regarding exercise, it is recommended to be in regular physical activity before the ascent.

References

1. Gallagher SA, Hackett PH. High-altitude illness. Emerg Med Clin North Am [Internet]. 2004;22(2):329–55. Available from: https://www.sciencedirect.com/science/article/pii/S073386270400015X
2. Hall JE. Guyton and hall textbook of medical physiology. 14th ed. Elsevier; 2021. p. 553–4.
3. Moore LG, Niermeyer S, Zamudio S. Human adaptation to high altitude: regional and life-cycle perspectives. Am J Phys Anthropol [Internet]. 1998;107(S27):25–64. https://doi.org/10.1002/(SICI)1096-8644(1998)107:27+%3C25::AID-AJPA3%3E3.0.CO.
4. Storz JF. Genes for high altitudes. Science (80-) [Internet]. 2010;329(5987):40–1. https://doi.org/10.1126/science.1192481.
5. Biscoe TJ, Purves MJ, Sampson SR. The frequency of nerve impulses in single carotid body chemoreceptor afferent fibres recorded in vivo with intact circulation. J Physiol [Internet]. 1970;208(1):121–31. https://doi.org/10.1113/jphysiol.1970.sp009109.
6. Costanzo LS. Physiology. In: Linda S, editor. Costanzo. 6th ed. Philadelphia, PA: Elsevier; 2018. p. 232–42.
7. Dempsey JA, Forster HV. Mediation of ventilatory adaptations. Physiol Rev [Internet]. 1982;62(1):262–346. https://doi.org/10.1152/physrev.1982.62.1.262.
8. Teppema LJ, Dahan A. The ventilatory response to hypoxia in mammals: mechanisms, measurement, and analysis. Physiol Rev [Internet]. 2010;90(2):675–754. https://doi.org/10.1152/physrev.00012.2009.
9. Bairam A, Uppari N, Mubayed S, Joseph V. In: Peers C, Kumar P, Wyatt C, Gauda E, Nurse CA, Prabhakar N, editors. An overview on the respiratory stimulant effects of caffeine and progesterone on response to hypoxia and apnea frequency in developing rats BT - arterial chemoreceptors in physiology and pathophysiology. Cham: Springer International Publishing; 2015. p. 211–20. https://doi.org/10.1007/978-3-319-18440-1_23.
10. Adrogué HJ, Madias NE. Secondary responses to altered Acid-Base status: the rules of engagement. J Am Soc Nephrol [Internet]. 2010;21(6):920–3. Available from: http://jasn.asnjournals.org/content/21/6/920.abstract
11. Krapf R, Beeler I, Hertner D, Hulter HN. Chronic respiratory alkalosis. N Engl J Med [Internet]. 1991;324(20):1394–401. https://doi.org/10.1056/NEJM199105163242003.
12. Gennari FJ, Goldstein MB, Schwartz WB. The nature of the renal adaptation to chronic hypocapnia. J Clin Invest [Internet]. 1972;51(7):1722–30. https://doi.org/10.1172/JCI106973.
13. Nishihara F, Shimada H, Saito S. Rate pressure product and oxygen saturation in tourists at approximately 3000 m above sea level. Int Arch Occup Environ Health. 1998;71(8):520–4.
14. Shah NM, Hussain S, Cooke M, O'Hara JP, Mellor A. Wilderness medicine at high altitude: recent developments in the field. Open access J Sport Med. 2015;6:319–28.
15. Dunham-Snary KJ, Wu D, Sykes EA, Thakrar A, Parlow LRG, Mewburn JD, et al. Hypoxic pulmonary vasoconstriction: from molecular mechanisms to medicine. Chest [Internet]. 2017;151(1):181–92. https://doi.org/10.1016/j.chest.2016.09.001.
16. Tameem A, Krovvidi VH. Cerebral physiology. Contin Educ Anaesthes Crit Care Pain. 2013;16(13):113–8.
17. Bärtsch P, Swenson ER. Clinical practice: acute high-altitude illnesses. N Engl J Med. 2013;368(24):2294–302.
18. Luks AM, Auerbach PS, Freer L, Grissom CK, Keyes LE, McIntosh SE, et al. Wilderness medical society clinical practice guidelines for the prevention and treatment of acute altitude illness: 2019 update. Wilderness Environ Med [Internet]. 2019;30(4):S3–18. https://doi.org/10.1016/j.wem.2019.04.006.
19. Bloch KE, Turk AJ, Maggiorini M, Hess T, Merz T, Bosch MM, et al. Effect of ascent protocol on Acute Mountain sickness and success at Muztagh Ata, 7546 m. High Alt Med Biol [Internet]. 2008;10(1):25–32. https://doi.org/10.1089/ham.2008.1043.
20. Beidleman BA, Fulco CS, Muza SR, Rock PB, Staab JE, Forte VA, et al. Effect of six days of staging on physiologic adjustments and Acute Mountain sickness during ascent to 4300 meters. High Alt Med Biol [Internet]. 2009;10(3):253–60. https://doi.org/10.1089/ham.2009.1004.

21. Richalet JP, Bittel J, Herry JP, Savourey G, Le Trong JL, Auvert JF, et al. Use of a hypobaric chamber for pre-acclimatization before climbing Mount Everest. Int J Sports Med. 1992;13(Suppl 1):S216–20.
22. Küpper T, Schöffl V. Preacclimatization in hypoxic chambers for high altitude sojourns. Sleep Breath. 2009;14:187–91.
23. Beidleman BA, Muza SR, Fulco CS, Cymerman A, Ditzler D, Stulz D, et al. Intermittent altitude exposures reduce acute mountain sickness at 4300 m. Clin Sci (Lond). 2004;106(3):321–8.
24. Wille M, Gatterer H, Mairer K, Philippe M, Schwarzenbacher H, Faulhaber M, et al. Short-term intermittent hypoxia reduces the severity of acute mountain sickness. Scand J Med Sci Sports. 2012;22(5):e79–85.
25. Schommer K, Wiesegart N, Menold E, Haas U, Lahr K, Buhl H, et al. Training in normobaric hypoxia and its effects on acute mountain sickness after rapid ascent to 4559 m. High Alt Med Biol. 2010;11(1):19–25.
26. Roeggla G, Roeggla H, Roeggla M, Binder M, Laggner AN. Effect of alcohol on acute ventilatory adaptation to mild hypoxia at moderate altitude. Ann Intern Med. 1995;122(12):925–7.
27. Schneider M, Bernasch D, Weymann J, Holle R, Bartsch P. Acute mountain sickness: influence of susceptibility, preexposure, and ascent rate. Med Sci Sports Exerc. 2002;34(12):1886–91.
28. Stellingwerff T, Peeling P, Garvican-Lewis LA, Hall R, Koivisto AE, Heikura IA, et al. Nutrition and altitude: strategies to enhance adaptation, improve performance and maintain health: a narrative review. Sports Med. 2019;49(Suppl 2):169–84.
29. Michalczyk M, Czuba M, Zydek G, Zając A, Langfort J. Dietary recommendations for cyclists during altitude training. Nutrients. 2016;8(6)
30. Simon-Schnass I, Pabst H. Influence of vitamin E on physical performance. Int J Vitam Nutr Res Int Zeitschrift fur Vitamin- und Ernahrungsforschung J Int Vitaminol Nutr. 1988;58(1):49–54.
31. Bailey DM, Davies B. Acute mountain sickness; prophylactic benefits of antioxidant vitamin supplementation at high altitude. High Alt Med Biol. 2001;2(1):21–9.
32. Baillie JK, Thompson AAR, Irving JB, Bates MGD, Sutherland AI, Macnee W, et al. Oral antioxidant supplementation does not prevent acute mountain sickness: double blind, randomized placebo-controlled trial. QJM. 2009;102(5):341–8.
33. Schmidt MC, Askew EW, Roberts DE, Prior RL, Ensign WYJ, Hesslink REJ. Oxidative stress in humans training in a cold, moderate altitude environment and their response to a phytochemical antioxidant supplement. Wilderness Environ Med. 2002;13(2):94–105.
34. Roach RC, Maes D, Sandoval D, Robergs RA, Icenogle M, Hinghofer-Szalkay H, et al. Exercise exacerbates acute mountain sickness at simulated high altitude. J Appl Physiol [Internet]. 2000;88(2):581–5. https://doi.org/10.1152/jappl.2000.88.2.581.

Chapter 6
Acid-Base Homeostasis at the High Altitude

Pradip Kumar Bhattacharya, Jay Prakash, and Anup Gohatre

A 40-year-old mountain climber was brought back from Camp 1 on Mt. Everest (6065 m) to Base Camp (5380 m) as he was complaining of shortness of breath and dry cough. Medical team at Base Camp evaluates him. He was having dyspnea at rest and pink, frothy sputum. Vitals: Temp = 97.8 ° F, HR = 130 bpm, BP = 158/90, RR = 36, SpO_2 = 80% on 6 L O_2 via facemask. He has diffuse bilateral crackles on lung auscultation. His ABG reveals: pH = 7.58, P_aCO_2 = 20, P_aO_2 = 40.

Let's first analyze the oxygenation part. For that, we will have to find out the A-a gradient (i.e., $P_AO_2 - P_aO_2$). P_AO_2 can be calculated by using alveolar gas equation. The alveolar gas equation is a formula used to approximate the 'partial pressure of oxygen in the alveolus (P_AO_2):

$$P_A O_2 = \left(P_B - P_{H2O}\right) FiO_2 - \left(P_a CO_2 \div R\right)$$

Where, P_B is the barometric pressure which changes with the altitude. For our case, at 5380 m, it will be 400 mmHg [1].

P. K. Bhattacharya (✉) · J. Prakash
Department of Critical Care Medicine, Rajendra Institute of Medical Sciences, Ranchi, Jharkhand, India

A. Gohatre
Indira Gandhi Institute of Medical Sciences, Patna, Bihar, India

© The Author(s), under exclusive license to Springer Nature Switzerland AG 2023
J. Hidalgo et al. (eds.), *High Altitude Medicine*,
https://doi.org/10.1007/978-3-031-35092-4_6

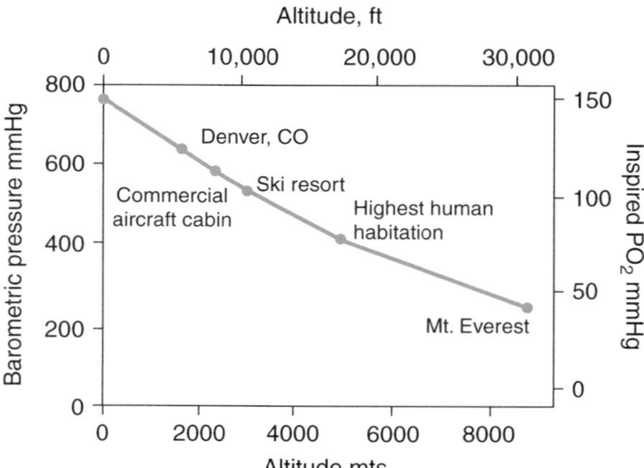

Relationship between altitude, barometric pressure and inspired PO₂ [2]

P_{H2O} is the water vapor pressure (usually 47 mmHg).

FiO_2 is the fractional concentration of inspired oxygen, which remains constant at 21% even at high altitudes,

P_aCO_2 is the partial pressure of carbon dioxide in blood, and R is the gas exchange ratio, i.e., 0.8.

Putting these values in the equation, we get $P_AO_2 = 116$. Therefore, A-a gradient will be $(116–40) = 76$. Is this normal for this age?

The approximate A-a gradient for 40 years is $= (40/4)/4 = 14$. So, there is hypoxemia with high A-a gradient. And the most likely cause in this case would be pulmonary edema, i.e., High Altitude Pulmonary Edema (HAPE) [3].

High altitude pulmonary edema (HAPE) is a noncardiogenic pulmonary edema which typically occurs in lowlanders who ascend rapidly to altitudes greater than 2500–3000 m. A nonproductive cough, dyspnea with exertion, and decreased exercise capacity are some of the early signs of HAPE. Dyspnea then develops while at rest. Cyanosis, tachycardia, tachypnea, and a high body temperature usually not reaching 38.5 °C are considered clinical signs. Initially, rales are distinct and situated over the middle lung areas. Exaggerated hypoxic pulmonary vasoconstriction and increased pulmonary artery pressure are the major causes of HAPE.

There are two different forms of the HAPE. One which is seen in unacclimatized lowlanders who ascends to high altitude and other which is seen in log-term residents of high altitude, who descend to low elevation for some time and then reascend [4].

Normal ABG Values at High Altitude

Mountaineers who ascend to high altitude, with the acclimatization show a hyperventilatory-induced respiratory alkalosis followed by renal compensation (bicarbonaturia) to return arterial blood pH (pHa) toward sea-level values. But indigenous highlanders usually have more acidic pH compared to lowlanders [5].

This changes in pH are significant enough to shift the P50 and therefor the oxygen dissociation curve to the left [6].

As a part of acclimatization hemoglobin level increases leading to increased oxygen carrying capacity of blood and eventually 2–3 DGP level in RBCs also increases over time leading to rightward shift of O2-Hb dissociation curve and improve oxygen offloading at the tissues.

One study has evaluated the ventilation and ABG by age and sex in an Andean population resident at high altitude (2640 m). They have found that, the mean PaO_2 in the whole group was 65.2 ± 5.6 mmHg, SpO_2 $92.4 \pm 2.3\%$, $PaCO_2$ 33.0 ± 2.9 mmHg and bicarbonate 21.7 ± 1.6 mEq/L with significant differences by age and sex [7].

Acclimatization in Lowlanders Visiting High Altitudes

As the person climbs from sea level to high altitude, both alveolar and arterial O2 pressure fall, resulting in development of hypoxemia. As a compensation for hypoxemia, alveolar ventilation increases, resulting in a slight reduction in pCO2. This stimulates the peripheral chemoreceptors located in carotid and aortic arch bodies, which send signals to medullary respiratory centers, resulting in progressive increase in ventilation.

But this hyperventilation does not continue forever because low pCO2 and low bicarbonate in cerebrospinal fluid seems to desensitize the peripheral chemoreceptors. Figure shows the mechanism of hypoxia-induced alveolar hyperventilation.

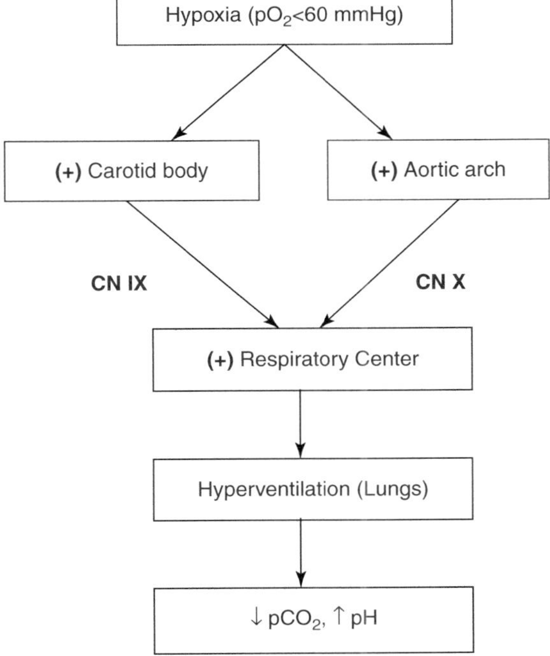

Therefore, it is observed that long-term residents living in high altitude areas maintain low alveolar ventilation and high pCO2 for any given pO2 level compared to short-term dwellers.

This decrease in PaCO2 induces a condition of respiratory alkalosis and a compensatory mechanism through acid retention and increased HCO3− excretion in the urine is elicited [8], which is only partially counterbalanced and this compensatory process results in a decrease in arterial blood pH (pHa) towards normal levels (pHa ∼ 7.4), known as a relative compensatory metabolic acidosis [9–11].

What If Acclimatization Is Inadequate?

The significance of the renal responsiveness through acid–base changes is well understood, but the timing of the reaction during gradual ascent and the degree of plasticity in this response are not well understood. A straightforward and accurate index to measure the renal response to exposure to chronic hypobaric hypoxia and persistent hypocapnia experienced during ascent to high altitude is also lacking, despite the HVR's unambiguous criteria.

An inadequate renal response to respiratory alkalosis may result in a sustained increase in blood pH, blunted HVR, decreased oxygen saturation and decreased cerebral blood flow, and all of these factors have been shown to affect acclimatization, as well as facilitate the onset and severity of acute mountain sickness symptoms [12, 13].

Can Acid-Base Changes and Acclimatization Be Predicted?

The majority of the available data consist of lumbar cerebrospinal fluid values [14], venous values [15] and/or rely on simulated altitudes in the laboratory [16] that do not take into account the realistic conditions encountered upon exposure to high altitude.

In 2018, based on the well described relationships between PaCO2 and HCO3−, a simple index of Renal Reactivity (RR) was developed, indexing the change in HCO3− against the relative change in PaCO2 during incremental ascent to altitude (Δ[HCO3−] a/ΔPaCO2). A strong negative correlation was found between RR and Δ pHa at all altitudes, with correlation coefficients (r) of −0.71, −0.98, −0.96 and − 0.97 at 3440, 3820, 4240 and 5160 m, respectively (all P < 0.001) [17]. This novel index that accurately quantifies renal acid-base compensation, will have laboratory, fieldwork and clinical applications. Using this index, authors have found that renal compensation increased and plateaued after 5 days of incremental altitude exposure, suggesting plasticity in renal acid-base compensation mechanisms.

The time-course and extent of plasticity in renal responsiveness will help in predicting severity of altitude illness or acclimatization at higher or more prolonged stays at altitude.

References

1. https://baillielab.net/critical_care/air_pressure
2. Paralikar SJ, Paralikar JH. High-altitude medicine. Indian J Occup Environ Med. 2010;14(1):6–12. https://doi.org/10.4103/0019-5278.64608.
3. Hackett PH, Roach RC. High-altitude illness. N Engl J Med. 2001;345(2):107–14. https://doi.org/10.1056/NEJM200107123450206.
4. Scoggin CH, Hyers TM, Reeves JT, Grover RF. High-altitude pulmonary edema in the children and young adults of Leadville. Colorado N Engl J Med. 1977;297(23):1269–72. https://doi.org/10.1056/NEJM197712082972309.
5. Figueroa-Mujica R, Foster GE, Bird JD, Champigneulle B, Stauffer E, Stone RM, et al. Acid-base balance at high altitude in lowlanders and indigenous highlanders. J Appl Physiol. 2022;132(2):575–80. https://doi.org/10.1152/japplphysiol.00757.2021.
6. Balaban DY, Duffin J, Preiss D, Mardimae A, Vesely A, Slessarev M, et al. The in-vivo oxy-haemoglobin dissociation curve at sea level and high altitude. Respir Physiol Neurobiol. 2013;186(1):45–52. https://doi.org/10.1016/j.resp.2012.12.011.
7. Gonzalez-Garcia M, Maldonado D, Barrero M, Casas A, Perez-Padilla R, Torres-Duque CA. Arterial blood gases and ventilation at rest by age and sex in an adult Andean population resident at high altitude. Eur J Appl Physiol. 2020;120(12):2729–36. https://doi.org/10.1007/s00421-020-04498-z.
8. Krapf R, Beeler I, Hertner D, Hulter HN. Chronic respiratory alkalosis. The effect of sustained hyperventilation on renal regulation of acid-base equilibrium. N Engl J Med. 1991;324(20):1394–401. https://doi.org/10.1056/NEJM199105163242003.
9. Samaja M, Mariani C, Prestini A, Cerretelli P. Acid-base balance and O2 transport at high altitude. Acta Physiol Scand. 1997;159(3):249–56. https://doi.org/10.1046/j.1365-201X.1997.574342000.x.
10. Steele AR, Ainslie PN, Stone R, Tymko K, Tymko C, Howe CA, et al. Global REACH 2018: characterizing Acid-Base balance over 21 days at 4,300 m in lowlanders. High Alt Med Biol. 2022;23(2):185–91. https://doi.org/10.1089/ham.2021.0115.
11. Swenson ER. Hypoxia and its Acid-Base consequences: from mountains to malignancy. Adv Exp Med Biol. 2016;903:301–23. https://doi.org/10.1007/978-1-4899-7678-9_21.
12. Forster HV, Dempsey JA, Chosy LW. Incomplete compensation of CSF [H+] in man during acclimatization to high altitude (48300 M). J Appl Physiol. 1975;38(6):1067–72. https://doi.org/10.1152/jappl.1975.38.6.1067.
13. Fan JL, Burgess KR, Basnyat R, Thomas KN, Peebles KC, Lucas SJ, et al. Influence of high altitude on cerebrovascular and ventilatory responsiveness to CO2. J Physiol. 2010;588(Pt 3):539–49. https://doi.org/10.1113/jphysiol.2009.184051.
14. Severinghaus JW, Mitchell RA, Richardson BW, Singer MM. Respiratory control at high altitude suggesting active transport regulation of CSF pH. J Appl Physiol. 1963;18(6):1155–66. https://doi.org/10.1152/jappl.1963.18.6.1155.
15. Shah MB, Braude D, Crandall CS, Kwack H, Rabinowitz L, Cumbo TA, et al. Changes in metabolic and hematologic laboratory values with ascent to altitude and the development of acute mountain sickness in Nepalese pilgrims. Wilderness Environ Med. 2006;17(3):171–7. https://doi.org/10.1580/pr43-04.
16. Ge RL, Simonson TS, Gordeuk V, Prchal JT, McClain DA. Metabolic aspects of high-altitude adaptation in Tibetans. Exp Physiol. 2015;100(11):1247–55. https://doi.org/10.1113/EP085292.
17. Zouboules SM, Lafave HC, O'Halloran KD, Brutsaert TD, Nysten HE, Nysten CE, et al. Renal reactivity: acid-base compensation during incremental ascent to high altitude. J Physiol. 2018;596(24):6191–203. https://doi.org/10.1113/JP276973.

Chapter 7
Cardiovascular Changes in High Altitude

Sharmili Sinha and Saurabh Debnath

Case Scenario

A well trained mountaineer travelled from a height of 1200 m to 2800 m by flight on Day1. Next 3 days (Day2–4) they climbed up to 5400 m. Where he was joined by two more well acclimatized mountaineers and they climbed up to 6900 m in next 2 days (Day5–6). The climb was steep and demanding. The following night the first mountaineer developed a rapidly worsening cough and shortness of breath. There were rales bilaterally with poor SpO2. Next morning, he expectorated increasing volumes of frothy and later bloody sputum. He was barely able to get out of the tent owing to shortness of breath. His friends who stayed out at high altitudes longer before the journey and was better acclimatized didn't have any symptoms.

What Is the Diagnosis and Underlying Pathophysiology?

The diagnosis is High altitude pulmonary edema (HAPE).

Pathophysiology-Exposure to high altitude environment poses unique and distinctive challenges to the human physiology. The difficulties faced could be of acute exposure, as experienced by hikers, mountaineers or rescue workers or they could

S. Sinha (✉)
Department Critical Care Medicine, Institution-Apollo Hospitals,
Bhubaneswar, Odisha, India

S. Debnath
Department Critical Care Medicine, Institution-AMRI Hospital, Mukundpur,
Kolkata, West Bengal, India

J. Hidalgo et al. (eds.), *High Altitude Medicine*,
https://doi.org/10.1007/978-3-031-35092-4_7

be of long term exposure to such habitat by people who live in such high altitudes. The main concern is related to hypoxia due to low atmospheric pressure and low partial pressure of oxygen (PatmO2). By definition high altitude hypoxia (HAH) means fall in arterial blood O2 saturation (SaO2) in the body at altitudes >2500 m [1]. At this level and moving upwards there is progressive lowering of barometric pressure with rarefied atmosphere. As a consequence the partial pressure of inspired oxygen in the atmosphere (PatmO2) is low, to the tune of between 20% and 60% at 2500 and 8000 m, respectively [2]. Less amount of oxygen is breathed in with each inspiration leading to less partial pressure of oxygen in alveolar air (PalvO2). Now, as the lung parenchyma is normal the alveolar – arterial oxygen gradient (Alv-a O2 gradient) is also normal or maintained, leading to lowering of pulmonary capillary oxygen partial pressure and subsequently low systemic arterial oxygen partial pressure (PaO2). The ensuing hypoxemic hypoxia is known as High Altitude Hypoxia (HAH) which affects almost all organ systems. Oxygen is the essential substrate for aerobic metabolism which generates maximum ATP which is absolutely important for cell survival. In order to offset the adverse effects of diminished oxygen delivery to cells of vital organ systems, major changes in adaptation are seen in mechanisms of oxygen trapping (respiratory system), carriage (blood) and distribution (cardiovascular system). In this chapter the cardiovascular changes in acute or chronic exposure to high altitude would be discussed.

What Is Acute High Altitude Hypoxia (HAH) and the Cardiovascular Response?

High altitude ascent leads to exposure to environment with progressive and nonlinear decline in barometric pressure and a reduction in ambient partial pressure of oxygen (PatmO2). This results in a decrease in the PO2 at every point along the oxygen transport cascade from inspired air to the alveolar space, arterial blood, the tissues, and the venous blood. Greater the elevation above sea level bigger is the decline in oxygen partial pressures across different points in the cascade. These decline in oxygen tension trigger a host of physiologic responses in the cardiovascular system over a period of minutes to weeks that enable the individual to adapt or compensate for the hypoxic environment.

$$DO2 = CO \times Hb \times SaO2 \left(\text{oxygen delivery equation} \right)$$

The Cardiac System

The low PaO2 for mechanisms explained above leads to lower hemoglobin saturation in arterial blood (SaO2), the predominant oxygen carrier. The net content of oxygen per unit volume of arterial blood (CaO2 = Hb x SaO2) is reduced. Initially the body tries to respond by increasing the flow (Cardiac output = Heart rate x Stroke volume) by increasing the heart rate (tachycardia) with little or no change in stroke volume. The increase in heart rate is related to increased sympathetic activity and vagal withdrawal [3]. Reeves et al. showed that for a given level of exercise, change in heart rate is greater at high altitude [4]. After a few days of acclimatization, stroke volume falls gradually through the first week and then tends to stabilize [5, 6]. The fall in stroke volume is associated with reduction in left ventricular dimensions and filling pressure, which in part may be a consequence of diuresis and reduction of plasma volume that decreases over the first weeks at high altitude by as much as 20% at 3800 to 4500 m [7]. Chemoreceptor stimulation along with increased release of atrial natriuretic peptide (ANP) and decreased synthesis of aldosterone are responsible for the initial loss of plasma volume whereas fluid shift from the extracellular to the intracellular compartment promotes it later on [8].

The parameters governing the cardiac function as well as cardiac output remains more or less unchanged as body slowly adapts and acclimatizes to the high altitude environment but it is accompanied by a decrease in maximal oxygen consumption (VO2max) in the tissues [9], which declines by roughly 1% per 100 m above 1500 m [10]. This in turn causes reductions in maximal cardiac output. This effect is modest in acute hypoxia but becomes substantial gradually with acclimatization. This is unique mechanism which is not explained by hypovolemia, acid-bases status, increased viscosity due to polycythemia, autonomic nervous system changes, or depressed systolic function. The reduction in maximal oxygen uptake at high altitudes is countered to some extent by the improved convective and diffusional oxygen transport systems at a lower maximal cardiac output. However, it is suggested that 10–25% of the loss in aerobic exercise capacity at high altitudes can be restored by interventions leading to pulmonary vasodilation such as oxygen support [11]. It could be a result of an improved maximum flow output by a relatively unloaded right ventricle. While resting cardiovascular yield is higher at high altitude as compared to sea level, at top exercise it is relatively lower [2, 9, 12]. These variables are aimed at supplying more oxygen at rest to the tissues and simultaneously restrict top exercise limit and oxygen utilization. Altitude exposure carries no identified risk of myocardial ischemia in healthy subjects but has to be considered as a potential cardiac stress in patients with previous cardiovascular compromise.

Evidence Contour-In an elegant study with Doppler echocardiography on healthy volunteers who have been exposed to acute short term (90 mins) HAH, Huez et al. demonstrated significantly increased HR, LVEF, isovolumic contraction wave velocity (ICV), acceleration (ICA), and systolic ejection wave velocity at the mitral annulus, indicating enhanced left ventricular systolic function. However, there was no change in right ventricular area shortening fraction, tricuspid annular plane systolic excursion (TAPSE), ICV, and ICA at the tricuspid annulus, indicating preserved right ventricular systolic function. Increase in isovolumic relaxation time (IRT) at both annuli also pointed towards an altered diastolic function of both ventricles [13].

Acute assent to high altitude and resultant hypoxia causes dilation of the epicardial coronary arteries, generating augmented myocardial blood flow which compensates for the reduced oxygen content of the blood [14] and also preserve the exercise-induced coronary flow reserve up to about 4500 m [10]. Malconian et al. demonstrated that in healthy young men, there was no myocardial ischemia on exercise during a simulated ascent to the summit of Mount Everest (8840 m) over 40 days [15].

Acute exposure to high altitude causes low PaO2 which is sensed by the carotid body chemo receptors, which causes an increase in the breathing rate and hyperventilation, which is perhaps the first response to HAH. Then the cardiovascular functions are modified in response to the short-term HAH. Ventilation and sympathetic activity are augmented, as demonstrated by increased urinary and plasma concentration of catecholamines [16] and skeletal muscle sympathetic activity [17]. Hypoxia directly affects the vascular tone of the pulmonary and systemic resistance vessels and increases ventilation and sympathetic activity via stimulation of the peripheral chemoreceptors [18]. Klaussen et al. showed that acutely breathing an inspired fraction of O2 (FiO2) of 0.12 caused 22% increase in cardiac output accompanied with 18% increase in heart rate and unchanged stroke volume, so the oxygen delivery to the tissues remained unchanged [5]. There is shift of sympatho-vagal balance towards more sympathetic and less parasympathetic activity [19]. Mazzeo et al. showed that in response to acute exposure to 4300 m (4 h), the arterial plasma epinephrine levels were significantly increased as compared to norepinephrine level. However, both epinephrine and norepinephrine concentrations were increased after 21 days of chronic exposure [16]. These findings provide evidence for a differential adaptive response between sympathetic neural activity and that of the adrenal medulla during high-altitude exposure.

The Pulmonary Vascular System

The concept of vasoconstriction in the pulmonary vasculature in response to hypoxia (HPV) was promulgated by Von Euler and Liljestrand in 1946 [20]. At low altitude this is helpful to preserve the V-Q matching and optimize gas exchange at the alveolo-capillary membrane in response to local hypoxia in a part of lungs such as in pneumonia or atelectasis. When the whole lung is exposed to hypoxia, as in HAH, HPV may be disadvantageous because it results in a substantial increase in pulmonary vascular resistance and pulmonary arterial pressure (PAP). However there is no change in pulmonary artery occlusion pressure (PAOP). This pattern is seen in chronic high altitude exposure and remains essentially unchanged with prolonged or lifelong high altitude stay. Exercise in acute as well as in chronic high-altitude exposure is associated with a brisk increase in pulmonary artery pressure.

The smooth muscle cells of the pulmonary arterial bed plays a major role in HPV and is independent of the endothelium, as demonstrated in experiments with pulmonary vascular rings denuded of endothelium and with isolated smooth cells from pulmonary arteries [20]. Although HPV is intrinsic to pulmonary smooth muscle cells, there are additional endothelium-dependent and independent factors which influence this response. Hypoxia also may increase PAP through endothelin and sympathetic activation, whereas HPV may be attenuated by increased synthesis of NO, hyperventilation improving alveolar PO2, and respiratory alkalosis [21].

High Altitude Pulmonary Edema (HAPE)

HAPE is a non-cardiogenic pulmonary edema that may occur in previously healthy individuals within the first 2–5 days after rapid ascent above 3000–4000 m. It was first described in South American high-altitude dwellers who returned from a sojourn at low altitude and subsequently in unacclimatized lowlanders [22]. Altitude, rate of ascent, and, most importantly individual susceptibility are the major determinants of HAPE in mountaineers and trekkers. The initial mechanism of HAPE is a lack of oxygen caused by the low air pressure at high altitudes. The detailed pathways of this oxygen shortage-induced HAPE are not known, but an excessive rise in pulmonary artery pressure (PAP) and vascular resistance (HPV) leading to increased microvascular pressures plays an important role. This enhanced hydrostatic stress causes dynamic changes in the permeability of the alveolar capillary barrier and induces a high permeability noninflammatory lung edema. This mechanism of high PAP doesn't fully explain the development of HAPE as not all high PAP lead to HAPE in high altitude. Decreased nitric oxide (NO) release and enhanced endothelin (ET) levels following acute high-altitude exposure may be responsible for exaggerated hypoxic pulmonary vasoconstriction in HAPE-susceptible individuals [23].

The Cerebro-Vascular System

The brain is the most oxygen-dependent organ in the body. With exposure to high altitude, there is a rise in cerebral blood flow (CBF) to compensate for low PaO2 and ensure an adequate supply of O2 to meet the demand of cerebral tissue [24]. However, this is gradually nullified to a fall to near sea level values within 1–3 weeks of acclimatization. The underlying mechanisms for regulating the CBF during short-term HAH are complex and is governed by the balance between low PaO2 (HAH) and hyperventilation induced low PaCO2 (low PaCO2 causes cerebral vasoconstriction) [25]. Low PaO2-to-PaCO2 ratio can explain 40% of the increase in brain blood flow upon arrival at high altitude (5050 m) [24]. The initial high CBF can be reversed by supplemental oxygen suggests a direct hypoxic effect. Other mechanisms that may contribute to raised CBF are increase in adenosine and nitric oxide level, which causes an increase in arterial diameter [26].

High Altitude Cerebral Edema (HACE)

High altitude cerebral edema (HACE) is a medical condition in which the intracranial pressure (ICP) is high due to accumulation of excess fluid in the brain as a direct consequence of ascending to high altitude and failing to acclimatize. The major cause of HACE is low PaO2 and resultant high CBF when the individual climbs to greater heights rapidly allowing less time for the body to adapt. It is most often a complication of acute mountain sickness (AMS) or high-altitude pulmonary edema (HAPE). It is a form of vasogenic edema [27]. HAH causes inflammation of endothelial lining intra-cerebral vasculature which along with raised hydrostatic pressure leads to leakage of fluid into the brain parenchyma. Furthermore, there could be impairment of the auto-regulation of cerebral blood flow and disruption of the integrity of the blood brain barrier due to HAH mediated release of certain neuromodulators such as vascular endothelial growth factor (VEGF) and calcitonin gene-related peptide (CGRP). Increased sympathetic nervous activity at high altitude may also play a role [27].

What Are the Long Term Adaptations at High Altitude?

People after acclimatization to high altitude and for those who live at such altitude show adaptive changes in the cardiovascular system to compensate for chronic exposure to High Altitude Hypoxia (HAH).

The Cardiac System

Post acclimatization the heart rate and arterial blood pressure may remain higher, but stroke volume is gradually decreased and the cardiac output returns to baseline after a longer hypoxic exposure [5]. Suarez et al. showed remarkably preserved contractility and excellent tolerance of the normal myocardium to long-term HAH [28]. Some of the adaptations are aimed at protection against ischemic heart disease. An epidemiological study reported that men residing at high altitude resulted in protection against death from ischemic heart disease [29]. The epidemiological observations on the cardio-protective effect of high altitude were confirmed in various experimental models [30–32]. It also protects the heart against ischemia induced arrhythmias, as was shown in rat models [33].

Cardiac structural changes also happens in response to sustained HAH as it leads to development of right ventricular hypertrophy (RVH). RVH is a beneficial adaptation that helps to counteract the increased afterload caused by persistent pulmonary hypertension and maintain a normal cardiac output [34]. Along with changes in right ventricular muscle mass there is marked change in cardiac protein profiling

[35]. Collagenous and non-collagenous proteins were significantly increased both in hypertrophic RV and non-hypertrophic LV, in rats exposed to intermittent high-altitude [36]. Cardiac enlargement may be the result of both an increase in the number of individual cell elements (hyperplasia) and an increase in their volume (hypertrophy).

The changes in response to long term HAH in the autonomic nervous system are different than in short term exposure to high altitude. Increase in plasma norepinephrine level is much more than epinephrine levels [37]. The resting heart rate remains increased, but the heart rate at maximal exercise is reduced at long-term HAH. There is reduced adrenergic receptor density. Experimental studies in rats exposed to 21 days of HAH found that there was a significant reduction in β-adrenergic receptor density [38] and a down regulation of α- and β-adrenergic receptor density in ventricular tissues [39].

Hemoglobin is the most important carrier of oxygen in the body. Prolonged exposure to HA lead to increased erythropoietin production resulting in increase in hemoglobin concentration increase [9]. Raised hemoglobin and RBC mass lead to increased viscosity which tempers down the cardiac output from initial raised levels in the long term.

The Pulmonary Vascular System

The most common and significant effect of chronic exposure to high altitude is development of pulmonary hypertension. Estimated prevalence of pulmonary hypertension amongst indwellers of high altitude ranged between 5% and 18% [40]. HPV induced increased pulmonary vascular pressure and resistance causes adaptation changes in the vascular structure and remodeling. The pulmonary vascular adaptations involve all elements of the vessel wall and include endothelial dysfunction, extension of smooth muscle into previously non-muscular vessels and adventitial thickening. High altitude induced pulmonary hypertension was only partially reversed by oxygen breathing, suggesting that pulmonary arteries structural remodeling plays a pivotal role in pulmonary hypertension during long-term HAH [41].

Intrinsic changes in the ionic balance and calcium homeostasis of pulmonary arterial smooth muscle cells (PASMCs) caused by long-term hypoxia have a major effect on PA remodeling. The membrane depolarization of PASMCs following the hypoxic inhibition of O2 sensitive K+ channels activated Ca2+ influx and elevated cytoplasmic ionized Ca2+ via voltage-gated Ca2+ channels. Changes in the transport of K+ and Ca2+ through their respective ion channels modulate these processes by affecting cell volume, membrane potential, gene transcription, apoptosis, and cell-cycle progression. The adaptation of these ion channels at high altitude appears to involve in pulmonary arteries remodeling [42]. Endothelin (ET)-1 is another important mediator of hypoxia-induced pulmonary vasoconstriction and vascular remodeling. Chronic hypoxia increases ET-1 gene transcription and peptide synthesis in cultured endothelial cells. ET-1 and its receptors are selectively upregulated in patients with primary pulmonary hypertension and in humans exposed to high altitude [43].

Dilation of the right ventricle due to increased pulmonary vascular resistance causes a pressure effect on the left side of the heart as the inter-ventricular septum deviates towards the left side leading to altered left ventricular structure and diastolic filling [44, 45]. In pathological forms of pulmonary hypertension, this may cause diastolic dysfunction of the left ventricle [46].

Conclusion

The changes in cardiovascular system can occur in response to acute and chronic exposure to high altitude. The pathophysiology involves multiple mechanisms. The acute responses include High Altitude Hypoxia (HAH) and High Altitude Pulmonary Edema (HAPE). The rate of development depends on the speed of ascent and extent of acclimatization. The main mechanisms of cardiovascular system adaptations to high altitude is variable and it depends on various factors like individual predisposition, the actual elevation, the rate of ascent, and the duration of exposure. The initial response to HAH exposure is hyperventilation and increase in sympathetic activity (which results partly from chemoreceptor reflexes and baroreceptor function) leading to increase in heart rate, systemic vascular resistance, blood pressure, cardiac output and pulmonary hypertension associated with pulmonary vasoconstriction. The significant reflection in chronic exposure to altitude is development of chronic pulmonary hypertension. Cardiovascular system gradually progress towards a compensatory and pathologic adaptation to HAH. Understanding these adaptive responses is crucial to monitor and reduce the development of adverse changes and also preserve the beneficial effects of the process of adaptation.

References

1. Moore LG, Charles SM, Julian CG. Humans at high altitude: hypoxia and fetal growth. Respir Physiol Neurobiol. 2011;178:181–90.
2. Bärtsch P, Gibbs JSR. Effect of Altitude on the Heart and the Lungs. Circulation. 2007;116:2191–202.
3. Koller EA, Drechsel S, Hess T, Macherel P, Boutellier U. Effects of atropine and propanolol on the respiratory, circulatory, and ECG responses to high altitude in man. Eur J Appl Physiol. 1988;57:163–72.
4. Reeves JT, Groves BM, Sutton JR, Wagner PD, Cymerman A, Malconian MK, Rock PB, Young PM, Houston CS. Operation Everest II: preservation of cardiac function at extreme altitude. J Appl Physiol. 1987;63:531–9.
5. Klausen K. Cardiac output in man in rest and work during and after acclimatization to 3,800 m. J Appl Physiol. 1966;21:609–16.
6. Alexander JK, Grover RF. Mechanism of reduced cardiac stroke volume at high altitude. Clin Cardiol. 1983;6:301–3.

7. Grover RF, Bärtsch P. Blood. In: Hornbein TF, Schoene RB, editors. High altitude: an exploration of human adaptation, vol. 161. New York, NY: Marcel Dekker Inc; 2001. p. 493–523.
8. Swenson ER. Renal function and fluid homeostasis. In: Hornbein TF, Schoene RB, editors. High altitude: an exploration of human adaptation, vol. 161. New York, NY: Marcel Dekker Inc; 2001. p. 525–68.
9. Naeije R. Physiological adaptation of the cardiovascular system to high altitude. Prog Cardiovasc Dis. 2010;52:456–66.
10. Wagner PD, Gale GE, Moon RE, Torre-Bueno JR, Stolp BW, Saltzman HA. Pulmonary gas exchange in humans exercising at sea level and simulated altitude. J Appl Physiol. 1986;61:260–70.
11. Ghofrani HA, Reichenberger F, Kohstall MG, et al. Sildenafil increased exercise capacity during hypoxia at low altitudes and at Mount Everest base camp: a randomized, double-blind, placebocontrolled crossover trial. Ann Intern Med. 2004;141:169–77.
12. Boos CJ, Mellor A, Begley J, Stacey M, Smith C, Hawkins A. The effects of exercise at high altitude on high-sensitivity cardiac troponin release and associated biventricular cardiac function. Clin Res Cardiol. 2014;103:291–9.
13. Huez S, Retailleau K, Unger P, Pavelescu A, Vachiery JL, Derumeaux G, et al. Right andleft ventricular adaptation to hypoxia: a tissue doppler imaging study. Am J Physiol Heart Circ Physiol. 2005;289:H1391–8. https://doi.org/10.1152/ajpheart.00332.2005.
14. Koepfli P, Wyss CA, Namdar M, Siegrist PT, Luscher TF, Camici PG, Kaufmann PA. Beta-adrenergic blockade and myocardial perfusion in coronary artery disease: differential effects in stenotic versus remote myocardial segments. Nucl Med. 2004;45:1626–31.
15. Malconian M, Rock P, Hultgren H, Donner H, Cymerman A, Groves B, Reeves J, Alexander J, Sutton J, Nitta M, Houston C. The electrocardiogram at rest and exercise during a simulated ascent of Mt Everest (operation Everest-II). Am J Cardiol. 1990;65:1475–80.
16. Mazzeo RS, Bender PR, Brooks GA, Butterfield GE, Groves BM, Sutton JR, Wolfel EE, Reeves JT. Arterial catecholamine responses during exercise with acute and chronic high-altitude exposure. Am J Phys. 1991;261:E419–24.
17. Hansen J, Sander M. Sympathetic neural overactivity in healthy humans after prolonged exposure to hypobaric hypoxia. J Physiol. 2003;546:921–9.
18. Heistad DD, Abboud FM. Circulatory adjustments to hypoxia. Circulation. 1980;61:463–70.
19. Princi T, Zupet P, Finderle Z, Accardo A. Linear and nonlinear assessment of heart rate variability in nonacclimatized middleaged subjects at different hypoxic levels. Biomed Sci Instrum. 2008;44:380–5.
20. Von Euler US, Liljestrand G. Observations on the pulmonary arterial blood pressure in the cat. Acta Physiol Scand. 1946;12:301–20. Olschewski A, Weir EK. Hypoxic pulmonary vasoconstriction and hypertension. In: Peacock A, Rubin LJ, eds. Pulmonary Diseases and Their Treatment. London, UK: Arnold; 2004:33–44.
21. Bärtsch P, Mairbäurl H, Maggiorini M, Swenson E. Physiological aspects of high-altitude pulmonary edema. J Appl Physiol. 2005;98:1101–10.
22. Houston CS. Acute pulmonary edema of high altitude. N Engl J Med. 1960;263:478–80.
23. Swenson ER, Bartsch P. High-altitude pulmonary edema. Compr Physiol. 2012;2:2753–73. https://doi.org/10.1002/cphy.c100029.
24. Lucas SJ, Burgess KR, Thomas KN, Donnelly J, Peebles KC, Lucas RA, et al. Alterations in cerebral blood flow and cerebrovascular reactivity during 14 days at 5050 m. J Physiol. 2011;589:741–53. https://doi.org/10.1113/jphysiol.2010.192534.
25. Ainslie PN, Ogoh S. Regulation of cerebral blood flow during chronic hypoxia: a matter of balance. Exp Physiol. 2010;95:251–62. https://doi.org/10.1113/expphysiol.2008.045575.
26. Wilson MH, Edsell ME, Davagnanam I, Hirani SP, Martin DS, Levett DZ, et al. Cerebral artery dilatation maintains cerebral oxygenation at extreme altitude and in acute hypoxia—an ultrasound and MRI study. J Cereb Blood Flow Metab. 2011;31:2019–29. https://doi.org/10.1038/jcbfm.2011.81.
27. Hackett PH, Roach RC. High altitude cerebral edema. High Alt Med Biol. 2004;5:136–46. https://doi.org/10.1089/1527029041352054.

28. Suarez J, Alexander JK, Houston CS. Enhanced left ventricular systolic performance at high altitude during operation Everest II. Am J Cardiol. 1987;60:137–42.
29. Mortimer EA Jr, Monson RR, McMahon B. Reduction in mortality from coronary heart disease in men residing at high altitude. N Engl J Med. 1977;296:581–5.
30. Turek Z, Kubat K, Ringnalda BEM. Experimental myocardial infarction in rats acclimated to simulated high altitude. Basic Res Cardiol. 1980;75:544–53.
31. Neckar J, Szarszoi O, Koten L, Papousek F, Ostadal B, Grover GJ, Kolar F. Effects of mitochondrial KATP modulators on cardioprotection induced by chronic high altitude hypoxia in rats. Cardiovasc Res. 2002;55:567–75. https://doi.org/10.1016/S0008-6363(02)00456-X.
32. Tajima M, Katayose D, Bessho M, Isoyama S. Acute ischaemic preconditioning and chronic hypoxia independently increase myocardial tolerance to ischaemia. Cardiovasc Res. 1994;28:312–9.
33. Asemu G, Papousek F, Ostadal B, Kolar F. Adaptation to high altitude hypoxia protects the rat heart against ischemia-induced arrhythmias. Involvement of mitochondrial K (ATP) channel. J Mol Cell Cardiol. 1999;31:1821–31.
34. Kolar F, Ostadal B. Right ventricular function in rats with hypoxic pulmonary hypertension. Pflugers Arch. 1991;419:121–6.
35. Ostadal B, Kolar F. Cardiac adaptation to chronic high-altitude hypoxia: beneficial and adverse effects. Respir Physiol Neurobiol. 2007;158:224–36. https://doi.org/10.1016/j.resp.2007.03.005.
36. Ostadal B, Mirejovska E, Hurych J, Pelouch V, Prochazka J. Effect of intermittent high altitude hypoxia on the synthesis of collagenous and non-collagenous proteins of the right and left ventricular myocardium. Cardiovasc Res. 1978;12:303–8.
37. Calbet JA. Chronic hypoxia increases blood pressure and noradrenaline spillover in healthy humans. J Physiol. 2003;551:379–86. https://doi.org/10.1113/jphysiol.2003.045112.
38. Kacimi R, Richalet JP, Corsin A, Abousahl I, Crozatier B. Hypoxia-induced downregulation of beta-adrenergic receptors in rat heart. J Appl Physiol. 1992;73:1377–82.
39. Leon-Velarde F, Bourin MC, Germack R, Mohammadi K, Crozatier B, Richalet JP. Differential alterations in cardiac adrenergic signaling in chronic hypoxia or norepinephrineinfusion. Am J Physiol Regul Integr Comp Physiol. 2001;280:R274–81.
40. Xu XQ, Jing ZC. High-altitude pulmonary hypertension. Eur Respir Rev. 2009;18:13–7. https://doi.org/10.1183/09059180.00011104.
41. Groves BM, Reeves JT, Sutton JR, Wagner PD, Cymerman A, Malconian MK, et al. Operation Everest II: elevated high-altitude pulmonary resistance unresponsive to oxygen. J Appl Physiol. 1987;63:521–30.
42. Remillard CV, Yuan JX. High altitude pulmonary hypertension: role of K+ and Ca2+ channels. High Alt Med Biol. 2005;6:133–46. https://doi.org/10.1089/ham.2005.6.133.
43. Chen YF, Oparil S. Endothelin and pulmonary hypertension. J Cardiovasc Pharmacol. 2000;35:S49–53.
44. Tanaka H, Tei C, Nakao S, Tahara M, Sakurai S, Kashima T, Kanehisa T. Diastolic bulging of the interventricular septum toward the left ventricle: an echocardiographic manifestation of negative interventricular pressure gradient between left and right ventricles during diastole. Circulation. 1980;62:558–63.
45. Louie EK, Rich S, Levitsky S, Brundage BH. Doppler echocardiographic demonstration of the differential effects of right ventricular pressure and volume overload on left ventricular geometry and filling. J Am Coll Cardiol. 1992;19:84–90.
46. Mahmud E, Raisinghani A, Hassankhani A, Sadeghi M, Strachan GM, Auger W, DeMaria AN, Blanchard DG. Correlation of left ventricular overload and pulmonary artery pressure in chronic thromboembolic pulmonary hypertension. J Am Coll Cardiol. 2002;40:318–24.

Chapter 8
Peripheral Tissue in High Altitude

Ranajit Chatterjee, Asif Iqbal, and Ahsina Jahan Lopa

Introduction

Acute Adjustments

At high altitude, acutely, the hypoxia is sensed by the peripheral chemoreceptors, which causes an increase in the respiratory rate (hyperventilation). However, hyperventilation also results in respiratory alkalosis due to the increase in the respiratory rate, resulting in carbon dioxide being removed from the body, which suppresses the respiratory centre from increasing the respiratory rate any further, to meet the oxygen demands.

It is also pertinent to note that, the peripheral chemoreceptors cause sympathetic nervous system (Autonomic Nervous System) stimulation, resulting in the heart rate to increase, while the stroke volume decreases, and digestion is impaired. Shortness of breath is a common occurrence, and tendency to micturate is also increased in the process.

The human body can adapt to high altitude through acute and chronic changes in the body via various acclimatization processes.

R. Chatterjee (✉)
Dept. of Anaesthesiology and Critical Care, Swami Dayanand Hospital, New Delhi, India

A. Iqbal
Apollo Hospital, Kolkata, India

A. J. Lopa
Brahmanberia Hospital, Brahmanbaria, Bangladesh

J. Hidalgo et al. (eds.), *High Altitude Medicine*,
https://doi.org/10.1007/978-3-031-35092-4_8

Along with respiratory alkalosis, the affects mentioned above, are the causes for the symptoms of altitude sickness, which worsen during increased physical activity, leading to higher oxygen demand at high altitudes (Involving more of anaerobic respiration compared to lower altitudes); But during acclimatization the effects of the same are much subdued, due to homeostasis.

Acclimatization

Acclimatization to higher altitude requires days and sometimes weeks. Gradually, the body starts compensating for the respiratory alkalosis by excreting bicarbonate ions through the kidneys, which allows for adequate respiration, through increased respiratory rate, to provide for adequate oxygenation without risking the deleterious effects of alkalosis. It takes about 4 days, at any given altitude, for acclimatization, and can be enhanced by drugs such as acetazolamide (which decreases fluid retention).

Staying well hydrated during acclimatization is important to minimize the effects of altitude sickness and also to counteract the effects of increased urination. The heart rate and respiratory rate, at rest, both remain elevated despite the acclimatization. While the heart rate at maximum activity level will be reduced than in normal conditions.

The marked difference brought about by acclimatization, that explains, why it makes high altitudes more comfortable for the body, is the increased levels of circulating red blood cells in the body, which improves the oxygen carrying capacity of haemoglobin. This is an adaptive response due to increased erythropotein synthesis in the kidneys (from hypoxia in the tissues) that act on the liver to increase erythrocyte (red blood cell) production.

Due to increased micturition the blood volume contracts, which also increases the haematocrit (concentration of haemoglobin in blood). This increase in the relative concentration of red blood cells in the blood remains for a few weeks, after one returns to lower altitudes. So those who acclimatize to higher altitudes will experience improved athletic performance at lower altitudes. Capillary density and tissue perfusion are also increased during acclimatization.

The physiological changes mentioned above, make high-altitude athletic training beneficial for athletes participating in various high end national and international competitions. Full haematological adaptation to high altitude, is said to be achieved, when the increase in red blood cells reaches a plateau and stops.

The duration for the full haematological adaptation to be manifested in the peripheral blood, can be approximated by multiplying the altitude in kilometres by 11.4 days. For example, to adapt to 4000 m (13,000 ft.) of altitude would require 45.6 days.

The upper altitude limit of this linear relationship has not been fully established, in part because, extremely high altitudes have such little oxygen concentration in air, that it would be fatal, regardless of acclimatization.

Acclimatization to High Altitude

The recent updates and developments, in our understanding of the molecular mechanisms of human responses to hypoxia/hypoxemia has focused on *hypoxia-inducible factor* (HIF). This transcription factor modulates the expression of hundreds of genes, including those involved in apoptosis, angiogenesis, metabolism, cell proliferation, and permeability processes. In chronic hypoxia, HIF activation by hypoxia has the positive effect of elevating oxygen delivery by boosting haemoglobin mass. However, HIF also plays a role in carotid body sensitivity to hypoxia, which in turn largely determines the ventilatory response to hypoxia. As the main regulator of response to hypoxia in humans, HIF has both beneficial and harmful effects at different stages during human exposure to hypoxia and in different cells in the body (Fig. 8.1).

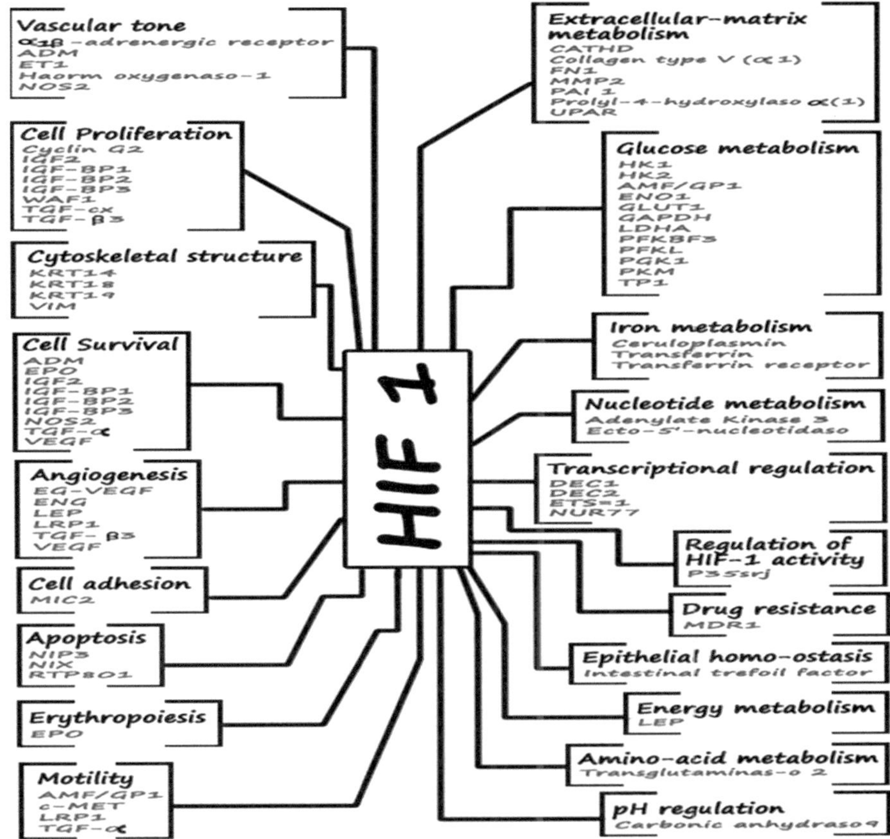

Fig. 8.1 Regulation of oxygen sensing by *hypoxia-inducible factor* (HIF)

HIF is produced constitutively, but in normoxiathe α subunit is degraded by the proteasome, which is dependent on oxygen. Hypoxic environment prevents hydroxylation of the α subunit, enabling the active HIF transcription complex to form at the hypoxia-response element (HRE) associated with HIF-regulated genes.

Systemic Circulation

Increased sympathetic activity on ascending heights causes an initial mild increase in blood pressure, moderate increases in heart rate and cardiac output, and increase in venous tone. Stroke volume comes down because of decreased plasma volume, which drops as much as 12% over the first 24 h, as a result of the: (1) Bicarbonate diuresis, (2) Shifting of fluid from the intravascular space, and (3) Suppression of aldosterone. Resting heart rate returns to near sea level values with acclimatization, except at extremely high altitudes. Maximal heart rate reached, follows a decline with maximal oxygen uptake and with increasing altitude. As the limits of hypoxic acclimatization are approached, maximal and resting heart rates tend to have similar values.

Pulmonary Circulation

On ascending to higher altitudes, a quick but variable increase in pulmonary vascular resistance (PVR) from hypoxic pulmonary vasoconstriction increases pulmonary artery pressure (PAP). Mild pulmonary hypertension is greatly aggravated by exercise, with PAP reaching near-systemic values, especially in persons with a prior history of HAPE. Administration of oxygen does not completely restore PAP values to sea level, likely because of vascular remodelling with medial hypertrophy. (PVR returns to normal within a few weeks after descent to lower altitudes).

Cerebral Circulation

Cerebral oxygen delivery, the product of arterial oxygen concentration and cerebral blood flow (CBF), is dependent on the balance between hypoxic vasodilation and hypocapnia-induced vasoconstriction. Despite hypocapnia, CBF increases when PaO2 is less than 60 mm Hg (altitude >2800 m [9186 feet]). In a classic study, CBF increased 24% on abrupt ascent to 3810 m (12,500 feet) and returned to normal over 3–5 days [6]. These findings have been confirmed by positron emission tomography (PET) and brain magnetic resonance imaging (MRI) studies showing both elevations in CBF in hypoxia in humans and striking heterogeneity of the CBF, with it rising up to 33% in the hypothalamus and 20% in the thalamus. Other areas showed no significant changes. Cerebral autoregulation, the process by which cerebral perfusion is maintained as blood pressure varies, is deranged in hypoxia. Interestingly, this occurs with acute ascent, after successful acclimatization, and in natives to high altitude.

Hematopoietic Responses to Altitude

Ever since the findings in 1890 by Viault that haemoglobin concentration was higher than normal, in animals living in the Andes, scientists have regarded the hematopoietic response to increase in altitude as an important component of the acclimatization process. On the other hand, haemoglobin values have shown to have no relationship with susceptibility to high-altitude illness. In response to hypoxemia, erythropoietin is synthesized by the kidneys and stimulates the bone marrow to produce red blood cells (RBCs). Erythropoietin is detectable in blood within 2 h of ascent; Nucleated immature RBCs can be found on a peripheral blood smear within days; And new RBCs are seen in the circulation in 4–5 days. Over weeks to months, the mass of RBCs increase in proportion to the degree of hypoxemia. Iron supplementation can be helpful; Women who take supplemental iron at high altitude approach the haematocrit values of men at altitude (Fig. 8.2). The field of erythropoietin and iron metabolism has exploded in recent years, with discovery of two new iron-regulating hormones, hepcidin and erythroferrone, and a novel, soluble erythropoietin receptor with function directly linked to performance at high altitude. How all these findings are integrated and their responses seen in a scenario of acclimatization to hypoxia remain to be determined, and is a matter of further research and study.

The increase in haemoglobin seen 1–2 days after ascent to a higher altitude is caused by haemoconcentration secondary to decreased plasma volume, rather than by a true increase in RBC mass. This results in a higher haemoglobin concentration at the cost of decreased blood volume, a scenario that might impair exercise

Fig. 8.2 Hematocrit changes on ascending to higher altitudes in men and in women with and without supplemental iron

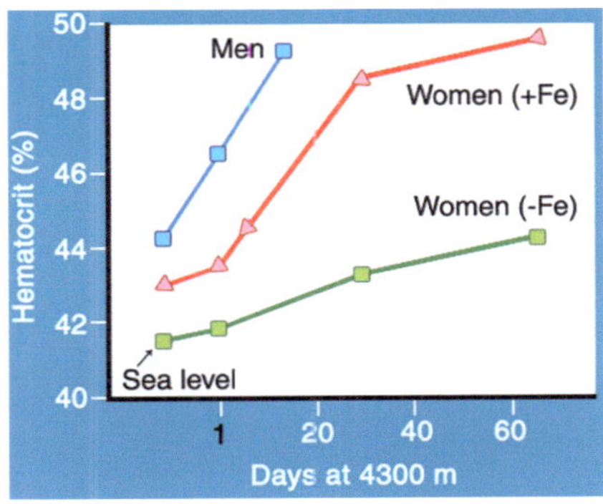

performance. Long-term acclimatization leads to an increase in plasma volume as well as in RBC mass, thereby increasing total blood volume. Overshoot of the hematopoietic response causes excessive polycythemia, which may impair oxygen transport because of increased blood viscosity.

Hematocrit changes on ascent to altitude in men and in women with (+Fe) and without (−Fe) supplemental iron.

Oxyhemoglobin Dissociation Curve

The oxygen dissociation curve (ODC) plays a crucial role in depicting the oxygen transport. The sigmoidal shape of the curve allows SaO2 to be well maintained up to 3000 m (9843 feet), despite significant decreases in PaO2 (see Fig. 8.3). Above 3000 m, small changes in PaO2 cause large changes in SaO2 (Fig. 8.3). Because PaO2 determines diffusion of oxygen from capillary to cell, small changes in PaO2 can have clinically significant effects. This is often bewildering for clinicians because SaO2 appears relatively well preserved. At high altitude, small changes in PaO2 lead to lower oxygen uptake that can have a deleterious effect on systemic hypoxemia, and thus on clinical status, while SaO2 may appear relatively unchanged.

Tissue Changes

The next thing in the oxygen transport chain is tissue oxygen transfer, which depends on capillary perfusion, diffusion distance, and driving pressure of oxygen from the capillary to the cell. Banchero [5] has shown that capillary density in dog skeletal muscle doubles in 3 weeks at PB of 435 mm Hg. A recent study in humans noted no change in capillary density or in gene expression thought to enhance muscle vascularity. Ou and Tenney revealed a 40% increase in mitochondrial number

Fig. 8.3 Oxygen-haemoglobin dissociation curve showing effect of 10–mm Hg decrement in arterial partial pressure of oxygen (PaO2) on arterial oxygen saturation (SaO2) at sea level *(A)* and near 4400 m

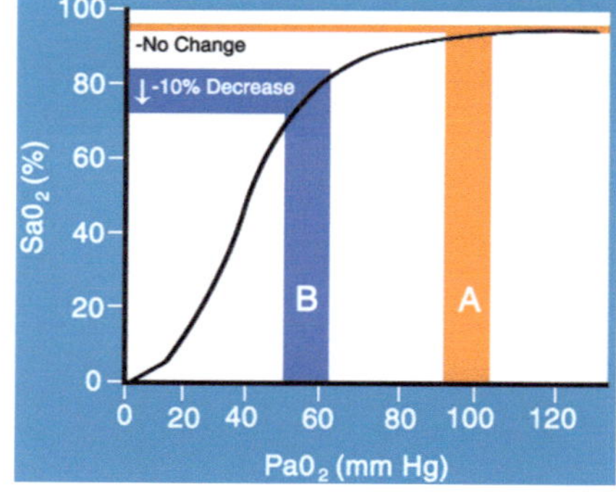

Table 8.1 Comparison of acclimatization, evolutionary adaptation and physiological responses to extreme altitude

Condition	Altitude	Physiological Features
Acclimatization to high altitude	Up to 5000 m	Hyperventilation Nearly complete renal compensation of the respiratory alkalosis Polycythermia Increase in intracellular oxidative enzymes Reduced intercapillary diffusion distances in some tissues
Evolutionary Adaptation	Up to 5000 m	Hyperventilation although this is less in best-adapted people Complete renal compensation Polycythemia although this is less in the best-adapted Changes in intracellular enzyme
Physiological response to extreme altitude	Up to 7000 m	Extreme hyperventilation Marked respiratory alkalosis Incomplete renal compensation Increased O_2-affinity of hemoglobin as a result of the alkalosis Very low maxima O_2 consumption Great reduction in anaerobic metabolism Relentless loss of weight and other evidence of progressive deterioration

but no change in mitochondrial size, whereas Oelz and colleagues showed that high-altitude climbers had normal mitochondrial density. A significant decrease in muscle size is often noted after high-altitude expeditions because of net energy deficit, resulting in increased capillary density and ratio of mitochondrial volume to contractile protein fraction as a result of the atrophy. Although there is no de novo synthesis of capillaries or mitochondria, the net result is a shortening of diffusion distance for oxygen (Table 8.1).

Physiologic Changes during Acclimatization to Maintain Tissue Oxygen (O2) Delivery

- Involuntary increase in ventilation
- Increased haemoglobin concentration
- Haemoconcentration because of decrease in plasma volume (within days)
- Increased red blood cell mass (2–3 weeks)
- Increased affinity of haemoglobin for O2
- Steep portion of O2 disassociation curve
- Leftward shift of O2 disassociation curve from decreased PCO2 and increased pH
- Increased tissue O2 extraction with lowering of mixed venous O2
- Decreased cardiac output

- Increased time for O2 diffusion from alveolus to capillary because of slower blood flow
- Attenuates rise in pulmonary artery and capillary pressure

The arterial oxygen content (CaO2) reflects the total number of oxygen molecules in arterial blood, both bound and unbound to haemoglobin. The greatest contributor to the maintenance of CaO2 during acclimatization is the increase in respiratory rate [1]. A drop in PO2 leads to hypoxic stimulation of peripheral chemo-receptors, primarily in the carotid and aortic bodies causing an increase in the depth and rate of breathing. This is known as the hypoxic ventilatory response. A reduction in PaCO2 leads to respiratory alkalosis, which, at sea level, would normally exert an inhibitory effect on respiration causing arterial PCO2 and pH to return to normal levels. However, at higher altitudes, this inhibitory effect is overridden by central medullary chemoreceptors, such that high rate of ventilation are maintained.

The persistent increase in the respiratory is because of the exit of HCO3 from the cerebrospinal fluid (CSF) with subsequent lowering of pH, which in turn stimulates the respiratory centre.

Acidification of the CSF is linked to decreased HCO3 reabsorption in the proximal tubule of the kidney, which is a compensatory response to chronic respiratory alkalosis. This renal response is fully manifested over the course of 2–3 days. In addition to the acid-base changes, increased ventilation is also driven by a sensitization of the carotid body to hypoxia during prolonged exposure to high altitude.

Changes in haemoglobin concentration and its affinity for oxygen also contribute to maintenance of CaO2 with respect to altitude. Within the first 1 to 2 days of exposure to higher altitudes, there is a rapid rise in haemoglobin concentration because haemoconcentration [4–6]. The decrease in plasma volume ranges from 15% to 25% and roughly correlates with the degree of altitude attained. Circulating levels of erythropoietin increases rapidly, with peak levels being attended at 48 h to 72 h after arrival to a higher altitude. This rise is short lived. The levels of erythropoietin tend to return towards baseline in 5–10 days [5]. Red cell mass begins to slowly increase, shortly after the rise in erythropoietin levels but it takes several weeks to fully manifest. For subjects who remain at a given altitude for periods of less than a week, the change in red cell mass is trivial and would not make any significant contribution to the acclimatization process.

In addition to the increase in haemoglobin concentrations, the acclimatization process leads to changes in factors that can shift the position of the oxygen disassociation curve leading to an either increase or decrease in oxygen affinity. The PaO2 at which haemoglobin is 50% saturated is called the P50. Increase in blood pH shifts the curve leftward, reflecting increased affinity of haemoglobin for oxygen, whereas accumulation of red cell 2,3-diphosphoglycerate shifts the curve rightward reflecting decreased affinity for oxygen (Fig. 8.4).

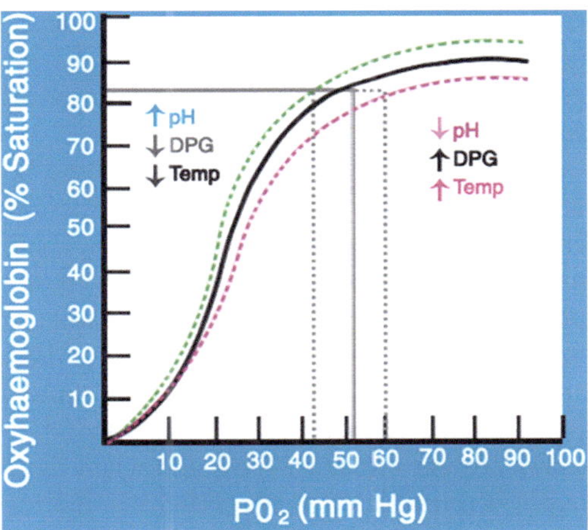

Fig. 8.4 Oxygen-hemoglobin dissociation curve

Renal Adaptations to High-Altitude Hypoxia

As described in the sections above, the initial response to high-altitude hypoxia is a respiratory alkalosis produced by an increase in the respiratory drive, leading to hyperventilation. Within minutes, the kidneys respond to the alkalosis with an increased excretion of bicarbonate ions; this renal effect can continue for hours or days and function to correct the alkalosis and return the pH of the serum toward a normal value.

The kidneys also respond to hypoxia by the increased synthesis of erythropoietin. Erythropoietin leads to an increase in red cell mass and the oxygen-carrying capacity of the blood (dissolved oxygen accounts for only about 2% of the oxygen-carrying capacity); However, it takes several days before an increased rate of erythrocyte production can be measured, and the process is not complete for weeks to months. For short-term ascents, the erythropoietin-mediated increase in red cell mass is of minor importance, although it is important for extended expeditions. The haematocrit, not the total haemoglobin, is increased during short-term ascents by a reduction in plasma volume caused by a hypoxia-mediated diuresis; the elevation in haematocrit increases the oxygen-carrying capacity per 100 mL of blood.

Metabolic Adaptation of Skeletal Muscle to High Altitude Hypoxia

Physiological adaptations that can improve oxygen delivery in hypoxic individuals are well known and include increased respiratory rate and cardiac output, erythropoiesis, and possibly enhanced vascularization of tissues. At increased altitude, however, despite normal oxygen content and delivery up to 7000 m above sea level, exercise capacity is dramatically reduced, and inter-individual variation in oxygen content does not correlate with exercise capacity. These findings support an important role for adaptive responses to a low arterial partial pressure of oxygen at the tissue level. In the hypoxic myocyte, adaptations might aim to improve local O_2 delivery by redistributing mitochondria within the cell to minimize O_2 diffusion gradients and also to limit ATP utilization by switching off non-essential cellular functions or to enhance ATP synthesis.

The master regulator for many of the body's adaptive responses is hypoxia-inducible factor 1 (HIF-1), a heterodimer transcription factor comprising HIF-1α and HIF-1β subunits. HIF-1α protein is continuously synthesized, and is predominantly regulated post-transcriptionally by the O_2-dependent hydroxylation of two proline residues by the prolyl-hydroxylase enzymes (PHD1–3). Hydroxylation promotes binding of the von Hippel-Lindau protein (VHL), leading to ubiquitination and proteasomal degradation. HIF-1α protein is thus stabilized in low concentrations of O_2, and accumulates spontaneously in the hypoxic cell. HIF-1β is constitutively present in the nucleus, and when dimerized with HIF-1α is able to bind to hypoxia response elements (HREs) in the regulatory region of a number of genes, thereby activating their transcription (Fig. 8.5). The levels of HIF-target genes are

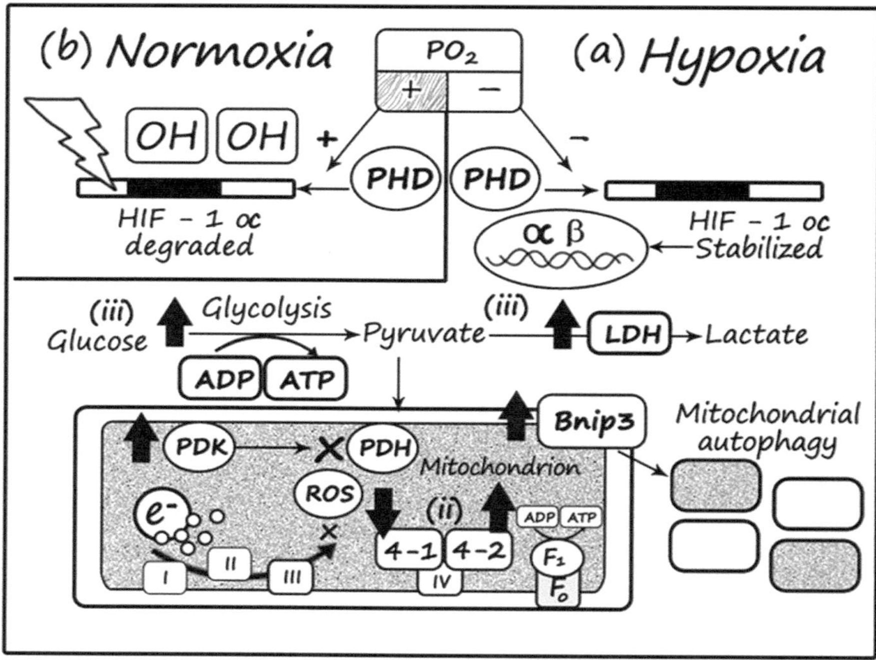

Fig. 8.5 Mechanisms of hypoxic adaptation. (**a**) In hypoxia, HIF-1α spontaneously accumulates and combines with HIF-1β in the nucleus to activate the transcription of hypoxia-responsive genes and driving a number of metabolic adaptations: (i) BNIP3 upregulation leads to mitochondrial autophagy; (ii) a subunit switch at cytochrome *c* oxidase (COX), complex IV of the electron transport chain, increases the efficiency of electron (e⁻) transfer, and attenuates reactive oxygen species (ROS) production; (iii) glycolytic enzymes and lactate dehydrogenase (LDH) are upregulated, increasing anaerobic ATP production and lactate; (iv) pyruvate dehydrogenase kinase (PDK) enzymes are upregulated, de-activating pyruvate dehydrogenase (PDH) and limiting the conversion of pyruvate to acetyl CoA. (**b**) In normoxia, hypoxia inducible factor-1α (HIF-1α) is degraded, following O_2-dependent hydroxylation by prolyl hydroxylase (PHD) enzymes

precisely controlled in response to cellular O_2 concentrations, and include those associated with improving O_2 delivery to muscle, such as vascular endothelial growth factor (VEGF) and erythropoietin (EPO), and many metabolic enzymes or regulators of metabolism, including all glycolytic enzymes, pyruvate dehydrogenase kinase 1 (PDK1), and subunit 4–2 of mitochondrial cytochrome *c* oxidase (COX).

Substrate Switches and Anaerobic Metabolism

The glucose transporter, GLUT1, which mediates non-insulin-stimulated glucose uptake by heart and skeletal muscle, is upregulated in hypoxia in a HIF-dependent manner, and protein levels of both GLUT1 and the insulin-stimulated glucose transporter, GLUT4, are increased in hypoxic rat skeletal muscle, although mRNA levels are unchanged. Curiously, no HRE has been identified in the *GLUT4* gene, although its expression patterns correlate with HIF-1 activity, perhaps suggesting that it is indirectly regulated by HIF-1α.

Measurement of metabolic enzyme activities in the skeletal muscle of rats housed in hypoxic-hypobaric chambers has suggested that shifts towards glycolysis are dependent on muscle type as well as activity levels.

In hypoxic epithelial cells, a dramatic reduction in levels of the fatty acid-activated transcription factor peroxisome proliferator-activated receptor (PPAR)α was mediated by HIF-1. PPARα activation increases the expression of a number of proteins associated with fatty acid oxidation, and is therefore a mechanism for a metabolic shift towards fat metabolism. Downregulation of the PPARα gene regulatory pathway and a number of PPARα target genes, including uncoupling protein 3 (*UCP3*), occurs in the hypoxic heart. In muscle fibres, however, it appears that the hypoxic response may be critically mediated by an up regulation of PPARα, which might promote anaerobic glycolysis by de-activating PDH via the up regulation of another pyruvate dehydrogenase kinase isoform, PDK4. PPARα activation could, however, increase inefficient fatty acid oxidation. Indeed, lipid metabolism in liver, and fatty acid uptake and oxidation in skeletal muscle increased in rats exposed to 10.5% O_2 for 3 months.

Furthermore, PPARα activation could activate mitochondrial uncoupling in hypoxic skeletal muscle by upregulation of UCP3, leading to relatively inefficient metabolism, and a recent study has shown that UCP3 is upregulated in hypoxic skeletal muscle via another PPARα-independent mechanism. Mitochondrial uncoupling by UCP3 can be activated by superoxide and may be an additional mechanism of antioxidant defence in the hypoxic cell, but at the cost of decreased metabolic efficiency, as protons re-enter the mitochondrial matrix independent of ATP synthesis. The regulation of mitochondrial efficiency, however, may occur independently of gene transcription mechanisms, and liver mitochondria from non-hypoxic acclimatized rats were found to have an improved phosphorylation efficiency and depressed uncoupling when respiration was measured under hypoxic conditions.

References

1. Zubieta-Calleja GR, Paulev P-E, Zubieta-Calleja L, Zubieta-Castillo G. Altitude adaptation through hematocrit change. J Physiol Pharmacol. 2007;58(Suppl 5(Pt 2)):811–8. ISSN 0867-5910
2. Zubieta-Castillo G, Zubieta-Calleja GR, Zubieta-Calleja L, Zubieta-Castillo N. Facts that prove that adaptation to life at extreme altitude (8842m) is possible. Adapt Biol Med. 2008;5(Suppl 5):348–55.
3. West JB. Highest permanent human habitation. High Alt Med Biol. 2002;3(4):401–7. https://doi.org/10.1089/15270290260512882. PMID 12631426
4. Auerbach P, Cushing T, Harris N. Auerbach's wilderness medicine. 7th ed. Elsevier; n.d. p. 3.
5. Auerbach P, Cushing T, Harris N. Auerbach's wilderness medicine. 7th ed. Elsevier; n.d. p. 5.
6. Severinghaus JW, Chiodi H, Eger EI, et al. Cerebral blood flow in man at high altitude: role of cerebrospinal fluid pH in normalization of flow in chronic hypoxia. Circ Res. 1966;19:274–82.

Chapter 9
Acute Mountain Sickness

Prithwis Bhattacharyya, Debasis Pradhan, and Prakash Deb

Case Presentation

A 45 years old non smoking healthy hiker, from an expedition group in the Himalayas, was scaling a 7000 meter (m) high mountain in Nepal. The team took 3 days to reach 4500 m by vehicle and spent there three nights. On routine check, the hiker did not show any altitude related signs and symptoms. Next day climb was of 500 m ascent over 12 kilometer (km) distance and weather remained quite snowy the whole day. On that day, his fluid intake and urine output got reduced. Hiker felt mild tiredness and had fragmented sleep. The next day, they reached next camp site at 5600 m which they achieved following a hike of 4.5 kilometer with further reduced intake and output. Weather remained harsh during both the days. On arrival at 5600 m, he complained of headache and incoordination, he had normal diet and took paracetamol and slept. Teammate complained of rapid and periodic breathing.

P. Bhattacharyya (✉)
Department of Critical Care Medicine, Trauma & Emergency Medicine, Pacific Medical College, Udaipur, Rajasthan, India

D. Pradhan
Anaesthesia, NHS Derby and Burton, Derby, UK

P. Deb
Department of Anaesthesiology, Critical Care & Pain Medicine, AIIMS, Guwahati, India

© The Author(s), under exclusive license to Springer Nature Switzerland AG 2023
J. Hidalgo et al. (eds.), *High Altitude Medicine*,
https://doi.org/10.1007/978-3-031-35092-4_9

At 2 o'clock in early morning, his pulse rate 130/min, regular, respiratory rate of 30/min, saturations (SpO_2) was 60%, his Lake Louise acute mountain sickness self-assessment questionnaire score (LLS) was 8. Then he was attended by the medical team at the well-equipped base clinic.

Q—What is the probable diagnosis? How is it self-reported? Main modalities of management? What happens if he continues to ascend untreated?

Ans—This is acute mountain sickness (AMS), one form of high altitude syndromes which includes acute hypoxia, AMS, high altitude pulmonary edema (HAPE), high altitude cerebral edema (HACE), high altitude retinopathy, bronchitis and others. It can be self-reported by using the Lake Louise acute mountain sickness self-assessment questionnaire score (LLS) which has been described in Table 9.2. Management includes no further ascend to higher sleeping altitude if symptomatic, plan to descend if symptomatic on medical management and descend with oxygen if there are symptoms of HAPE or HACE. If untreated, he will progress to moderate to severe AMS, HAPE and or HACE [1–3].

Introduction

As the altitude increases the atmospheric pressure decreases leading to fall in the partial pressure of oxygen in the inspired air and alveoli which leads to decreased partial pressure in the arterial blood while the inspired oxygen concentration being 21% at all the levels of troposphere. Alveolar gas equation explains this part of the physiology quite well, $PAO_2 = PiO_2$ ($PACO_2/R$), $PIO_2 = FiO_2$ ($P_{ATM} - P_{H2O}$), PAO_2 = partial pressure of oxygen in alveolus, PiO_2 = partial pressure of oxygen in inspired air, $PACO_2$ = partial pressure of carbon dioxide in alveolus, R = respiratory quotient, FiO_2 = Fraction of oxygen in inspired air, P_{ATM} = atmospheric pressure, P_{H2O} = standard vapour pressure (SVP) of water at 37 °C. Altitude can be classified into intermediate, high, very high and extreme altitude (Table 9.1) [1].

Hypobaric hypoxia directly leads to various presentations such as acute hypoxia, AMS, HAPE, HACE, retinopathy, peripheral oedema, sleeping problems and a group of neurologic syndromes. Each of these clinical manifestations has distinctive pattern and phenotype while sharing the same fundamental aetiology of hypobaric hypoxia. All are presented with similar history of rapid ascent with or without appropriate acclimatisation, and respond to the same management strategy of descent and various forms of oxygen therapy. Sleeping altitude plays a critical role in the pathophysiology of altitude illness, because hypoxemia is maximal during sleep [1, 2].

AMS is a syndrome characterized by headache along with combination of nausea or vomiting, dizziness, fatigue, or sleep disturbance [1]. While AMS is very uncommon under 2500 m, but at 3000 m it affects upto 75% of non-acclimated climbers [4]. The reported incidences of AMS among the climbers are 40% and 70% while trekking Mount Everest and Mount Rainier respectively (higher in later

Table 9.1 Stages of altitude, its physiologic effect and clinical impact [1, 2]

Altitude	Height in meters (Feet)	Physiologic effect	Clinical impact
Intermediate	1520–2440 (5000–8000)	Increased alveolar ventilation Decreased exercise performance No major impact on arterial oxygen transport	Rapid ascent leads to transient mild symptoms Moderate to severe illness- uncommon
High	2440–4270 (8000–14,000)	Decreased arterial oxygen saturation (SaO$_2$) Hypoxemia during exertion and sleep	Rapid decline with smaller ascent Individuals with comorbidities becomes symptomatic
Very high	4270–5490 (14,000–18,000)	Further decrease in SaO$_2$ Hypoxemia at rest Can avoid changes with a period of acclimatisation	Chances of altitude illness high Increased risk of HAPE and HACE
Extreme	>5490 (>18,000)	Severe hypoxemia and hypocapnia Physiological derangements supersede benefits of acclimatization	Complete acclimatization not possible Longer stays lead to gradual deterioration Limited physiologic reserve Incapacitated individual dependent on others for survival

group due to rapidity of ascent) [1]. Certain phenotypes with blunted ventilatory response to hypoxia have a high threshold to develop AMS. Cardiovascular training status and gender have little influence on attack rates. While children have similar tendency as adults, those >50 years of age tend to have less tendency to develop AMS. Obesity related nocturnal oxygen desaturation appears to increase the risk of AMS [5]. People with history of AMS are at greater risk than those who have tolerated similar trips in the past. Pre-existing diseases can increase AMS risk by magnifying the effects of the hypoxia. Common comorbidities such as anaemia (reduced oxygen-carrying capacity of the blood) and chronic obstructive pulmonary disease (reduced degree of oxygenation occurring in the lungs) increases the risk of AMS by exaggerating the effects of hypobaric hypoxia [4].

Pathophysiology

Following acute exposure to hypobaric hypoxia AMS can develop within 4–8 h whereas HACE and HAPE typically occur 2–4 days after exposure [2] Though the exact etiopathogenesis of AMS is unclear, hypobaric hypoxia plays a major role. Hypoxia induced cerebral vasodilation increases cerebral blood flow and cerebral blood volume which lead to mild AMS. Persons who progress to HACE, have increased T2 signal on MRI and this finding may support above aetiopathogenesis.

Another cause of AMS and HACE can be leaky blood–brain barrier (BBB) due to loss of autoregulation (caused by hypoxia) leading to overperfusion and or increased permeability caused by inflammatory mediators [1]. Hypoxia induces the release vascular endothelial growth factor, nitric oxide, reactive cytokines, and free radicals, which in turn mediate brain endothelial permeability [2]. Individuals with strong anti-inflammatory response will have less disruption of BBB and are resistant to develop AMS [6]. The benefits of dexamethasone in the treatment of AMS also supports the vasogenic hypothesis [1]. With increasing severity, cytotoxic oedema sets in secondary to ischaemia from the ongoing hemodynamic changes, inflammatory mediators, vasogenic oedema and increased blood volume to intracranial ratio [7]. Tight fit hypothesis, proposed three decades ago, suggests increased susceptibility to develop AMS and HACE in individuals with decreased intracranial compliance. Individuals with decreased CSF buffering capacity will have lower intracranial compliance. Such individuals will have greater rise in intracranial pressure in response to hypoxia related increased intracranial blood volume and cerebral oedema. The findings of lumbar puncture, MRI brain and serial optic nerve sheath diameter supports the tight fit hypothesis [2].

Diagnosis

As per the Lake Louise Consensus, diagnosis of AMS is made when a person in the setting of recent altitude gain, presents with headache and at least one of the following symptoms: gastrointestinal (GI) (anorexia, nausea or vomiting), fatigue or weakness, dizziness or light headedness, difficulty sleeping. HACE is considered as the "end stage" or severe AMS and is diagnosed in the setting of recent altitude gain presenting with either presence of change in mental status and or ataxia in a person with AMS or presence of both mental status change and ataxia in a person without AMS. Lake Louise AMS self-questionnaire (Table 9.2) can be used to self-report and plan the management based on the severity [3].

Mild AMS has similar presentation to that of hangover (Ethanol) with constitutional symptoms such as lassitude and weakness. Headaches are usually bifrontal and worsen with exertion, bending over, or Valsalva manoeuvre. GI symptoms include anorexia, nausea, and sometimes vomiting (especially in children). The person with AMS can be irritable and often wants to be left alone. The Lake Louise AMS self-report questionnaire (Table 9.2) can be helpful in following the severity of the illness. Mild AMS has nonspecific physical findings with variable heart rate and blood pressure within the normal range, although postural hypotension may be present. The percent SaO_2 correlates poorly with the diagnosis of AMS. On auscultation localized rales are heard in 20% of persons with AMS. Fundoscopy findings include venous tortuosity and dilatation, and retinal haemorrhages at altitudes >5000 m (>16,400 feet) and in those with HAPE and HACE. Facial and peripheral oedema may be present. Optic nerve sheath diameter increases with altitude due to oedema but rarely correlate with AMS

Table 9.2 Lake Louise AMS self-questionnaire[a] [3]

Symptom	Score	Description
Headache	0	No headache
	1	Mild headache
	2	Moderate headache
	3	Severe headache, incapacitating
GI symptoms	0	No symptoms
	1	Poor appetite or nausea
	2	Moderate nausea or vomiting
	3	Severe nausea and vomiting, incapacitating
Fatigue/weakness	0	Not tired or weak at all
	1	Mild fatigue or weakness
	2	Moderate fatigue or weakness
	3	Severe fatigue or weakness, incapacitating
Dizzy/light-headedness	0	No dizziness/light-headedness
	1	Mild dizziness/light-headedness
	2	Moderate dizziness/light-headedness
	3	Severely light-headed, fainting/passing out
Difficulty sleeping	0	Slept well
	1	Did not sleep as well as usual
	2	Woke many times, poor night's sleep
	3	Could not sleep at all

Classification of AMS based on the score: mild- 2–4, moderate 5–9, severe 10–15
[a]AMS is diagnosed when there is headache plus one or more of the other symptoms

development [8]. Severe headache accompanied by vomiting and decreased urine output indicated further progression of AMS. Victim requires assistance in eating and dressing due to lassitude. Onset of ataxia or altered level of consciousness marks the progression to HACE. Coma may ensue within 12 h if treatment is delayed. AMS in preverbal children is a diagnosis of exclusion due to difficulty in diagnosis [9].

AMS is a clinical diagnosis in the high altitude setting based on the presence of headache with or without other typical presentations and this does not have specific investigations [4]. The differential diagnosis in this setting includes but not limited to tension headache, migraine, dehydration, caffeine withdrawal, viral illness, CNS infections (meningitis, encephalitis), carbon monoxide (CO) poisoning, alcohol intoxication/ toxidrome, hypothermia, gastroenteritis, intracranial pathology such as mass, hemorrhage, aneurysm, venous sinus thrombosis, acute angle closure glaucoma. CO poisoning is not very uncommon in high altitude cold climate settings and may have similar presentation to that of AMS. Decreased oxyhemoglobin level in CO poisoning exacerbate the hypobaric hypoxia of high altitude. In climbers with a personal or family history of migraine, hypoxia may trigger an acute attack of migraine [10, 11]. Headache due to AMS resolves within 10–15 min of oxygen therapy as compared to non-AMS headache and helps in ruling out others [1].

Management

Successful management of AMS includes early diagnosis, careful observation, prevention of further progression, symptomatic management and acclimatization. Fundamentals of AMS treatment are (a) if symptomatic, do not ascend to a higher sleeping altitude, (b) if no improvement or worsening of symptoms with ongoing treatment, descend to a lower altitude, (c) in presence of HACE or HAPE, plan immediate descent and treatment [1].

Oxygen Therapy and Descent

Mild AMS is usually self-limited, does not need oxygen supplementation and a halt in ascent followed by 12–36 h of acclimatization provides good relief. Remarkably, a drop in sleeping altitude of only 300 to 1000 m (980 to 3280 feet, even upto 500 feet is usually effective) in ameliorating symptoms. If descent is not feasible, to simulate descent, patient is inserted into the fabric chamber (Gamow® bags) and manual or automated pump achieves a pressure of 0.9 kg/2.5 cm^2 (2 lb./in^2) which is equivalent to a drop in altitude of 1500 m (4920 feet). Effective ventilation to avoid CO_2 accumulation and oxygen depletion is achieved by valve system. Oxygen supplementation quickly relieves headache and dizziness. Nocturnal administration of low-flow oxygen (0.5–1 L/min) is particularly helpful. Severe AMS and HACE warrants both, immediate descent and oxygen therapy [1].

Acetazolamide

Acetazolamide, a renal tubular carbonic anhydrase inhibitor, decreases renal reabsorption of bicarbonate, leading to bicarbonate diuresis and metabolic acidosis which stimulates ventilation. This hyper ventilatory response increases PaO_2, reduces harmful effects of hypobaric hypoxia and improves sleep by reducing nocturnal periodic breathing. Other beneficial effects are diuresis leading to decrease in fluid retention, decrease in CSF volume and intracranial pressure, maintenance of cerebral blood flow despite greater hypocapnia, relaxation of smooth muscles, and upregulation of fluid resorption in the lungs (beneficial effect in HAPE) [1, 2]. Acetazolamide accelerates acclimatization and, if given early in the development of AMS, may rapidly resolve symptoms [2]. The treatment regimens for AMS are mentioned in table. Adverse effects occur more commonly with higher doses, which include peripheral paresthesias, polyuria, and sometimes nausea, drowsiness, tinnitus, transient myopia and dysgeusia (altering flavour of carbonated beverages). Although it carries low cross-reactivity in individuals with sulfa antibiotic allergy, acetazolamide should be avoided in such situations. Also it should be avoided in pregnancy and lactation. Treatment should be continued until the symptoms of AMS resolve. It need to be restarted if symptoms reappear [1, 2].

Table 9.3 Medications for AMS [1]

Acetazolamide	
Prevention of AMS	125–250 mg PO twice a day beginning 24 h before ascent and continuing during ascent and for at least 48 h after arrival at highest altitude
Treatment of AMS	250 mg PO every 8–12 h
Paediatric AMS	5 mg/kg/day PO in divided doses every 8–12 h
Periodic breathing	125 mg PO 4 h before bedtime
Dexamethasone	
Treatment of AMS	4 mg every 6 h PO, IM or IV

Dexamethasone

Dexamethasone known to decrease inflammatory properties, reduce cerebral blood flow, and block the action of vascular endothelial growth factor. Reduction of AMS symptoms may be the result of these and or its euphoric effects [2]. Dexamethasone is quite effective treatment for AMS (Table 9.3), but is best reserved for moderate to severe AMS because of its potential side effects. Dexamethasone does not aid in acclimatization, some rebound symptoms may follow discontinuation. A short taper period may prevent rebound. Its prophylactic use is preserved for cases of emergency rapid ascent (professionals involved in mountain search and rescue operations). It is often clinically beneficial to use simultaneously with acetazolamide (to hasten acclimatization), in patients with acetazolamide intolerance (to allow dose reduction of acetazolamide). A brief course of dexamethasone along with acetazolamide helps in symptomatic relief and facilitate descent. Side effects include but not limited to gastrointestinal irritation, gastritis, esophagitis, mood alteration and gastroesophageal reflux [1, 2].

Antiemetics and Analgesics

Prescriptions for altitude related headache can include acetaminophen (650–1000 mg) or ibuprofen (600–800 mg) or aspirin (650 mg) [1]. Use of narcotics for treatment of headache should be avoided because of depression of the hypoxic ventilatory response (HVR) and respiratory drive during sleep [2]. Ondansetron, 4–8 mg as orally disintegrating tablets every 4–6 h, effectively treats nausea and vomiting associated with AMS and should be the first-line antiemetic in this setting [1]. Antiemetics such as prochlorperazine stimulates HVR [2].

Improve Sleep Quality

Periodic breathing causes frequent night time awakening. Before bedtime, acetazolamide, 62.5–125 mg, improves sleep oxygenation and reduces apnoeic periods, thereby improves sleep quality. Other safe hypnotics that do not cause respiratory depression include zolpidem, zopiclone, and diphenhydramine [1]. Benzodiazepines should be avoided as it decreases ventilation during sleep [2].

Prevention

Gradual or staged ascent with adequate time for acclimatization is the best method of prevention, however time constraints make such recommendations unrealistic. Sleeping altitude is very critical and first night should not be spent at an altitude higher than 2800 m (9200 feet). Mountaineers and trekkers should avoid abrupt ascent to sleeping altitudes over 3000 m (9840 feet) and allow two nights for each 1000 m (3230 feet) gain in camp altitude starting at 3000 m (9840 feet). For every 3000 to 5000 feet of altitude gain above 10,000 feet, one extra night of acclimatization (sleeping at the same altitude) should be allowed. Also, the principle of "climb high and sleep low" helps (Climbing to higher altitude during day time followed by return to a lower sleeping altitude). Other preventive measures include avoiding overexertion (mild to moderate exercise helps in acclimatization), alcohol, and respiratory depressants. Adequate hydration, preferably by using balance salt solutions, aiming for relatively clear and normal urine output is recommended [1, 2].

Prophylactic acetazolamide benefits those with a history of AMS and those with forced rapid ascent to a sleeping altitude above 2500 m. For prophylactic use, acetazolamide (250 mg twice daily, can be reduced to 125 mg to avoid side effects) should be started 24 h before the ascent and should be continued for the first 2 days. It can be restarted on reappearance of symptoms. Acetazolamide reduces the symptoms of AMS by approximately 75% in persons ascending rapidly to sleeping altitudes of >2500 m (>8200 ft) [12]. Dexamethasone is an alternative to prevent AMS for those with anaphylaxis to sulfa, the doses are 2 mg every 6 h or 4 mg PO every 12 h, starting the day of ascent and continuing for the first 2 days at altitude [1, 13].

Several promising recent studies suggest that over-the-counter analgesics such as ibuprofen and acetaminophen are effective for AMS prevention. Among individuals climbing above 3800 m (>12,000 feet), ibuprofen was shown to reduce the incidence of AMS from 69% to 43% [14]. Ibuprofen may exacerbate high-altitude gastropathy found in some, theoretically leading to GI bleeding [15, 16]. When acetaminophen was compared to ibuprofen, both medicines performed similarly in reducing incidence of AMS [17].

Although gradual ascent and acclimatisation are the most effective means of preventing altitude illness, this strategy is not always feasible. Numerous pre-acclimatization protocols use intermittent exposure either to hypobaric hypoxia by use of hypobaric chambers or normobaric hypoxia through commercially available low-oxygen tents or breathing masks. Even though many of these strategies induce physiologic responses suggestive of acclimatization, only a few are able to demonstrate a significant decrease in AMS incidence [18, 19]. An efficient and effective pre-acclimatization strategy is yet to be determined.

References

1. Davis C, Eifling KP. High-altitude disorders. In: Tintinalli JE, Ma OJ, Yealy DM, Meckler GD, Stapczynski JS, Cline DM, Thomas SH, editors. Tintinalli's emergency medicine—A comprehensive study guide. 9th ed. New York: Elsevier; 2020. p. 1376–83.
2. Harris NS. High-altitude medicine. In: Walls RM, Hockberger RS, Gausche-Hill M, Bakes K, Kaji AH, Baren JM, VanRooyen M, Erickson TB, Zane RD, Jagoda AS, editors. Rosen's emergency medicine: concepts and clinical practice. 9th ed. Philadelphia: Elsevier; 2018. p. 1787–800.
3. Roach RC, Hackett PH, Oelz O, Bärtsch P, Luks AM, MacInnis MJ, Baillie JK, Lake Louise AMS Score Consensus Committee. The 2018 Lake Louise acute mountain sickness score. High Alt Med Biol. 2018;19(1):4–6.
4. Prince TS, Thurman J, Huebner K. Acute Mountain Sickness. [Updated 2022 Jul 12]. In: StatPearls [Internet]. Treasure Island (FL): StatPearls Publishing; 2022. Available from: https://www.ncbi.nlm.nih.gov/books/NBK430716/
5. Ri-Li G, Chase PJ, Witkowski S, Wyrick BL, Stone JA, Levine BD, Babb TG. Obesity: associations with acute mountain sickness. Ann Intern Med. 2003;139(4):253–7.
6. Julian CG, Subudhi AW, Wilson MJ, Dimmen AC, Pecha T, Roach RC. Acute mountain sickness, inflammation, and permeability: new insights from a blood biomarker study. J Appl Physiol. 2011;111(2):392–9.
7. Baneke A. What role does the blood brain barrier play in acute mountain sickness? Travel Med Infect Dis. 2010;8(4):257–62.
8. Schatz A, Guggenberger V, Fischer MD, Schommer K, Bartz-Schmidt KU, Gekeler F, Willmann G. Optic nerve oedema at high altitude occurs independent of acute mountain sickness. Br J Ophthalmol. 2019;103(5):692–8.
9. Yaron M, Waldman N, Niermeyer S, Nicholas R, Honigman B. The diagnosis of acute mountain sickness in preverbal children. Arch Pediatr Adolesc Med. 1998;152(7):683–7.
10. Davis C, Reno E, Maa E, Roach R. History of migraine predicts headache at high altitude. High Alt Med Biol. 2016;17(4):300–4.
11. Hackett P, Rennie D, Levine H. The incidence, importance, and prophylaxis of acute mountain sickness. Lancet. 1976;308(7996):1149–55.
12. Her Y, Kil MS, Park JH, Kim CW, Kim SS. Stevens–Johnson syndrome induced by acetazolamide. J Dermatol. 2011;38(3):272–5.
13. Luks AM, Auerbach PS, Freer L, Grissom CK, Keyes LE, McIntosh SE, Rodway GW, Schoene RB, Zafren K, Hackett PH. Wilderness medical society clinical practice guidelines for the prevention and treatment of acute altitude illness: 2019 update. Wilderness Environ Med. 2019;30(4):S3–18.
14. Lipman GS, Kanaan NC, Holck PS, Constance BB, Gertsch JH, PAINS Group. Ibuprofen prevents altitude illness: a randomized controlled trial for prevention of altitude illness with nonsteroidal anti-inflammatories. Ann Emerg Med. 2012;59(6):484–90
15. Fruehauf H, Erb A, Maggiorini M, Lutz TA, Schwizer W, Fried M, Fox MR, Goetze O. T1080 Unsedated transnasal esophago-gastroduodenoscopy at 4559 M (14957 ft)-endo-

scopic findings in healthy mountaineers after rapid ascent to high altitude. Gastroenterology. 2010;5(138):S-483.
16. Wu TY, Ding SQ, Liu JL, Jia JH, Dai RC, Zhu DC, Liang BZ, Qi DT, Sun YF. High-altitude gastrointestinal bleeding: an observation in Qinghai-Tibetan railroad construction workers on Mountain Tanggula. World J Gastroenterol: WJG. 2007;13(5):774.
17. Kanaan NC, Peterson AL, Pun M, Holck PS, Starling J, Basyal B, Freeman TF, Gehner JR, Keyes L, Levin DR, O'Leary CJ. Prophylactic acetaminophen or ibuprofen result in equivalent acute mountain sickness incidence at high altitude: a prospective randomized trial. Wilderness Environ Med. 2017;28(2):72–8.
18. Muza SR, Beidleman BA, Fulco CS. Altitude preexposure recommendations for inducing acclimatization. High Alt Med Biol. 2010;11(2):87–92.
19. Fulco CS, Beidleman BA, Muza SR. Effectiveness of preacclimatization strategies for high-altitude exposure. Exerc Sport Sci Rev. 2013;41(1):55–63.

Chapter 10
Chronic Mountain Sickness (Monge's Disease)

Ranajit Chatterjee (Chattopadhyay) and Nishant Kumar

A 40-year-old engineer overseeing a hydroelectric plant in the Tibetan plateau born and brought up in the Peruvian Andean mountains complained of headache, insomnia, loss of appetite, loss of concentration, burning sensation in hands and bone and muscle pains. He complained of increasing breathlessness and dilatation of veins on his hands and feet.

What Is the Diagnosis?

The person is most likely suffering from chronic mountain sickness.

Eponym

Monge's Disease.

R. Chatterjee (Chattopadhyay)
Dept. of Anaesthesiology and Critical Care, Swami Dayanand Hospital, New Delhi, India

N. Kumar (✉)
Department of Anaesthesiology and Critical Care, Lady Hardinge Medical College &
Associated Hospitals, New Delhi, India

© The Author(s), under exclusive license to Springer Nature Switzerland AG 2023
J. Hidalgo et al. (eds.), *High Altitude Medicine*,
https://doi.org/10.1007/978-3-031-35092-4_10

Historical Terms

High altitude excessive polycythemia or erythrocytosis.
Excessive erythrocytosis.
High altitude pathologic erythrocytosis.

Definition

Chronic mountain sickness (CMS) has been defined as a clinical syndrome occurring in natives or residents residing above 2500 m altitude for prolonged periods. It develops gradually and is characterised by excessive erythrocytosis, hypoxia, pulmonary hypertension leading to cor- pulmonale and congestive heart failure [1] most likely due to loss of 'adaptation' to high altitude [2].

The clinical picture disappears gradually on descent to lower altitudes but reappears on reascent to altitude above 2500 metres [1].

Historical Aspect

First described by Charles Monge in 1928 as 'Erythremia of high altitude' [3], chronic mountain sickness, an entirely different entity from acute mountain sickness, is due to failure of an individual to fully acclimatise or loss of acclimatisation after living asymptomatically for years at a high altitude.

While the most common features are due to excessive erythrocytosis or polycythemia vera, fibrosis of lungs, neurologic and psychiatric forms have also been described [2].

Monge has described two stages of mountain sickness: sub-acute and chronic which are distinct from acute altitude sickness [2].

Epidemiology

Distribution and Ethnicity

More than 140 million people reside permanently at high altitude, mainly in the Andes (Peru, Bolivia, Argentina: South America), Himalayas (Tibet, India, Nepal, China and Bhutan) and East African Highlands (Ethiopia). However, not all are affected. The incidence of the disease varies from 5–33% based on altitude and ethnicity [4].

CMS has been extensively studied in the Andean population. This could be due to the fact that most of the high-altitude permanent settlements including the highest city in the world (La Rinconada 5100–5300 m) lie in this region [4]. The highest incidence of 33.7% has been reported from the mining town of Cerro de Pasco in Central Peru (4300 m) in population aged 60-69 years, which was found to be only 6.8% in the younger age group (20–29 years) [5, 6]. In Bolivia, where two-thirds of the population resides above 3000 m, the incidence is only 8–10% [7].

However, the prevalence of CMS in residents of Tibet (0.91–1.2%) are much lower and the native population has been well adapted over the years despite living at an average higher altitude than the Andean population [6]. The Chinese Han migrants living in the same region have a higher prevalence of 5.6%-17.8% indicating that ethnicity plays an important role in etiology [6, 8, 9].

Prevalence of high altitude cor- pulmonale from Tien Shan and Pamir mountains (3000–4200 m) in Kyrgyzstan has been reported to be 4.6% in the male population [5].

Studies from India (Himachal Pradesh and Ladakh) record a prevalence of 6.17%-28.7% [10, 11] and 6.87% respectively [12].

The CMS prevalence in the East African mountains has been studied the least. Studies in Ethiopian highlands have reported no cases of CMS and appear to be most adapted for life at HA [13–15].

Aetiology

The most accepted aetiology of CMS is loss or malfunction of the adaptive process of acclimatisation, which refers to the physiological changes (excessive eryhthrocytosis) occurring in the human body in response to the decrease in PO_{2atm} with increase in altitude above sea level. This starts at >2500 m but is most evident at 4000 m and above, above the sea level.

Pathophysiology

The response to constant exposure to hypobaric hypoxia is alveolar hypoxia, hypoxemia and resultant polycythemia which develops over a period of time. This is generally what occurs when a someone ascends from sea level to altitudes above 2500 m. There is an acute adaptation, the failure of which is termed acute mountain sickness, and then there are biological homeostatic adaptations which are found in natives or after long stay at these altitudes. Inability to achieve the homeostasis/ adaptation or subsequent loss in individuals who have been well adapted is termed as chronic mountain sickness [2]. Let us look at the changes that occur in natives which help them survive in the rarefied environment under constant hypoxic conditions.

The underlying cause of CMS has always been associated with an increase in erythrocytic count or as measured clinically, haemoglobin. However, as Monge himself has clarified, this is more of a misinterpretation and what he referred to was a clinical syndrome rather than just a rise in RBCs [2]. The increase in Hb is also associated with the altitude [10], duration spent at that altitude [16–18], age [5, 6, 19] and underlying genetic composition [20–23]. It is reasonable to deduce that increasing Hb levels would increase the oxygen content of the blood and thus ameliorate the prevailing hypoxic conditions. Recent studies seem to challenge this concept [4, 7, 24]. With an increasing Hb, there appears to be a plateau phase beyond which a further increase does not improve pO_2 and in fact is detrimental because of increased viscosity and volume leads to congestive symptoms, the cardiac output is variable and oxygen extraction increases. This affects the pulmonary blood flow and V/Q relationship resulting in impaired pulmonary gas exchange. The arterial hypoxemia that ensues, further propagates erythropoiesis leading to a vicious cycle and further increasing the symptoms. This also forms the basis of early treatment of phlebotomy and hemodilution which cause a dramatic reduction in symptoms. That is why all risk scores and initial treatment modalities rely on the Hb levels and an Hb >21 g/dl has been associated with an increased risk of developing CMS [7]. An association between cobalt toxicity and excessive erythrocytosis has been suggested by Jefferson et al. [25] A recent study by Hancco et al. seems to refute this fact. They found an incidence of 44% for excessive erythrocytosis and a prevalence of 26% for CMS in a population residing at >5000 m in La Rinconada, Peru, however, individuals with excessive erythrocytosis reported less severe symptoms than those with lower haematocrit [4].

Hypoxia and hypercapnia have been identified as the root underlying features in CMS. Alveolar hypoventilation predominates along with V/Q mismatch and widened alveolar-arterial pO_2 gradient [26].

Hyperventilation in response to hypoxia is stimulated by carotid bodies but this hypoxic ventilation response (HVR) is blunted in these patients. Although no change in structure or function of the carotid bodies has been found, experimental studies denote more of a central mechanism for this response or only a marginal contribution of the peripheral chemoreceptors. The time constant for peripheral response to an increase in CO_2 is similar in HA and CMS individuals, however, the central response is much slower in CMS [27].

The central chemoreceptors respond to changes in CO_2 and H^+ ions. The sensitivity of these cells to CO_2 in presence of hypoxia is greatest in HA dwellers as compared to sea level inhabitants and those suffering from CMS. This indicates that the ventilatory response elicited in response to increase in CO_2 would be highest in HA individuals, but is blunted in those with CMS thus leading to further hypoxia and the characteristic symptoms. This is due to the fact that the central chemoreceptors in CMS operate around the resting CO_2 levels, which are closer to individuals residing at sea levels as is also the case with HCO_3^- and pH levels [27].

The CMS individuals show a lower basal sympathetic vasomotor activity which may be mediated due to a high circulating blood volume seen in response to chronic hypoxia as described above [28]. A previous study has demonstrated the same effect in HA native Sherpa population when compared to the acclimatized low landers [29].

The vagal tone tends to be increased in HA natives with heart rates often resembling those of athletes at sea level [5]. The interesting fact in CMS is the inability to increase the heart rate in response to increased oxygen demand which is preserved in natives without the disease and is the cause of many of the symptoms associated with the disease [30]. In fact, as described by Monge, there is an inappropriate paradoxical bradycardia when oxygen demand is increased, and a reflex tachycardia after cessation which also results in resolution of symptoms [2]. There are changes in rhythm, sinus arrhythmia is accentuated and shortening of PR interval, inverted P waves, ST-T abnormalities, atrial and ventricular premature contractions consistent with a hypoxic myocardium. This occurs despite the fact that noradrenaline and adrenaline levels are higher in CMS patients than in native HA dwellers [27].

The arterial pressure in CMS is similar to those of HA natives. They respond well to the orthostatic stress, but the sympathetic response is less with smaller increase in heart rate as described above. The venous pressure on the other hand is increased, probably due to high viscosity and increased blood volume which manifests as dilated and tortuous veins.

Cerebral blood flow and autoregulation remain similar in CMS, HA natives and lowlanders. However, on descent to sea level, CMS individuals show a larger fall in cerebral blood flow with little change in resistance. As explained above, this due to a higher set point which normalises on descent [31].

Despite an almost of a century of research, the exact pathophysiology remains elusive and only the altered homeostasis in afflicted individuals has been studied with much speculation and hypothesis.

Pathogenesis of High Altitude Pulmonary Hypertension (HAPH)

High altitude pulmonary hypertension has been described as a distinct form of CMS from the beginning. The consensus statement on chronic and high altitude diseases in 2005 has classified CMS as a consequence of excessive erythrocytosis, with or without the presence of HAPH (other than that commensurate with altitude), often seen in older individuals, while the latter, sometimes described as subacute CMS, has been described in children and young adults without the presence of excessive erythrocytosis [1].

Adaptation to high altitude (hypobaric hypoxia) mandates changes in the oxygen storage, delivery and utilisation. While pulmonary hypertension is a reasonable end point explanation of chronic hypoxia, the study of Tibetan natives who have been residing at HA since centuries, revealed normal pulmonary artery pressures (PAP) and minimal hypoxic pulmonary vascular reactivity. They also had higher SaO2 and lower Hb levels as compared to Han immigrants and Andeans, and could be assumed to have reached complete adaptation [8].

Therefore, development of HAPH would indicate incomplete adaptation for compatibility with life at HA. While mild and moderate forms often fare well, severe disease mandates early management.

The newborns at sea level and HA show similar anatomical and physiological characteristics with a right ventricular hypertrophy and similar PAP. However, while the right heart preponderance regresses rapidly at sea level, the hypertrophy and increased PAP, pulmonary vascular resistance persist in natives of HA due to delayed remodelling of the distal pulmonary vasculature. There is a delayed closure of ductus arteriosus and results in an increased incidence of patent ductus arteriosus [5].

The underlying cause of development of pulmonary hypertension in HA natives is the proliferation of smooth muscle cells in the distal pulmonary artery and arterioles, which increases the vascular resistance. In addition, secondary factors such as hypervolemia, polycythemia and increased blood viscosity further promote vasoconstriction, thus aggravating pulmonary hypertension [5, 32].

Recently association between iron levels and pulmonary circulation in response to hypoxia has been shown. It was found that iron infusion prior to induced hypoxia abolished or reduced the rise in pulmonary artery pressures, conversely, chelation of iron with deferoxamine increased PAP. Smith and colleagues demonstrated a rise in PAP due to phlebotomy as a treatment of CMS, whereas, iron administration reduced PAP [33, 34]. However, like the elusive pathophysiology of CMS, extensive research is required to fully understand the mechanisms for the development of HAPH.

Risk Factors

Age

The incidence of CMS increases with increasing age. The cause is an excessive erythrocytosis occurring in response to hypoventilation which is accentuated with increasing age. There is no change in ventilatory rates in adults upto 69 years of age at sea level, however, the PaO_2 decreases with age. Since this decline lies on the plateau of the HbO_2 dissociation curve, the hypoxemia is not noticeable and does not induce a polycythemic response, which is reversed in CMS [19].

Altitude

High altitude has been defined as a height of 2500 m or more above sea level. At this level the atmosphere starts thinning and the PO_2 starts decreasing. Most cases of CMS have been reported from areas well above 3000 m, with the incidence and severity increasing with altitude. In fact, most severe cases have been reported at altitudes above 4000 m. This could also be due to the fact that the symptoms being milder at lower altitudes, many remain undiagnosed, thus undermining the exact extent of the disease and its public health implications.

Gender

To say that CMS affects mainly males would not be untrue. Literature is replete with observations and case reports that cite only males. The incidence of signs suggestive of cor-pulmonale was much higher in Kyrgyz males (23%) as compared to females (6%) [5]. Epidemiological studies from India though found no association of the disease with gender [10, 11]. The reason for male predilection could be the natural protection young females beget due to the effect of hormones on ventilation and natural phlebotomies experienced during menstruation [9, 35, 36].

Ethnicity

As has been discussed earlier, the Ethiopians living at altitudes above 3000 m seem immune to the disease, while the Tibetans and Sherpas are the best adapted. The immigrant Chinese Han males, on the other hand, have a much higher incidence in the same region and altitudes. This could be an evolutionary change as these regions have been inhabited for more than 2000 years. The least adapted and the highest incidence is to be found in the Andean population of Peru and Bolivia.

Duration of Stay

So, when do we call this disease to be chronic? Is there a cut off for time spent at high altitude before it can be considered that the individual has lost his adaptation?

While most authors consider a period of having spent asymptomatic 5 years or more at high altitude before the new symptoms are noted, periods as less as 2 months without symptoms have been attributed to be deemed sufficient for the probable diagnosis of CMS [18].

With prolonged exposure to low PaO2, erythrocytosis in susceptible individuals is bound to increase, thus there is a direct linear relationship between the duration of stay and incidence and severity of the disease.

Genetics

Since there is wide variation in the incidence and maladaptation to high altitude among various ethnicities, a possible genetic change or mutation seems probable to either offer protection or make an individual more susceptible to the disease.

CBARA1, VAV3, ARNT2 and THRB, CIC, LIPE and PAFAHIB3 are associated with adaptation in Ethiopians [23].

Specific single nucleotide polymorphism (SNP) in the EPAS1 and EGLN1 genes are responsible for a lower Hb concentration in Tibetans, thus offering protection against the development of disease [22, 37–39]. Products of this gene Hypoxia Inducible Factor 2 (HIF2), GATA and Prolyl Hydroxylase Domain 2 (PHD2) regulate erythropoiesis at the transcriptional level [40].

Since the incidence is highest in the Andean population, and the individuals with the disease exhibit heritable and familial character, genetic mechanism might be at play. ANP32D, SENP1, G allele NOS3 and vascular endothelial growth factor (VGEF) loci may be responsible for the disease [21, 23, 40]. Whole gene sequencing of those suffering with and without CMS were studied in ten Andean individuals each. An SNP in the SENP1 gene may be responsible for the increased incidence in this population. This SNP induced a significant upregulation of SENP1 in CMS individual cells in the presence of hypoxia as compared to non CMS cells [21]. SENP1 mediated deSUMOylation regulates activation of GATA1. CMS cells produce higher levels of VGEF, Bcl-xL and more than tenfold deSUMOylated GATA1 and GATA 1 inducible genes S1c4a1 and Alas 2 in the presence of hypoxia which promote erythrocytosis, as compared to SUMOylated GATA1 and its repressive genes cMyc and cKit in non-CMS cells. Therefore, the SNP in Andeans probably is pro-erythrocytic rather than protective as in Tibetans and Ethiopians [21–23].

Clinical Features

CMS is usually preceded by a subacute illness, which may not necessarily follow acute mountain sickness. The consensus statement on high altitude diseases recognises the development of right sided cardiac changes that occur with prolonged hypoxia as a separate entity called as high-altitude pulmonary hypertension (HAPH). Historical terms include CMS of the vascular type, high altitude heart disease, hypoxic cor-pulmonale, infant subacute mountain sickness, paediatric high altitude heart disease and adult subacute mountain sickness. Clinical symptoms include dyspnoea, cough, cyanosis, sleep disturbance, irritability and other signs of right heart failure [1].

The earliest symptoms include a decline in the routine work capacity. Minor illnesses are poorly tolerated and recovery is prolonged. Symptoms are exaggerated in pregnancy and miscarriages are frequent. The incidence of infertility is higher.

The symptoms may develop slowly and include fatigue, cyanosis after increased exertion, mental lethargy, confusion, dizziness, headaches, congestion of the mucous membranes especially the conjunctiva, poor appetite, weight loss and decreased sleep which may be alleviated by decreased exertion and rest. However, the non-reversibility of these symptoms heralds the onset of CMS.

The clinical features of CMS include those mentioned for the subacute disease, only these are accentuated with minimal exertion, even on routine work. Cyanosis is usually permanent and clubbing is evident. Dilated peripheral veins, paraesthesias, nausea, vomiting, vertigo, alterations of memory, tachypnoea and dyspnoea are usually present. Moderate haemoptysis and epistaxis are common [2]. Other manifestations associated with CMS include restless leg syndrome (both share oxygen alteration as a trait) [41] and orthopaedic complaints like muscle and joint pain (due to hyperuricemia), burning of hand and feet [42]. Features and symptoms of pulmonary hypertension or heart failure are not mandatory for diagnosis of CMS [1].

HAPH

The clinical symptoms are those of right heart failure and include dyspnoea, cough, cyanosis, sleep disturbances and irritability.

Exclusion criteria include:

- Other causes of pulmonary hypertension including persistent pulmonary hypertension of the newborn
- Chronic pulmonary diseases resulting in cor pulmonale
- Other cardiovascular diseases complicated with pulmonary hypertension [1].

Diagnosis

Clinical features with polycythemia (Hb $\geq$ 21 g/dl in males or $\geq$ 19 g/ dl in females) and a high degree of suspicion remain the cornerstone of diagnosis. Exclusion criteria include:

- Chronic pulmonary diseases
- Chronic medical conditions predisposing to hypoxia
- Abnormal pulmonary function tests
- Persons living below an altitude of 2500 m

The Qinghai CMS score provides the basis of diagnosis and severity of the disease. It includes signs, symptoms and Hb levels at the altitude of residence. It includes 8 parameters with a score ranging from 0–3, giving a minimum score of 0 and a maximum of 24. A score of 0-5 denotes the absence of disease, whereas 6–10 is categorised as mild, 11–14 as moderate and > 15 as severe [1]. The parameters include:

A. Breathlessness	
a. No breathlessness/palpitations	0
b. Mild breathlessness/palpitations	1
c. Moderate breathlessness/palpitations	2
d. Severe breathlessness/palpitations	3
B. Sleep disturbance	
a. Slept as well as usual	0
b. Did not sleep as well as usual	1
c. Woke many times, poor night's sleep	2
d. Could not sleep at all	3
C. Cyanosis	
a. No cyanosis	0
b. Mild cyanosis	1
c. Moderate cyanosis	2
d. Severe cyanosis	3
D. Dilatation of veins	
a. No dilatation of veins	0
b. Mild dilatation of veins	1
c. Moderate dilatation of veins	2
d. Severe dilatation of veins	3
E. Paraesthesia	
a. No paraesthesia	0
b. Mild paraesthesia	1
c. Moderate paraesthesia	2
d. Severe paraesthesia	3
F. Headache	
a. No headache	0
b. Mild headache symptoms	1
c. Moderate headache	2
d. Severe headache, incapacitating	3
G. Tinnitus	
a. No tinnitus	0
b. Mild tinnitus	1
c. Moderate tinnitus	2
d. Severe tinnitus	3
H. Haemoglobin (Hb)	
a. Males: 18–21 g/dl	0
> 21 g/dl	3
b. Females: 16-19 g/dl	0
> 19 g/dl	3

Recent Advances

Proteomic analysis has been utilised to identify differentially expressed proteins and three potential plasma biomarkers: Haemoglobin β chain (Hb-β), thioredexin-1 (TRX1) and phosphoglycerate kinase 1 (PGK1) are increased in patients with CMS [43]. Certain mediators of inflammation IL-1 β, IL-2, IL-3, TNFα, MCP-1 and IL-16 promote development of polycythemia via oxidative stress and positive feedback in response to hypoxia [44]. Identification and modulation of these plasma biomarkers may prove beneficial in recognition, prevention and treatment of CMS.

HAPH

The diagnosis may be difficult to differentiate from CMS without investigations. The investigations include: Xray Chest, ECG, 2D echocardiography and definitive by cardiac catheterisation and determination of pulmonary artery pressures.

The screening of HAPH is based on echocardiographic estimation of systolic pulmonary artery pressure of >50 mmHg (Mean > 30 mmHg). This is calculated by the peak velocity of the regurgitant tricuspid jet using Bernoulli's equation and adding estimated right atrial pressure. For confirmation of the diagnosis and exclusion of pulmonary hypertension due to heart diseases, invasive pulmonary artery pressure measurement is advised [1].

Chest X ray: increased cardiac size, enlarged right atrium and ventricle and prominent pulmonary arteries.
ECG is suggestive of a right axis deviation and evidence of marked right ventricle hypertrophy.
2D Echocardiography: Signs of right ventricular hypertrophy and/ or failure.
Cardiac catheterisation: Mean PAP >30 mmHg or a systolic PAP >50 mmHg measured at the altitude of residence.
Infants (up to 6 months): Mean PAP > 50 mmHg or a systolic PAP >65 mmHg.
Children 1–5 years: Mean PAP > 45 mmHg or a systolic PAP >58 mmHg
Children 6–14 years: Mean PAP > 28 mmHg or a systolic PAP >41 mmHg [1]

Management

Non Pharmacologic

The ideal treatment is return to low altitude, preferably sea level as the underlying cause is hypoxia.

Phlebotomy with or without isovolemic haemodilution to reduce haematocrit has been practiced as a treatment since recognition of disease, with latter providing longer lasting benefit [45].

Physical exercise and breathing techniques may reduce blood erythropoietin [46].

Tibetan herbs such as *Rhodiola* may alleviate sleep symptoms [1].

Pharmacologic

Symptomatic treatment can be provided by a high inspired fraction of oxygen, but is short lived.

Medroxyprogesterone (20–60 mg/day for 10 weeks) improved tidal volume, minute ventilation, lowered $PaCO_2$, raised PaO_2, SaO_2 and decreased haematocrit. This could be the explanation for relatively low incidence of CMS in females due to natural progesterone.

Acetazolamide (250 mg/day for 3 weeks) causes acidosis which shifts the O_2-Hb affinity curve to the right, releasing more O_2 to the tissues resulting in increased ventilation, and a parallel drop in erythropoietin and haematocrit leading to elimination of symptoms.

Almitrine stimulates aortic and carotid chemoreceptors. Oral administration of 3 mg/kg/day increased PaO_2, pH and respiratory rate. A dose of 1 mg/kg/day for 4 weeks reduced haematocrit most likely due to improved ventilation during sleep.

Patients suffering from HAPH may benefit from Nifedepin (25–30 mg/12 hrly), Nitric oxide (40 ppm for 15 min), Nitric oxide (15 ppm) with 50% oxygen, prostaglandins and phosphodiesterase inhibitors such as sildenafil. Newer modalities include endothelin receptor antagonists.

Areas of interest and future research include angiotensin converting enzyme inhibitors (ACE I) or angiotensin II receptor antagonists. They increase renal blood flow, inhibit sodium reabsorption in renal tubular cells with fall in oxygen consumption leading to increased erythropoietin production and blockade of effect of angiotensin II on erythropoiesis.

Methylxanthines including theophylline and pentoxifylline reduce blood viscosity and may improve blood flow and tissue oxygenation thus decreasing erythropoiesis. Although this effect has been seen in post transplanted kidneys, this remains unconfirmed in recent studies.

Blunting of ventilatory response to hypoxia may be due to increased levels of dopamine. Dopaminergic blockade (domperidone 40 mg, single dose) increased the slope of isocapnic ventilation as a function of SaO_2 and can be explored as a treatment of CMS [46].

Excessive erythrocytosis has been shown not to be suitable for acclimatization and a 'suitably optimal' Hb has been hypothesised at 15.8 g/dl for resting and 16.9 g/dl for a young, iron sufficient Andean man, with V_{O2max} of 55 ml/kg/min such that neither the oxygen carrying capacity is decreased nor the symptoms of CMS appear. However, this remains theoretical concept which may be explored further [7].

References

1. Leon-Velarde F, Maggiorini M, Reeves JT, Aldshev A, Asmus I, Bernardi L, et al. Consensus statement on chronic and subacute high altitude diseases. High Alt Med Biol. 2005;6:147–53.
2. Monge C. Chronic Mountain sickness. Physiol Rev. 1943;23:166–84.
3. Monge C. La enfermedad de los Andes. Sindromes eritremicos. 1928;11:76.
4. Hancco I, Bailly S, Baillieul S, Doutreleau S, Germain M, Pépin JL, et al. Dissociation between polycythemia and symptoms of chronic mountain sickness in dwellers of the highest city in the world. SSRN Electron J https://doi.org/10.2139/ssrn.3474515.
5. Penaloza D, Arias-Stella J. The heart and pulmonary circulation at high altitudes: healthy highlanders, and chronic mountain sickness. Circulation. 2007;115:1132–46.
6. Pasha MA, Newman JH. High altitude disorders: pulmonary hypertension: pulmonary vascular disease: the global perspective. Chest. 2010;137:3S–9S.
7. Vargas E, Spielvogel H. Chronic Mountain sickness, optimal hemoglobin, and heart disease. High Alt Med Biol. 2006;7:138–49.
8. Jiang C, Chen J, Liu F, Luo Y, Xu G, Shen HY, et al. Chronic mountain sickness in Chinese Han males who migrated to the Qinghai-Tibetan plateau: application and evaluation of diagnostic criteria for chronic mountain sickness. BMC Public Health. 2014;14:701–11.
9. Wu T, Li W, Li Y, Ri-Li G, Cheng Q, Wang S, et al. Epidemiology of chronic mountain sickness: ten years' study in Qinghai-Tibet. In: Ohno H, Kobayashi T, Masuyama S, Matsumoto NM, editors. Progress in mountain medicine and high altitude physiology. Japan: Press committee of the 3rd world congress on mountain medicine and high altitude physiology; 1998. p. 120–5.
10. Sahota IS, Panwar NS. Prevalence of chronic mountain sickness in high altitude districts of Himachal Pradesh. Indian J Occup Environ Med. 2013;17:94–100.
11. Negi PC, Asotra S, V RK, Marwah R, Kandoria A, Ganju NK, et al. Epidemiological study of chronic mountain sickness in natives of Spiti Valley in the Greater Himalayas. High Alt Med Biol. 2013;14:220–9.
12. Norboo T, Saiyed HN, Angchuk PT, Tsering P, Angchuk ST, et al. Mini review of high altitude health problems in Ladakh. Biomed Pharmacother. 2004;58:220–5.
13. Appenzeller O, Claydon VE, Gulli G, Qualls C, Slessarev M, Zenebe G, et al. Cerebral vasodilatation to exogenous NO is a measure of fitness for life at high altitude. Stroke. 2006;37:1754–8.
14. Beall CM. High altitude adaptations. Lancet. 2003;362:S14–5.
15. Hainsworth R, Drinkhill MJ. Cardiovascular adjustments for life at high altitude. Respir Physiol Neurobiol. 2007;158:204–11.
16. Monge C, Leon-Velarde F, Arregui A. Increasing prevalence of excessive erythrocytosis with age among healthy high-altitude miners. N Engl J Med. 1989;321:1271.
17. De Ferrari A, Miranda J, Gilman R. Prevalence, clinical profile, iron status, and subject specific traits for excessive erythrocytosis in Andean adults living permanently at 3825 meters above sea level. Chest. 2014;146:1327–36.
18. Khan DI. Extreme altitude chronic mountain sickness misdiagnosed as high altitude cerebral edema. Int J Travel Med Glob Health. 2016;4:132–4.
19. Sime F, Monge C, Whittembury J. Age as a cause of chronic mountain sickness (Monge's disease). Int J Biometeorol. 1975;19:93–8.
20. Mejia OM, Prchal JT, Leon-Velarde F, Hurtado A, Stockton DW. Genetic association analysis of chronic mountain sickness in an Andean high-altitude population. Red Cell Disorder. 2005;90:13–8.
21. Zhou D, Udpa N, Ronen R, Stobdan T, Liang J, Appenzeller O, et al. Whole genome sequencing uncovers the genetic basis of chronic mountain sickness in Andean highlanders. Am J Hum Genet. 2013;93:452–62.
22. Villafuerte FC. New genetic and physiological factors for excessive erythrocytosis and chronic mountain sickness. J Appl Physiol. 2015;119:1481–6.

23. Azad P, Zhao HW, Cabrales PJ, Ronen R, Zhou D, Pousen O, et al. Senp 1 drives hypoxia – induced polycythemia via GATA1 and Bcl-Xl IN SUBJECTS WITH Monge's disease. J Exp Med. 2016;213:2729–44.
24. Oberholzer L, Lundby C, Stauffer E, Ulliel-Roche M, Hancco I, Pichon A, et al. Reevaluation of excessive erythrocytosis in diagnosing chronic mountain sickness in men from the world's highest city. Blood. 2020;136:1884–8.
25. Jefferson JA, Escudero E, Hurtado ME, Pando J, Tapia R, Swnson ER, et al. Excessive erythrocytosis, chronic mountain sickness, and serum cobalt levels. Lancet. 2002;359:407–8.
26. Kryger MH, Grover RF. Chronic mountain sickness. Sem Resp Med. 1983;5:164–8.
27. Leon-Velarde F, Villafuerte FC, Richalet JP. Chronic mountain sickness and the heart. Prog Cardiovasc Dis. 2010;52:540–9.
28. Simpson L, Meah V, Steele A, Gasho C, Howe C, Dawkins T, et al. Global REACH 2018: Andean highlanders, chronic mountain sickness and the integrative regulation of resting blood pressure. Exp Physiol. 2021;106:104–16.
29. Simpson LL, Busch SA, Oliver SJ, Ainslie PN, Stembridge M, Moore JP, et al. Baroreflex control of sympathetic vasomotor activity and resting arterial pressure at high altitude: insight from Lowlanders and Sherpa. J Physiol. 2019;597:2379–90.
30. Claydon VE, Norcliffe LJ, Moore JP, et al. Cardiovascular responses to orthostatic stress in healthy altitude dwellers, and altitude residents with chronic mountain sickness. Exp Physiol. 2005;90:103–10.
31. Norcliffe LJ, Riviera-Ch M, Claydon VE, et al. Cerebrovascular responses to hypoxia and hypocapnia in high altitude dwellers. J Physiol. 2005;566:287–94.
32. Ge RL, Helun G. Current concept of chronic mountain sickness: pulmonary hypertension-related high altitude heart disease. Wilder Environ Med. 2001;12:190–4.
33. Smith TG, Balanos GM, Croft QP, Talbot NP, Dorrington KL, Ratcliffe PJ, Robbins PA. The increase in pulmonary arterial pressure caused by hypoxia depends on iron status. J Physiol. 2008;586:5999–6005.
34. Patrician A, Dawkins T, Coombs GB, Stacey B, Gasho C, Gibbons T, Howe CA, Tremblay JC, Stone R, Tymko K, Tymko C, Akins JD, Hoiland RL, Vizcardo-Galindo GA, Figueroa-Mujíca R, Villafuerte FC, Bailey DM, Stembridge M, Anholm JD, Tymko MM, Ainslie PN. Global research expedition on altitude-related chronic health 2018 iron infusion at high altitude reduces hypoxic pulmonary vasoconstriction equally in both lowlanders and healthy Andean highlanders. Chest. 2022;16:1022–35.
35. Leon-Velarde F, Ramos MA, Hernandez JA, De Idiaquez D, Munoz LS, Gaffo A, Cordova S, Durand D, Monge C. The role of menopause in the development of chronic mountain sickness. Am J Phys. 1997;272:R90–4.
36. Leon-Velarde F, Rivera-Chira M, Tapia R, Huicho L, Monge CC. Relationship of ovarian hormones to hypoxemia in women residents of 4,300 m. Am J Physiol Regul Integr Comp Physiol. 2001;280:R488–93.
37. Beall CM, Cavalleri GL, Deng L, Elston RC, Gao Y, Knight J, Li C, et al. Natural selection on EPAS1 (HIF2alpha) associated with low hemoglobin concentration in Tibetan highlanders. Proc Natl Acad Sci U S A. 2010;107:11459–64.
38. Simonson TS, Yang Y, Huff CD, Yun H, Qin G, Witherspoon DJ, et al. Genetic evidence for high-altitude adaptation in Tibet. Science. 2010;329:72–5.
39. Yi X, Liang Y, Huerta-Sanchez E, Jin X, Cuo ZX, Pool JE, et al. Sequencing of 50 human exomes reveals adaptation to high altitude. Science. 2010;329:75–8.
40. Leon-Velarde F, Mejia O. Gene expression in chronic high altitude diseases. High Alt Med Biol. 2008;9:130–9.
41. Vizcarra-Escobar D, Mendiola-Yamasato A, Risco-Rocca J, Mariños-Velarde A, Juárez-Belaunde A, Anculle-Arauco V, et al. Is restless legs syndrome associated with chronic mountain sickness? Sleep Med. 2015;16:976–80.

42. Karaytug K, Ekinci M, Yücekul A. Unnoticed etiology in orthopedic complaints: chronic mountain sickness. J Ist Faculty Med. 2022;85:98–104.
43. Zhang P, Li Z, Yang F, Ji L, Yang Y, Liu C, et al. Novel insights into plasma biomarker candidates in patients with chronic mountain sickness based on proteomics. Biosci Rep. 2021;41:BSR20202219. https://doi.org/10.1042/BSR20202219.
44. Yi H, Yu Q, Zeng D, Shen Z, Li J, Zhu L, et al. Serum inflammatory factor profiles in the pathogenesis of high-altitude polycythemia and mechanisms of acclimation to high altitudes. Mediat Inflamm. 2021;2021:8844438. https://doi.org/10.1155/2021/8844438.
45. Rivera-Ch M, Leon-Velarde F, Huicho L. Treatment of chronic mountain sickness: critical reappraisal of an old problem. Respir Physiol Neurobiol. 2007;158:251–65.
46. Villafuerte FC, Corante N. Chronic mountain sickness: clinical aspects, etiology, management, and treatment. High Alt Biol. 2016;17:61–9.

Chapter 11
Management of High-Altitude Cerebral Edema and High-Altitude Pulmonary Edema

Gentle Sunder Shrestha, Sabin Bhandari, Rajesh Chandra Mishra, and Ahsina Jahan Lopa

Case Presentation

A 25-year-old male with no prior co-morbidities, residing at 300 m above the sea level decided to go to Annapurna circuit for vacation. On the fifth day of his ascent to Thorong-la pass which is at 5416 m above the sea level, he started having generalized headache associated with vertigo, nausea, and vomiting, progressively worsening over the next 24 h when he was observed to have an unsteady gait by his friends. Within the next few hours, he was found to be drowsy and not responding to verbal commands. He was then heli-rescued within the next few hours to our hospital at Kathmandu. On arrival to our hospital, he was found to have a pulse of 96/min, blood pressure of 142/72 mm Hg, respiratory rate of 32/min and SpO_2 77% in ambient air. Neurologically he was found to be disoriented with non-coherent talks and had bilateral positive Babinski sign. Chest examination revealed bilateral basal crepitations. Other systemic examination was normal. Fundus examination revealed papilledema.

G. S. Shrestha (✉)
Department of Critical Care Medicine, Tribhuvan University Teaching Hospital, Kathmandu, Nepal

S. Bhandari
DM Critical Care Medicine Resident, Department of Critical Care Medicine, Tribhuvan University Teaching Hospital, Kathmandu, Nepal

R. C. Mishra
Consultant Intensivist and Internist, Khyati Multi-Speciality Hospital, Ahmedabad, India

A. J. Lopa
MH Samorita Hospital and Medical College, Dhaka, Bangladesh

© The Author(s), under exclusive license to Springer Nature Switzerland AG 2023
J. Hidalgo et al. (eds.), *High Altitude Medicine*,
https://doi.org/10.1007/978-3-031-35092-4_11

Q1: What are your differentials from the history and findings of physical examination?
A:

1. Acute Mountain Sickness/High altitude cerebral edema/High altitude pulmonary edema
2. Right sided stroke
3. Sub-arachnoid hemorrhage
4. Central nervous system infections
5. Hypothermia
6. Seizures
7. Transient Ischemic attack
8. Brain tumor
9. Myocardial infarction
10. Pulmonary embolism
11. Pneumonia with MODS
12. Hyperventilation syndrome

Q2: What further tests would you like to do?
A: **Lab investigations - helpful**

1. Random blood sugar level

   - Hypoglycemia and exhaustion may be the cause of low GCS

2. ABG

   - With increasing altitude, there is a decrease in atmospheric pressure, resulting in a lower PAO_2 and, consequently, a lower PaO_2, as explained by the alveolar gas equation

     - $PAO_2 = FiO_2 (Patm - PH_2O) - (PaCO_2/R)$

   - Thus, a low PaO_2 is expected at such a high altitude of Thorong La Pass, as is low SpO_2. However, A-a gradient will help us distinguish if pulmonary edema is present.
   - Low PaO_2 and normal A-a gradient implies hypoxia due to high altitude, whereas, Low PaO_2 and elevated A-a gradient implies pulmonary edema
   - Mild respiratory alkalosis may be present due to hyperventilation secondary to hypoxia

3. CBC

   - Haemoglobin concentrations may be high due to a fall in the plasma volume as a result of dehydration
   - White blood cell count may be elevated in the setting of HACE

4. RFT

   - To rule out kidneys as a cause of dys-electrolytemias or altered sensorium

5. LFT

   - To rule out liver as a cause of altered sensorium

6. ECG and bedside ECHO

   - To rule out myocardial infarction, left ventricular dysfunction and assessment of volume status

7. Chest X-ray

   - To rule out pulmonary edema and possible pneumonia

8. Non contrast CT head

   - To rule out other causes of fall in GCS

Investigations – less helpful (but may be needed if first line of investigations are not helpful in establishing the diagnosis or the patient does not respond to the initial treatment)

1. Lumbar puncture

   - To rule out CNS infections

2. EEG

   - To rule out seizure as a cause of altered sensorium and possible toad's palsy

3. CT angiography with venogram

   - If there is suspicion of Cerebral venous sinus thrombosis as a cause of altered sensorium

4. MRI brain

   - To rule out other pathologies as a cause of altered sensorium

His hematological and biochemical parameters were within normal limits (hemoglobin 14 g/dL, total leucocyte count 10,500/µL, differential leucocytes polymorphs 65%, lymphocytes 32%, blood sugar random 100 mg/dL, urea/creatinine 28/1.0 mg/dL, total/direct bilirubin – 1/0.2 mg/dl, SGOT/SGPT-34/42 mg/dl, protein/albumin- 6.3/4.6 gm/dl, cultures negative). ECG showed normal sinus rate and rhythm without ST changes. Chest radiograph revealed fluffy perihilar opacities in bilateral lung fields suggestive of pulmonary edema (Fig. 11.1). Optic nerve sheath diameter (ONSD) was 6 mm in the right eye and 6.2 mm in the left eye. Non-contrast CT scan (NCCT) of the brain showed diffuse cerebral edema involving white matter of bilateral cerebral hemispheres with accentuation of grey–white matter differentiation, mass effect in the form of the effacement of the overlying sulci and compression of the lateral ventricles and third ventricle (Fig. 11.2). EEG was normal.

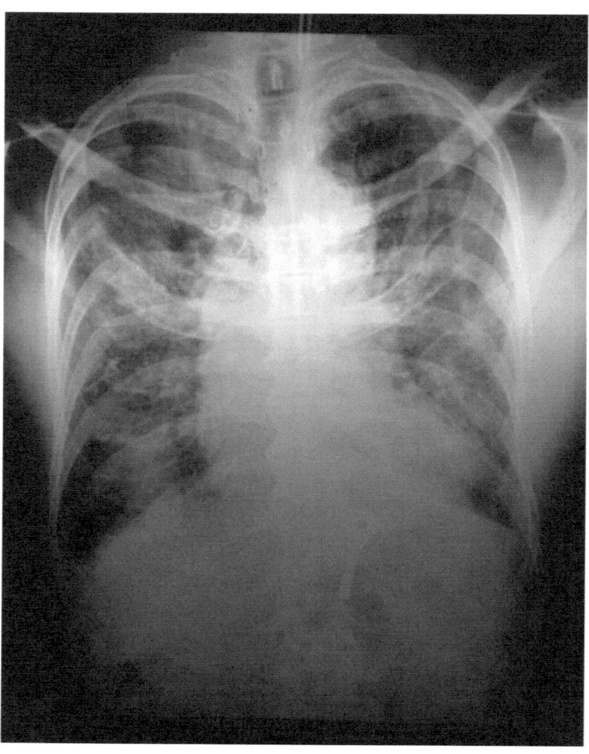

Fig. 11.1 Chest radiograph revealing fluffy perihilar opacities in bilateral lung fields suggestive of pulmonary edema

Q3: What is your provisional diagnosis?

A: High altitude cerebral edema with high altitude pulmonary edema.

Q4: How did you come to this conclusion?

A: Unacclimatized individuals are at risk of high-altitude illness when they ascend rapidly to altitudes above 2500 m [1]. HACE has been reported at around 2500 m in patients with concurrent HAPE [2]. The patient is young, without prior co-morbidities, who had been residing at an altitude of 300 m and has rapidly ascended to an altitude of 5416 m in five days. He has presented initially with clinical features of acute mountain sickness viz., headache, nausea and vomiting which has progressed to signs of HACE viz., ataxia and progressive decline of mental function and consciousness. This transition takes time ranging from 12 h to three days, however HACE develops faster in patients with HAPE, most likely as a result of severe hypoxemia as seen in this case [3]. The presence of papill-edema in the eyes and positive Babinski sign has been reported in HACE [4]. Similarly the findings of non-contrast CT head has further supported the diagno-sis. The findings of hypoxia and chest x-ray points out towards acute pulmonary edema. There are negative findings of hematological and biochemical parameters along with negative ECG and EEG findings to suggest alternative diagnosis. Thus, the history, clinical and investigations points towards the diagnosis of HACE and HAPE.

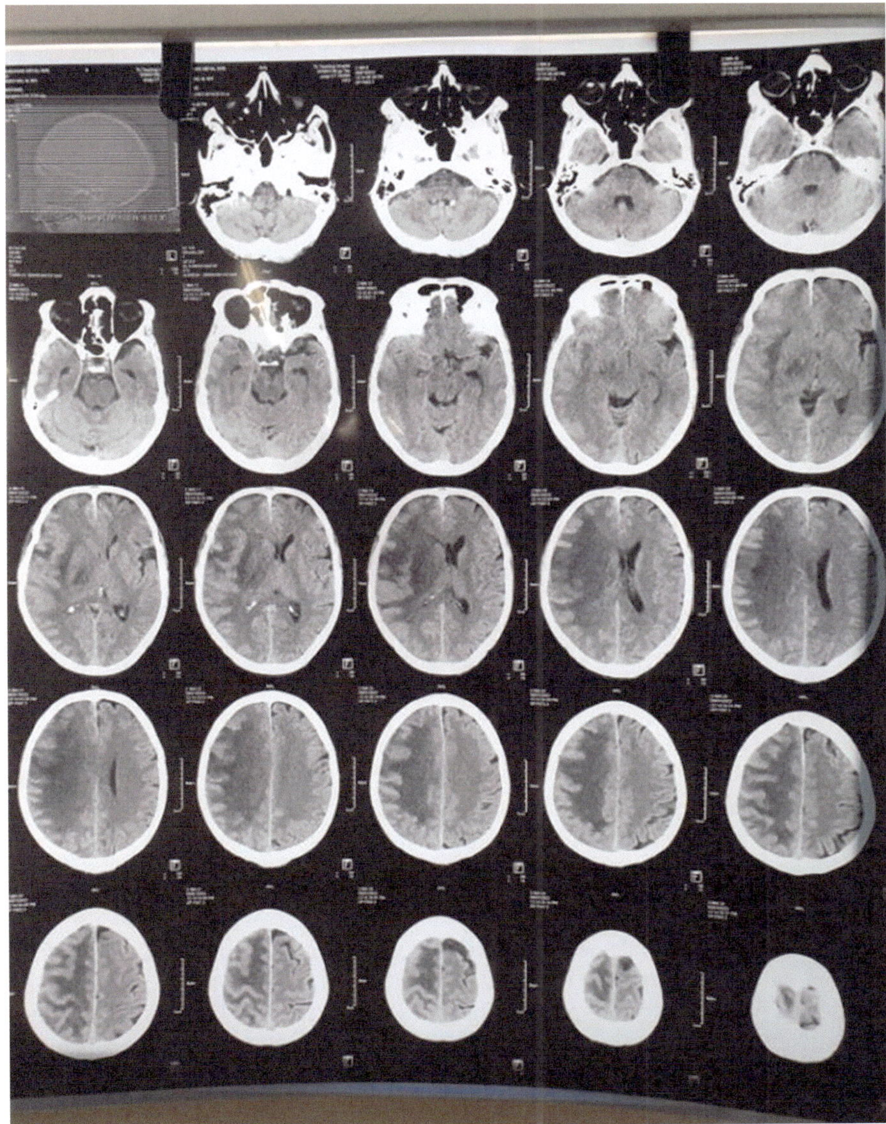

Fig. 11.2 Non-contrast CT scan (NCCT) of the brain showed diffuse cerebral edema involving white matter of bilateral cerebral hemispheres with accentuation of grey–white matter differentiation, mass effect in the form of the effacement of the overlying sulci and compression of the lateral ventricles and third ventricle

Q5: Do you know of any scoring systems to identify Acute Mountain Sickness/ HACE/ HAPE?

A: Lake Louise AMS Score has been the most widely used scoring system for research (Table 11.1). Other tools to diagnose AMS includes Acute Mountain

Table 11.1 The Lake Louise Acute Mountain Sickness Scoring System [2] [8]

Symptoms	Severity	Points
Headache	None at all	0
	Mild headache	1
	Moderate headache	2
	Severe headache, incapacitating	3
Gastrointestinal symptoms	Good appetite	0
	Poor appetite or nausea	1
	Moderate nausea or vomiting	2
	Severe nausea and vomiting, incapacitating	3
Fatigue and/or weakness	Not tired or weak	0
	Mild fatigue/weakness	1
	Moderate fatigue/weakness	2
	Severe fatigue/weakness, incapacitating	3
Dizziness/light-headedness	No dizziness/light-headedness	0
	Mild dizziness/light-headedness	1
	Moderate dizziness/light-headedness	2
	Severe dizziness/light-headedness, incapacitating	3
Difficulty sleeping	Slept as well as usual	0
	Did not sleep as well as usual	1
	Woke many times, poor sleep	2
	Could not sleep at all	3

A total score of 3 to 5 indicates mild AMS
A score of 6 or more signifies severe AMS

Sickness-Cerebral Score, Visual Analog Scale for the Overall Feeling of Mountain Sickness and Clinical Functional Score (CFS).

Q6: How will you manage the case of HACE and HAPE?
A:

1. ***Descent:*** Immediate descent at the first suspicion of HACE, while the patient is still ambulatory, is the gold standard treatment in those who develop HACE. A descent of approximately 1000 m is usually lifesaving [5]. Other treatment options should not delay descent, rather, it should be reserved for situations where descent is not possible or may be delayed [6].
2. ***Supplemental oxygen:*** Oxygen delivered by face mask or preferably non-rebreathing mask to maintain peripheral capillary oxygen saturation (SpO_2) > 90% is recommended [1]. It should however be noted that at high altitude PAO_2 is low and consequently PaO_2 and SpO_2 shows lower values that may be normal for that patient at that altitude.
3. ***Hyperbaric therapy:*** Portable hyperbaric chambers (such as the Gamow bag) should be used for patients with severe AMS or HACE when descent is delayed or not possible and supplemental oxygen is not available [1]. However, symptoms may recur when individuals are removed from the chamber, thus, use of a portable hyperbaric chamber should not delay descent in situations where descent is required such as in the case of HACE and HAPE.

4. ***Dexamethasone:*** Though studies are lacking supporting the use of dexamethasone for HACE, its use has been recommended based upon extensive clinical experience. The recommended initial dose is 8 to 10 mg orally, intramuscularly, or intravenously (IV), followed by 4 mg every six hours until symptoms resolve. The pediatric dose is 0.15 mg/kg/dose every 6 h [1]. The mechanism by which dexamethasone works is unclear, however, reduction in vascular permeability, inflammatory pathway inhibition, antioxidant balance, aquaporin-4 channel (AQP4) modulation and sympathetic blockade have all been proposed to help in the prevention and treatment of high-altitude cerebral edema [7].

Evidence Contour

1. **Acetazolamide:** Acetazolamide has been shown to accelerate acclimatization to high altitude. Similarly multiple trials have established a role for acetazolamide in prevention of AMS [8–11]. However few studies have rigorously assessed the effectiveness of acetazolamide in the treatment (rather than prophylaxis) of AMS. A small study used acetazolamide for AMS and found it to be effective [12], however, the diuretic effect of acetazolamide might provoke hypotension in the intravascularly depleted patient, and the added stimulus to ventilation might worsen dyspnea. Hence, it is not recommended for the treatment for HACE and HAPE [1].
2. **Diuretics:** Many patients with AMS and HAPE have intravascular volume depletion and the use of diuretics in such patients may worsen the volume status further, hence diuretics should not be used for the treatment of HAPE [1].
3. **Nonsteroidal anti-inflammatory drugs and acetaminophen:** Acetaminophen, and ibuprofen has been found to relieve headache at high altitude but it is unclear whether they are useful as prophylaxis or treatment of AMS, HACE and HAPE [13, 14]. These drugs can be used to treat headache at high altitude but are not recommended for the prevention and treatment of HACE and HAPE [1].
4. **Nifedipine:** Extensive clinical experience and one randomized study has shown that Nifedipine in a dose of 30 mg of the extended-release preparation administered every 12 h is effective in preventing HAPE in susceptible people [15]. Similarly, though a single, nonrandomized, unblinded study found nifedipine useful for HAPE treatment when oxygen or descent was not available, another observational study of individuals with HAPE reported that nifedipine offered no advantage when used as an adjunct to oxygen and descent [16, 17]. Thus, nifedipine can be used for HAPE prevention in HAPE-susceptible people and as an adjunct to treatment when descent is impossible or delayed and reliable access to supplemental oxygen or portable hyperbaric therapy is unavailable [1].
5. **Phosphodiesterase inhibitors:** Tadalafil and sildenafil are phosphodiesterase-5 (PDE-5) inhibitors that augment the pulmonary vasodilatory effects of nitric oxide and thus cause pulmonary vasodilation and decrease pulmonary artery pressure. Though there is a strong physiologic rationale for using phosphodiesterase inhibitors in HAPE, supported by evidences for its use as prophylaxis for HAPE, however, no systematic study has examined the role of tadalafil or

sildenafil in HAPE treatment as either mono- or adjunctive therapy [18, 19]. Tadalafil and sildenafil can be used for HAPE prevention in known susceptible individuals who are not candidates for nifedipine as well as for the treatment of HAPE when descent is impossible or delayed, access to supplemental oxygen or portable hyperbaric therapy is impossible, and nifedipine is unavailable [1].

6. **Ginkgo biloba:** Ginkgo biloba is an herbal extract preparation with variable compositions. Though some small studies have suggested the effectiveness of ginkgo biloba at reducing the symptoms of AMS in adults, larger trials have failed to demonstrate the benefit [20–22]. Ginkgo biloba has not been recommended for AMS prevention and treatment [1].

7. **Beta agonist:** Barring few case reports of beta-agonist use in HAPE treatment [23], no data exists to support the use of beta agonists for HAPE, hence there is no recommendation in its use [1].

Q7: What ventilatory strategy would you consider in such patients?
A: Role of Continuous positive airway pressure

CPAP increases transmural pressure across alveolar walls which increases alveolar volume and thus leads to an improvement in ventilation-perfusion matching and gas exchange [1]. However, there are no controlled studies to show improvement in patient outcomes with the use of CPAP or EPAP compared to oxygen alone or in conjunction with medications in patients who have developed AMS or HAPE. Few reports have shown that CPAP can be used as an adjunct for treating HAPE [24, 25], and since the risks associated with the therapy is low, CPAP or EPAP can be considered an adjunct to oxygen administration, provided the patient has normal mental status and can tolerate the mask [1].

Since this patient has hypoxemia (SpO_2–77%) at our center, which is at a level higher than sea level, but not high enough to level SpO_2 of 77% as normal, a trial of CPAP can be given if his saturation cannot be maintained with nasal cannula/face mask/venturi mask. However, his GCS has to be monitored continuously and ABG repeated to monitor improvement in hypoxia. Once the hypoxemia improves and the patient becomes fully conscious, he can be taken off CPAP and kept in nasal cannula/face mask/venturi mask. However, if his GCS falls further or he cannot tolerate the mask, CPAP should be discontinued and consideration should be given for endotracheal intubation and mechanical ventilation.

Role of Mechanical Ventilation

The management of patients with HACE who require mechanical ventilation can be challenging. Though intubation and short-term hyperventilation is a possible therapeutic option in patients with cerebral edema who have clinically significant ICP elevation, these patients are likely to have a respiratory alkalosis, and overventilation could cause cerebral ischemia. Oxygen alone markedly decreases cerebral blood flow and ICP at high altitude, thus providing high FiO_2 might be detrimental. The optimal PEEP and tidal volume are another controversial aspect in the ventilatory management of such patients. In a recent survey by ESICM, most clinicians utilize a tidal volume of 6–8 ml/kg and low PEEP than suggested by ARDS Net in patients with severe traumatic brain injury [26].

Since there are no systematic studies regarding ventilatory settings in patients with HACE and HAPE, evidences and recommendations are lacking. A general approach would be to utilize lung protective ventilation with a target PaO_2 80–120 mm Hg, target $PaCO_2$ 35–45 mm Hg, use the low PEEP/FiO_2 table of ARDS Net protocol and titrate the settings according to the response of the patient [27].

This patient had rapidly descended via heli-rescue and brought to our center. He was given oxygen via face-mask initially which improved his SpO_2 improved to 86%, however, his SpO_2 was not maintained in the target range, hence CPAP of 10 cm H2O was started which improved his SpO_2 to 94%. He was started on Inj Dexamethasone 4 mg iv every six hourly, tab nifedipine 30 mg ever 12 hourly and Inj paracetamol 1 gm iv every 6 hourly. His cognitive functions started improving within 6 h. On second day of admission, CPAP was stopped and he was put on face-mask. However, his ataxia improved slowly, and by the fourth day of hospitalization, his chest was clear and his gait was normal. Repeat chest radiograph on the fourth day of admission showed complete resolution of the opacities. A repeat NCCT-head performed on the fourth day also showed that the white matter edema had subsided with decreased mass effect and the grey–white matter differentiation was seen to be normal. He was discharged on the tenth day.

The following definitions on the diagnosis of altitude illness were adopted at the 1991 International Hypoxia Symposium, held at Lake Louise in Alberta, Canada [28].

Acute Mountain sickness (AMS)	In the setting of a recent gain in altitude, the presence of headache and at least one of the following symptoms: 1. Gastrointestinal 2. Fatigue or weakness 3. Dizziness or lightheadedness 4. Difficulty sleeping
HIGH ALTITUDE CEREBRAL EDEMA (HACE)	Can be considered "end stage" or severe AMS. In the setting of a recent gain in altitude, either: 1. The presence of a change in mental status and/or ataxia in a person with AMS 2. Or, the presence of both mental status changes and ataxia in a person without AMS
HIGH ALTITUDE PULMONARY EDEMA (HAPE)	In the setting of a recent gain in altitude, the presence of the following: Symptoms: At least two of: 1. Dyspnea at rest 2. Cough 3. Weakness or decreased exercise performance 4. Chest tightness or congestion Signs: At least two of: 1. Crackles or wheezing in at least one lung field 2. Central cyanosis 3. Tachypnea 4. Tachycardia

References

1. Luks AM, Auerbach PS, Freer L, Grissom CK, Keyes LE, McIntosh SE, et al. Wilderness medical society clinical practice guidelines for the prevention and treatment of acute altitude illness: 2019 update. Wilderness Environ Med. 2019;30(4):S3–18.
2. Hackett PH, Yarnell PR, Weiland DA, Reynard KB. Acute and evolving MRI of high-altitude cerebral edema: microbleeds, edema, and pathophysiology. AJNR Am J Neuroradiol. 2019;40(3):464–9.
3. Hackett P, Luks AM, Lawley JS, Roach RC. high altitude medicine and pathophysiology. In: Auerbach PA, editor. Wilderness medicine. 7th ed. Philadelphia: Elsevier; 2017. p. 8–28.
4. Dickinson JG. High altitude cerebral edema: cerebral acute mountain sickness. Seminars Respir Med. 1983;5(2):151–8.
5. Hackett PH, Roach RC. High altitude cerebral edema. High Alt Med Biol. 2004;5(2):136–46.
6. Zelmanovich R, Pierre K, Felisma P, Cole D, Goldman M, Lucke-Wold B. High altitude cerebral Edema: improving treatment options. Biologics. 2022;2(1):81–91.
7. Swenson ER. Pharmacology of acute mountain sickness: old drugs and newer thinking. J Appl Physiol. 2016;120(2):204–15.
8. Forwand SA, Landowne M, Follansbee JN, Hansen JE. Effect of acetazolamide on acute mountain sickness. N Engl J Med. 1968;279(16):839–45.
9. Basnyat B, Gertsch JH, Holck PS, Johnson EW, Luks AM, Donham BP, et al. Acetazolamide 125 mg BD is not significantly different from 375 mg BD in the prevention of acute mountain sickness: the prophylactic acetazolamide dosage comparison for efficacy (PACE) trial. High Alt Med Biol. 2006;7(1):17–27.
10. van Patot MC, Leadbetter G 3rd, Keyes LE, Maakestad KM, Olson S, Hackett PH. Prophylactic low-dose acetazolamide reduces the incidence and severity of acute mountain sickness. High Alt Med Biol. 2008;9(4):289–93.
11. Low EV, Avery AJ, Gupta V, Schedlbauer A, Grocott MP. Identifying the lowest effective dose of acetazolamide for the prophylaxis of acute mountain sickness: systematic review and meta-analysis. BMJ. 2012;345:e6779.
12. Grissom CK, Roach RC, Sarnquist FH, Hackett PH. Acetazolamide in the treatment of acute mountain sickness: clinical efficacy and effect on gas exchange. Ann Intern Med. 1992;116(6):461–5.
13. Harris NS, Wenzel RP, Thomas SH. High altitude headache: efficacy of acetaminophen vs. ibuprofen in a randomized, controlled trial. J Emerg Med. 2003;24(4):383–7.
14. Gertsch JH, Corbett B, Holck PS, Mulcahy A, Watts M, Stillwagon NT, et al. Altitude sickness in climbers and efficacy of NSAIDs trial (ASCENT): randomized, controlled trial of ibuprofen versus placebo for prevention of altitude illness. Wilderness Environ Med. 2012;23(4):307–15.
15. Bartsch P, Maggiorini M, Ritter M, Noti C, Vock P, Oelz O. Prevention of high-altitude pulmonary edema by nifedipine. N Engl J Med. 1991;325(18):1284–9.
16. Oelz O, Maggiorini M, Ritter M, Waber U, Jenni R, Vock P, et al. Nifedipine for high altitude pulmonary oedema. Lancet. 1989;2(8674):1241–4.
17. Deshwal R, Iqbal M, Basnet S. Nifedipine for the treatment of high-altitude pulmonary edema. Wilderness Environ Med. 2012;23(1):7–10.
18. Maggiorini M, Brunner-La Rocca HP, Peth S, Fischler M, Böhm T, Bernheim A, Kiencke S, et al. Both tadalafil and dexamethasone may reduce the incidence of high-altitude pulmonary edema: a randomized trial. Ann Intern Med. 2006;145(7):497–506.
19. Bates MG, Thompson AA, Baillie JK. Phosphodiesterase type 5 inhibitors in the treatment and prevention of high altitude pulmonary edema. Curr Opin Investig Drugs. 2007;8(3):226–31.
20. Seupaul RA, Welch JL, Malka ST, Emmett TW. Pharmacologic prophylaxis for acute mountain sickness: a systematic shortcut review. Ann Emerg Med. 2012;59(4):307–17.

21. Gertsch JH, Basnyat B, Johnson EW, Onopa J, Holck PS. Randomised, double blind, placebo controlled comparison of ginkgo biloba and acetazolamide for prevention of acute mountain sickness among Himalayan trekkers: the prevention of high altitude illness trial (PHAIT). BMJ. 2004;328(7443):797.
22. Chow T, Browne V, Heileson HL, Wallace D, Anholm J, Green SM. Ginkgo biloba and acetazolamide prophylaxis for acute mountain sickness: a randomized, placebo-controlled trial. Arch Intern Med. 2005;165(3):296–301.
23. Fagenholz PJ, Gutman JA, Murray AF, Harris NS. Treatment of high altitude pulmonary edema at 4240 m in Nepal. High Alt Med Biol. 2007;8(2):139–46.
24. Johnson PL, Johnson CC, Poudyal P, Regmi N, Walmsley MA, Basnyat B. Continuous positive airway pressure treatment for acute mountain sickness at 4240 m in the Nepal Himalaya. High Alt Med Biol. 2013;14(3):230–3.
25. Walmsley M. Continuous positive airway pressure as adjunct treatment of acute altitude illness. High Alt Med Biol. 2013;14(4):405–7.
26. Picetti E, Pelosi P, Taccone FS, Citerio G, Mancebo J, Robba C. VENTILatOry strategies in patients with severe traumatic brain injury: the VENTILO survey of the European Society of Intensive Care Medicine (ESICM). Crit Care. 2020;24(1):158.
27. Robba C, Poole D, McNett M, Asehnoune K, Bösel J, Bruder N, et al. Mechanical ventilation in patients with acute brain injury: recommendations of the European Society of Intensive Care Medicine consensus. Intensive Care Med. 2020;46(12):2397–410.
28. Hackett PH, Oelz O. The Lake Louise consensus on the definition and quantification of altitude illness. Hypoxia and mountain medicine. 1992:327–30.

Chapter 12
Excessive Erythrocytosis and Chronic Mountain Sickness

Andrés Velázquez García, Vanessa Fonseca Ferrer, Gerald Marín García, and Gloria M. Rodriguez-Vega

Living at high altitudes requires a physiological adaptation process to be able to adjust to the hypoxic environment above 2500 m. Erythropoiesis is a well-known response to hypoxic states, where this stimulus elicits a chain of events leading to the eventual increase in erythrocytes count improving oxygen delivery. When erythropoiesis produces an exaggerated response to hypoxia the result may be pathological. This combination, excessive erythrocytosis (EE) & hypoxemia are the major features of a syndrome known as "Chronic Mountain Sickness" (CMS) [1]. Excessive erythropoiesis and CMS represent a progressive incapacitating syndrome with high prevalence in highlanders living above 2500. This chapter aims to present a clinical scenario of this syndrome, define and discuss the epidemiology, risk factors, diagnosis, effects on other systems and current evidenced-based therapeutic approaches.

The Case

A 55-year-old dwell miner presents to the local Emergency Department (ED) with a chief complain of progressive shortness of breath, headache, difficulty concentrating and having difficulty sleeping. Upon questioning he also reports intermittent palpitations and recent decreased tolerance to exercise. He has lived in the Andeans Zone for the past 25 years. He denies recent travel, upper respiratory infections,

A. V. Velázquez García · V. F. Ferrer · G. M. García
Department of Pulmonary and Critical Care Medicine, VA Caribbean Health Care System, San Juan, Puerto Rico
e-mail: vanessa.fonseca-ferrer@va.gov; gerald.marin@upr.edu

G. M. Rodriguez-Vega (✉)
Department of Critical Care Medicine, HIMA San Pablo-Caguas, Caguas, Puerto Rico

J. Hidalgo et al. (eds.), *High Altitude Medicine*,
https://doi.org/10.1007/978-3-031-35092-4_12

abdominal pain, nausea, vomits, chest pain, visual changes, or cough. Patient has been previously healthy and does not have pertinent past medical history. He does reports that his late father, who also worked as a miner and lived at La Rinconada, suffered from some chronic sickness that had to do something with oxygenation and blood concentration. Patient reports that symptoms have been worsening for the past month or so, and he first notice them about 2 months ago. Despite 8 h of sleep daily he complains of daily somnolence and persistent headache. He used to run a mile every morning but for the past year and a half he has reduce his workout due to intolerance. Denies alcohol, tobacco, or any other toxic habit. Physical exam pertinent for digital clubbing, peripheral cyanosis, tenderness to palpation of the joints mild to moderate tachypnea. Vitals as follows: BP 174/92 mmHg – HR 92 – RR 22 – Sat 87%. Labs pertinent for:

Hgb: 22 g/dL.
Hct: 67%.
Creatinine: 1.4; K: 4.0; Na 138; Cl 102; HCO3 24; BUN 20; GLU 225.
ABGS: 7.4/36/55/23.2/0/87%/RA.
ECG: LVH changes, no conduction delays, no acute ischemic changes. P-pulmonale also present.
CXRAY: Unremarkable, No signs of congestion, no effusion, no pneumothorax, no consolidations. Right heart border seems dilated. (Discuss basic laboratory work up CBC w diff, CMP, ABGs ECG and chest imaging maybe and ECHO.)

What Is the Next Step in Diagnosis?

Definition

It is well known that the partial pressure of oxygen in inspired air decreases as elevation above sea level increases. Residents of high altitudes (highlanders) develop numerous physiologic responses to adjust to the hypobaric environment. Within the many responses, there is a particular increase in hemoglobin (Hb) concentration and pulmonary artery pressure [1] . It has been observed that in severely hypoxic residents a large increase in Hb concentration may be associated with fatal illness. This large increment in Hb has been coined as excessive erythrocytosis. In conjunction with severe hypoxemia, are the hallmark of chronic mountain sickness (CMS).

Excessive erythrocytosis is defined as two standard deviations above mean Hb concentration value of the highlander population at the altitude of residence [2, 3] . Based on epidemiological studies in the different highlander population studies in South America (Andean), Asia (Tibetan & Sherpa), and East Africa (Ethiopian), the cut-off values for EE are Hb >19 g/dL for women and Hb >21 g/dL for men [1, 2, 4, 5]. According to current international consensus statement CMS & EE are define as a clinical syndrome that occurs to native or long-life resident above 2500 meters. It is characterized by EE (females Hb 19 g/dL; males Hb >21 g/dL), severe hypoxemia and in some cases moderate to severe pulmonary hypertension, which may evolve to COR pulmonale and congestive heart failure [1]. For it to be defined as primary CMS there should not be a previous diagnosis of chronic pulmonary disease (COPD, asthma, emphysema, chronic bronchitis, bronchiectasis, cystic fibrosis, lung cancer, etc.) or other chronic medical conditions that worsen the hypoxemia. If any off the previous conditions is present, diagnosis of Secondary CMS should be made [1].

This definition is not without its controversies. Recent studies conducted in dwellers from La Rinconada, the highest city on the world (5100–5300 m) [4], suggest that these international cutoff values should be reconsider based on their observation of lower prevalence of EE according to their calculations in based of the population under study.

The diagnosis is made by the combination of the presence of EE and a minimum score based on the following symptoms: breathlessness, palpitations, sleep disturbances, cyanosis, dilation of veins, paresthesia, headache, and tinnitus [1, 2, 4] . CMS severity is determined by the Qinghai Scored, that is based on Hb concentration and on the presence and extent by the previously mentioned agreed by the international consensus. A numeric value is given to each of the mentioned symptoms accordingly to its presence and the extent of them. CMS final severity is determined by the sum of the assigned values, and then classified as follow: 0–5 Absent, Mild 6–10, Moderate 11–14, and Severe >15 [1, 4].

Epidemiology

The prevalence of EE and CMS worldwide has shown to be variable among studied regions and population of highlanders. Approximately 140 million individuals reside at high altitude (>2500 m) worldwide, the largest populations being found in South America (Andean), central Asia (Tibetan and Sherpa), and East Africa [4, 5]. The variability difference could be related to many factors. These include time residing at high altitude, recent migration, age, sex, body habitus, etc. This variability may represent different level of adaptation to high altitude living conditions, meaning that not only hypoxia and EE are involved in the development of the disease.

The lowest prevalence is found in Tibetans from Qinghai, China with a CMS of around 1.2%; whereas in Han immigrants, it was approximately 5.6% in the same city. (Wu et al., 1998). The prevalence values of CMS in the three mainly evaluated locations in the Andes are: Puno in Perú 6%; in La Paz, Bolivia 5.2%; Cerro de Pasco, Perú 15.4% in men between 30–39 years, and 33% by the 60 years of age [2, 6–8]. Altitude has also been related to changes in prevalence, since an increment in altitude has been associated with increased percentage of prevalence among highlanders. In the Tibetan plateau (2261–2980 m) CMS was found in 1.05% of the population; at 3128–3980 m, in 3.75%; and at 400–5226 m, in 11.73%. A study in India between 2350 and 3000 m no cases were reported; but, between 3000–4150 m, the prevalence of CMS&EE was 13.3% [2].

Physiology and Pathophysiology of EE & CMS

Under hypoxic conditions specialized stem cells in the kidney increase the production and secretion of erythropoietin (EPO), the main physiological regulator of erythrocyte production. Erythropoietin gene expression is a complex process, with many transcription factor interactions, mainly regulated by the transcription factor complex hypoxia-inducible factor (HIF-1). Is the expression of this TF complex in response to hypoxic conditions, in combination with others, that will be responsible for the increased EPO in the blood that will eventually result in a higher erythrocytes concentration in the blood stream. This ability of the body to adapt and respond to hypoxic conditions is one of the studied adaptations present in the highlander populations, as a mechanism to acclimatization to their low oxygen containing environment.

The exact pathogenesis of EE behind it still unclear [9]. However recent genetic and functional studies in highlanders have brought to light important information about the pathogenesis of EE & CMS [10] The transcription process elicited in response to hypoxia is mainly controlled by the downstream events in Hypoxia-Inducible Factor (HEF-1) cascade. Under non-hypoxic conditions HIF-alpha undergoes hydroxylation, ubiquitination, and eventual degradation. In contrast, with hypoxic conditions, HIF-alpha is readily available and promote the expression of at least one hundred genes associated with increased oxygen delivery to hypoxic tissues. HIF is the one responsible for the increased expression of EPO that is seen in blood under low partial pressure of oxygen conditions [11]. The increased concentration in blood EPO is believed to be the responsible for the eventual development of inadequate erythropoiesis that leads to developing the EE present in CMS.

Classically has been thought that higher blood availability of EPO was translated to a higher level of EPO-EPOR binding and this was the cause of an inadequate erythropoiesis and eventual EE. However, recent discovery of the existence of a soluble EPO-R (sEPOR), have changed the latter perspective. Andean Highlanders population studies showed that decreased blood concentration of S-EPOR and higher EPO/S-EPOR ratio, were associated with higher Hb concentrations and higher incidence of EE. These findings suggest that not only the amount of EPO in blood is responsible for the response to hypoxia and eventual development of EE [12].

The recent discovered single-nucleotide polymorphism (SNP) in the Sentrin-specific Protease 1 (SENP1) gene, present in Andean highlanders and his differential expression in patients with and without CMS have made its gene product a study interest due to his potential role in the control of erythropoiesis. HIF-1 and GATA function is mainly regulated by the protease encoded by the SENP1 gene. These transcription factors are well known to be relevant in the mounted response to hypoxic conditions by increasing the expression of EPO and EPO receptors. SENP1, through the protease it encodes, might have an erythropoietic role in EE&CMS through the modulation of EPO and EPOR expression [10] It was observed, that in Andean Highlanders the increased expression of the SNP SENP1 was associated with an exaggerated erythropoiesis and development of CMS [10, V13]. Different physiological patterns in the EPO-EPOR system and different degrees in erythropoietic response among Andean highlander was described by Villafuerte et al., 1015, findings that suggest various levels of adaptation to high-altitude hypoxia. Based in the previously discussed studies, the functional and phenotypic differences observed between healthy highlanders, those with CMS, and the ones observed in highlanders with CMS, suggest that the adaptative response to high-altitude hypoxia involves multiple physiological and genetic control mechanisms.

Risk Factors and Comorbidities

Even though hypoxia is believed to be the main promoter of excessive editorial many other risk factors have been related with increased risk of developing EE and CMS. Studies have demonstrated a higher likelihood of developing CMS in those with family history of CMS or those with a reduce response to hypoxia stimulus [2]. Higher prevalence in men than women a postmenopausal woman has shown higher prevalence than premenopausal woman [2, 13]. Increase age and BMI has also been associated with higher rates of developing the disease [1, 2, 6]. A recent study showed that EE was associated with three times higher (>20%) estimated risk of developing a cardiovascular event in 10 years when compared with healthy Andean Highlanders [14]. Studies have shown association between diabetes mellitus, dyslipidemia, hypertension and insulin resistance and suffering from EE. Hypertension associated with excessive erythrocytosis was also recently reported in Andean highlanders [14]. The exact mechanism behind the association between EE and the increased CVR, metabolic abnormalities and other comorbidities associated with higher cardiovascular risk remains unclear. Excessive Erythrocytosis leads to higher blood viscosity, hypervolemia, hyperviscosity syndrome, and an increased risk of thromboembolic events. Further studies regarding the exact mechanism of EE association with the previously described cardiovascular and metabolic derangements is needed, because it could lead to a better understanding of the process and how to prevent these effects.

Back to our Case Now that you have made an accurate diagnosis, what is the next step in therapy?

Treatment

Despite EE and CMS's high and their incapacitating natural history that could lead to congestive heart failure, pulmonary hypertension and Cor Pulmonale, no long-term pharmacological therapeutic regimen has been stablished [15]. Current therapeutic approaches used for EE and CMS are centered around a Hb goal, erythrocyte count reduction, increasing blood oxygenation levels, and symptomatic relief. Therapy can be divided into two groups: Nonpharmacological and pharmacological.

Non-pharmacological Treatment

The most effective therapeutic approach reported is relocation to lower altitude. This is based on studies that showed progressive normalization in blood oxygenation, erythrocyte count, and resolution of symptoms related to CMS once this occurred. Due to the negative social, economic, and psychological impact that it represents, relocation is not always a therapeutic option for highlanders [1, 2, 5, 15].

Phlebotomy has been the most used method utilized for therapy against high altitude polycythemia. Its function is to effectively decrease the Hb, and erythrocyte count by decreasing blood volume. Another method studied was phlebotomy with isovolumetric replenishment to avoid the loss of volume, and possible provide a dilution effect. Even though superiority of one over the other has not been stablished and appropriately studied, it has been observed a longer period of symptomatic improvement with the volume repletion approach [1, 2]. The drawback of phlebotomy is that it only provides a temporary improvement in symptoms with an eventual return of symptoms and the need of frequent phlebotomies for symptomatic control.

Oxygen supplementation has been associated with improvement in blood oxygen saturation and decreased erythrocytosis, and better exercise tolerance reported by Andean's highlanders [1, 5]. This therapy is limited cost of home oxygen therapy and the unpractical nature, as an unsustainable amount of oxygen would be needed in the highlander populations [2, 5].

Pharmacological

One of the pharmacological agents studied as possible therapy were the ACE inhibitors [16]. ACE inhibitors has been effective when giving to treat the secondary polycythemia that follows renal transplantation, which is sustained by an increased in erythropoietin activity. Proposed mechanism for the ACE-I's effect in erythropoiesis is by increased renal blood flow, decreased sodium re-absorption, and thus lowering oxygen supplementation. Also, have been proposed that it might have its effect by a direct interruption of the angiotensin II might have on erythroid precursors [16]. Enalapril 5 mg/day therapy was given to thirteen highlanders living on Calixto of la Paz, Bolivia, and they were routinely monitored for treatment compliance over a 2-year period. Baseline blood pressure, urine protein content, packed red cell volume, and hemoglobin levels were documented and compared with the follow up results to see any change over time. This was also done to 13 control patient who did not receive any therapy. After 2 years the observed outcome showed reduction in Hb (2.4 g/dL at 1 year and 4.3 g/dL at 2 yeas), Hct (3.9% at 1 year and 6.7% at 2 years) and proteinuria (74.1 mg/24 h at 1 year and 110.9 mg/24 h at 2 years) [2, 16].

Very limited studies have used respiratory stimulants as medroxyprogesterone and as therapeutic agents for EE and CMS. These have shown decrease in Hct and improvement of blood oxygen saturation. However, there is no clinical evidence of their safety and efficacy, adverse effects and the lack of adequately controlled placebo-treated group. Therefore, they have not been implemented as treatment of EE and CMS [15].

The most promising therapeutic agent studied is acetazolamide (ACZ). Two randomized, double-blind, placebo-controlled studies assessed the efficacy and safety of acetazolamide treatment in CMS patients from Cerro de Pasco [15]. They assigned, in a random-blinded fashion, a total of 28 male patients with CMS in to three different groups based on the therapy that was going to be provided: placebo, ACZ 250 mg/Day, and ACZ 500 mg/Day. They compared baseline Hct, serum EPO, serum transferrin and ferritin levels with those obtained after 3 weeks of therapy. Results showed, in the 2 ACZ treated groups (250 and 500 mg/Day), decreased in Hct by 7.1% and 6.7% serum EPO decreased by 67% and 50%, serum transferrin decreased by 11.4% and 3.4%, and increased serum ferritin by 540% and 134% respectively. Treatment also increased mean nocturnal saturation by 4.3% and 5.1% and decreased mean nocturnal heart rate by 11% and 4% for ACZ 250 and 500 mg [15]. The effect of ACZ in decreasing EPO serum concentration was mainly attributed to the improvement in ventilation and $SpO2$ induced by its use. The induced metabolic acidosis induced by ACZ causes an increase in respiratory rate and decrease hypoventilation episodes which translate to the observed improvement in ventilation and saturation. ACZ therapy seems safe and efficient, but additional trials should analyze the possible long-term adverse effects caused by its chronic use [2].

References

1. Leon-Velarde F, Maggiorini M, Reeves JT, Aldashev A, Asmus I, et al. Consensus statement on chronic and subacute high-altitude diseases. High Alt Med Biol. 2005;6(2):147–57.
2. Villafuerte F, Corante N. Chronic Mountain sickness: clinical aspects, Etiology, management, and treatment. High Alt Med Biol. 2016;17(2):61–9.
3. Monge C, Leon-Valverde F, Arregui A. Increasing prevalence of excessive erythrocytosis with age among healthy high-altitude miners. N Engl J Med. 1989;321(18):1271.
4. Hancco I, et al. Excessive erythrocytosis and Chronic Mountain sickness in dwellers of the highest City in the world. Front Physiol. 2020;11(773):1–13.
5. West JB. Physiological effects of chronic hypoxia. N Engl J Med. 2017;376(20):1965–71.
6. De Ferrari A, Miranda J, Gilman R. Prevalence, clinical profile, iron status, and subject-specific traits for excessive erythrocytosis in Andean adults living permanently at 3825 meters above sea level. Chest. 2014;146:1327–36.
7. Spielvogel, et al. Poliglobulia y ejercicio muscular. Gaceta del. Thorax. 1981;XIII(48):4–11.
8. Monge C, Leon-Velarde F, Arregui A. Increasing prevalence of excessive erythrocytosis with age among healthy high-altitude miners. N Engl J Med. 1989;321:1271.

9. Spicuzza, et al. Sleep-related hypoxemia and excessive erythrocytosis in Andeans high-altitude natives. Eur Respir J. 2004;23:41–6.
10. Villafuerte F. New genetic and physiological factors for excessive erythrocytosis and Chronic Mountain sickness. J Appl Physiol. 2015;119(12):1481–6.
11. Pham K, Parikh K, Heinrich E. Hypoxia and inflammation: insights from high-altitude physiology. Front Physiol. 2021;12:676782.
12. Villafuerte, et al. Decrease plasma soluble erythropoietin receptor in high-altitude excessive erythrocytosis and Chronic Mountain sickness. J Appl Physiol. 2014;117:1356–62.
13. Leon-Valverde, et al. Relationship of ovarian hormones to hypoxemia in women residents of 4,300m. Am J Physiol Regul Integr Comp Physiol. 2001;280:R488–93.
14. Corante N, et al. Excessive erythrocytosis and cardiovascular risk in Andean highlanders. High Alt med & Biol. 2018;19(3):221–31.
15. Richalet J, Rivera M, Bouchet P, et al. Acetazolamide: a treatment for Chronic Mountain sickness. Am J Respir Crit Care Med. 2005;172:1427–33.
16. Plata R, et al. Angiotensin-converting-enzyme inhibition therapy in altitude polycythemia: a prospective randomized trial. Lancet. 2002;359:663–6.

Chapter 13
High-Altitude Cerebral Edema

Sabrina Da Re Gutierrez, Jorge Sinclair Avila,
Jorge Enrique Sinclair De Frías, and Jorge Hidalgo

The Case

A 33-year-old male with no medical history, resident in a coastal country, arrives by plane to the city of La Paz at 3600 m.a.s.l. for tourism. Thirty-six hours after his arrival, he presented mild headache, which later evolved into oppressive-type holocranial headache of moderate intensity, nausea, and drowsiness. The patient is inmediatly transferred from the Hotel to the Hospital. It was done to him arterial blood gas, that reports pH:7.32, $PaCO_2$: 40 mmHg, PaO_2: 50 mmHg, HCO3: 24 mMol/L, BE: +2, SatO2: 85%, and a simple brain CT scan is performed, showing effacement of sulci.

Treatment was started with supplemental oxygen at 4 L/min., head position at 30°, dexamethasone, antiemetic (ondansetron), acetazolamide, paracetamol-based analgesia and parenteral hydration. The evolution in the following 48 h was favorable, returning to the country of origin.

S. D. R. Gutierrez (✉)
Department of Intensive Care Medicine, Materno Infantil Hospital, La Paz, Bolivia

J. Sinclair Avila
Critical Care Department, Hospital Punta Pacífica, Panama City, Panama

J. De Frías
Department of Physiology, University of Panama, Panama City, Panama

J. Hidalgo
Department of Critical Care, Belize Healthcare Parners, Belize City, Belize

J. Hidalgo et al. (eds.), *High Altitude Medicine*,
https://doi.org/10.1007/978-3-031-35092-4_13

Although most people who increase to high altitude suffer a physiological response without major compromise of the general state, in the present case the patient suffered an infrequent complication such as high-altitude cerebral edema between 0.5 to 1.8% of cases [1] -0.5 al 1% according to Zelmanovich *et al* [2]- This pathology can evolve to death if it is not treated in a timely manner. Although most authors point out that HACE occurs at altitudes above 4000 m.a.s.l. our patient developed HACE at a lower altitude, fortunately he did not develop ataxia or coma, conditions that have a worse prognosis and an early fatal outcome. It is important for people rising to high altitudes to recognize the symptoms of Acute Mountain Sickness (AMS) and High Altitude Cerebral Edema (HACE).

Introduction

Acute mountain sickness known in Bolivia as altitude sickness or *"Sorojchi"* (from Quechua *suruqchi o suruqch'i*), it is the lack of adaptation of the organism to the decrease in barometric pressure when increasing altitude. "High altitude" is predicated on territories that are above 2500 m.a.s.l. [3, 4]. Imray et al. they categorize altitude as high (1500 to 3500 m.a.s.l.), very high (3500 to 5500 m.a.s.l.) and extreme (above 5500 m.a.s.l.) [4].

Lafuente et al. explain the increased prevalence of HACE due to the increased displacement of people to and from high altitude regions, points out that around 140 million people live at altitudes above 2500 m.a.s.l. [5]. Luks indicates that the human being inhabiting these territories, physiologically, experiences a decrease in barometric pressure that causes, in turn, a decrease in the partial pressure of O_2 between the alveoli and the pulmonary capillary, slowing down the rate of diffusion of O_2 through the alveolar/capillary membrane [6].

Evidence indicates that, reciprocally, the human body adapts to hypobaric hypoxia:

1. Increasing respiratory rate/tidal volume generating respiratory alkalosis and increasing sympathetic activity with increased resting heart rate/cardiac output/ blood pressure [3]
2. Constricting the bed of the pulmonary artery.
3. Increasing urinary sodium loss and increasing diuresis (Aksel et al. show that cardiac output decreases due to high-altitude diuresis, reducing the delivery of O_2 to the tissues) [3].
4. Increasing the concentration of hemoglobin (Luks specifies that this phenomenon begins between 24 and 48 h after the application of hypobaric hypoxia [6].
5. Greater aggregation of red cells [3].

Adaptation is not immediate, it takes time [3]. The rapid subjection of the human body to high altitude impedes adaptation and causes High Altitude Illness (HAI). Furthermore, Aksel et al. point out that adaptation depends on the altitude and the duration of exposure to it, taking from hours to weeks [3].

Now, Aksel et al. point out that HAI is a group of syndromes, namely:

1. Acute mountain sickness (AMS).
2. High altitud cerebral edema (HACE).
3. High altitude pulmonary edema (HAPE).

Likewise, they emphasize that the pathophysiology of the cause of HAI is partially -well- known, but treatment plans are mostly based on low-quality evidence [3].

Pathogeny

Acute Mountain Sickness (Ams)

Results of Aksel et al. indicate that the partial pressure of O_2 is 90–100 mmHg at sea level, 65–80 mmHg at 1610 m.a.s.l., 45–70 mmHg at 2440 m.a.s.l., 42–53 mmHg at 3660 m.a.s.l. and less than 50 mmHg at 5300 m.a.s.l. [3].

Considering that low PaO_2 and high $PaCO_2$ can cause high cerebral blood flow with increased intracranial volume/pressure, Luks posits that blunted ventilatory response could be related to AMS, in this vein, he proposes the "tight fit" hypothesis (based on the Monro-Kellie doctrine) which states that people with a higher ratio of cerebrospinal fluid to blood/volume of brain tissue are better able to compensate for the cerebral edema or increased intracranial blood volume. Additionally, Luks points out that subjects with a smaller intracranial volume may have an increased risk of AMS [6].

In another hypothesis, Dekker et al. propose that the decrease in PaO_2 activates compensatory physiological mechanisms to maintain the delivery of O_2 to the tissues, the most important are: 1) increased respiratory/cardiac rate and 2) increased erythropoietin/erythrocyte production. Thus, they question the validity of the "tight fit" theory, emphasizing that it does not explain the cause of the edema [7].

Results of Dekker et al. also show that:

1. A physiological predisposition to hypoxemia could contribute to edema.
2. A hydrostatic effect due to the relative inability of the venous system (hypoxia-dependent) to drain the increased cerebral blood flow can cause edema, which, in turn, can impair venous drainage and worsen venous/intracranial hypertension.
3. The functioning of factors that alter vascular permeability ("hypoxia-inducible factor 1" and vascular endothelial growth factor) are the clearest cause of edema [7].

Dekker et al. propose that hypoxia-induced cerebral vasodilation, increased intracranial pressure, and disruption of the blood-brain barrier cause molecular processes, capillary leakage, microhemorrhages, and cerebral edema [7].

High Altitude Cerebral Edema (HACE)

HACE is an encephalopathy, probably occurs above 2500 m.a.s.l. The evidence indicates that it affects 0.5–1% of subjects with HACE and, above 4500 m.a.s.l., 5% of non-adapted subjects. In contrast, Luks points out that less than 1% of subjects above 3000 m.a.s.l. become ill, evidence shows that it is potentially fatal if not promptly diagnosed/treated [6].

Delving into the pathophysiology, one of the first neurological consequences of hypoxemia is dilation of the cerebral arteries and increased blood flow to the brain to maintain O_2 supply [8]. Dilation of the middle cerebral artery occurs almost instantaneously during induction of hypoxemia and progressively dilates over 4–6 h. In addition, generalized dilation of intracranial/extracranial arteries and dilation of intracranial veins occurs [8].

The evidence explains that there is an inverse relationship between atmospheric pressure, PaO_2 and altitude. When ascending, chemoreceptors in the carotid body detect the decrease in PaO_2. Hypobaric hypoxia produces a neurohumoral and hemodynamic response that increases capillary pressure and causes cerebral edema [5].

In a similar sense, Britze et al. describe that peripheral and central chemoreceptors detects changes in O_2 pressure, CO_2 pressure, blood pH and temperature, triggering compensatory autonomic responses [9]. In this way, hypoxemia:

1. It causes increased ventilation, sympathetic activity, and blood pressure [9]. Britze et al. emphasize that short-term reductions in atmospheric pressure do not necessarily lead to reduced O_2 saturation in the peripheral circulation and especially in brain tissue [9]. Lafuente et al. indicate that CO_2 and O_2 influence cerebral blood flow, hypoxia causes vasodilation and increases cerebral blood flow [5]. They relate that at 3048 m.a.s.l. the O_2 saturation is at least 90%, but at 6100 m.a.s.l. it decreases to less than 70% and at higher altitudes it decreases progressively.
2. If the partial pressure of arterial oxygen (PaO_2) falls below 8 kPa (60 mmHg), the peripheral chemosensors in the carotid/aortic bodies increase their rate of activation [9].
3. The afferent fibers of the glossopharyngeal nerve of the carotid bodies and the vagal afferent fibers of the aortic bodies transmit this information to the nucleus of the solitary tract (NTS), from which they contact neurons that project to the paraventricular nucleus (PVN) of the hypothalamus [9].

   The stimulation of these respiratory centers (ventral respiratory group -VRG- and dorsal respiratory group -DRG-) causes greater ventilation through the phrenic nerves/diaphragm [9]. Like Britze et al., Lafuente et al. explain that the decrease in O_2 pressure perceived by peripheral chemoreceptors increases alveolar ventilation more or less 1.65 times and total ventilation 5 times [9, 5]. Increased ventilation expels large amounts of CO_2 causing hypocapnea and increased pH in body fluids [5].

4. Neurons of the PVN also project to the autonomic regulatory center of the medulla oblongata (rostral ventrolateral). Here, they connect with the neurons projected to the intermediolateral nucleus (IML) of the spinal cord and activate the efferent sympathetic nerves, causing an increase in heart rate [9].

On the role of intracranial hypertension and the "tight fit" hypothesis, Lafuente et al. point out that intracranial hypertension secondary to hypobaric hypoxia was reputed to be the main cause of HACE. Both the affected cerebral blood flow and the existence of central venous insufficiency would produce cerebral edema; this could be secondary to pulmonary hypertension caused by vasoconstriction of the pulmonary bed that would affect cerebral venous return. The "tight fit" hypothesis proposes that the existence of anatomical variations would obstruct venous return, worsening intracranial hypertension and consequently cerebral edema, explaining why some people would develop AMS or HACE and others would not [5]. Lafuente et al. add that these variations could be apparent only after hypoxia (stressor) acts and this would explain the susceptibility of some people to AMS or HACE. The decrease in available O2 increases capillary permeability causing passage of liquid that disables the sodium/potassium pumps. This causes neurons to swell due to loss of cell volume control mechanisms, causing massive infarction or death due to brain herniation. Additionally, they state that the increase in systemic arterial pressure and cerebral blood flow at high altitude were demonstrated in numerous studies. They point that this causes an increase in intracranial hydrostatic pressure as in hypertensive encephalopathy, worsened by obstruction of the sinovenous egress flow [5].

Cerebral venous/arterial dilation increases blood volume (the compensatory phenomenon is based on the absorption and/or translocation of cerebrospinal fluid -CSF-), decreasing intracranial distensibility, causing increased intracranial pressure [8].

In relation to the role of redox activation in the trigemino-vascular system (TVS), Lafuente et al. explain that the AMS and the HACE have classically been considered one the continuation of the other. The HACE as the final phase of the AMS. Instead, traditional theories state that AMS and HACE are secondary to vasogenic extracellular edema due to blood-brain barrier disruption and consequent intracranial hypertension. Thus, the proposed redox activation hypothesis aims to explain AMS based on oxidative damage. It suggests that mild vasogenic edema may be an adaptive physiological response to altitude hypoxemia, causing a succession of events secondary to oxidative stress, which would activate TVS [5].

A study focused on the molecular determinants of blood-brain barrier damage, showing that there was no damage to neuroglia components, but their authors did not detect changes in protein concentrations in cerebrospinal fluid, neurospecific enolase in serum or S100b (astrocytic protein considered a specific marker of the integrity of the blood-brain barrier) [5].

The presence of high-altitude cerebral edema may be an adaptive phenomenon with respect to hypoxia. Increased extracellular space may buffer excess neurotransmitters (e.g. glutamate and glycine), protecting neurons from N-methyl-D-aspartate receptor activation, and may also buffer extracellular K+ preventing brain depolarization [5].

Cerebral white matter blood flow is low (even in normoxia), therefore, increased intracranial pressure compresses small white matter capillaries affecting O_2 delivery, disrupting O_2 dependent ion homeostasis and membrane potentials, resulting in intracellular edema in most individuals [8].

The increase in O_2 free radicals could decrease the Na+/K + -ATPase function. This would explain the redistribution of fluid and astrocytic edema without the need for any volume increase. Consequently, this hypothesis indicates that AMS can be considered an "ionopathy" where free radicals cause ion channel malfunction, generating different clinical courses depending on their distribution and activity [5]. For Lafuente et al. hypoxic inactivation of the Na+/K+ pump in the blood-brain barrier would explain the expansion of extracellular fluid without any damage to the blood-brain barrier. The water that enters the astrocytes would be the same that would be in the extracellular space during the extracellular edema present in hypoxia, in this way, the volume available for redistribution would not cause a significant cerebral edema, which could explain the symptoms of AMS [5]. Data have failed to demonstrate that intracranial hypertension caused by High-Altitude brain edema underlies AMS symptoms. On the contrary, there is evidence that the redox activity of TVS causes the symptoms, that is, in hypoxia, the depletion of mitochondrial O_2 generates hydroxyl radicals (OH). The radicals would depress hypoxic ventilatory control and cause neurovascular endothelial dysfunction. Hypoxia in AMS alters systemic free radical metabolism. Redox imbalance alters dynamic brain autoregulation independently of blood-brain barrier damage [5].

Astrocytic swelling activates p47 NADPH-dependent oxidase (phox) and causes "oxidative osmotic stress". As a result, the increase in NO in the brain directly activates TVS and causes membrane destabilization by lipid peroxidation, local activation of hypoxia-inducible factor 1 alpha (HIF-1α) and Vascular Endothelial Growth Factor (VEGF), as well as the release of free radicals [5, 10]. Recent research shows the involvement of the lymphatic system of the brain in the formation of HACE, the increase in the expression of water channels aquaporin-4 (AQP-4) (main component of the lymphatic system) in astrocytes was associated with the development of HACE in animals exposed to hypobaric hypoxia [11].

Lafuente et al. state that the observations failed to detect an increase in the peptide related to the calcitonin gene ("migraine molecule") -this would indicate the absence of sustained TVS activation or acute delivery of calcitonin gene- related peptide in perivascular trigeminal nerve fibers. The latter could not be detected in cerebrospinal fluid since it does not cause dysfunction of the blood-brain barrier [5]. Paramagnetic electron resonance spectroscopy results obtained from an AMS patient showed increased OH radicals and production of lipid-derived free radicals in cerebrospinal fluid. In addition, prophylaxis with dietary antioxidants, vitamins, and the relationship between net brain production of free radical-mediated lipid peroxidants in hypoxia and symptoms of AMS favors the redox hypothesis [5]. The evidence allows us to conclude that HACE would be an extreme form of oxidative osmotic stress, with severe dysfunction of the blood-brain barrier, cerebral capillary failure "due to stress" and extravasation of erythrocytes, which would explain the microbleeding in the genu and splenium of the corpus callosum demonstrated by highly sensitive magnetic resonance imaging of sensitivity weighting in patients with HACE. These microbleeds are not observable in AMS, supporting the theory that edema and blood-brain barrier disruption are minor. Hemosiderin deposits cannot be removed across the blood-brain barrier, which is why they can be used to diagnose HACE even after years of recovery. Consequently, microbleeds could manifest a blood-brain barrier disorder during HACE but not in AMS [5].

Clinic

The evidence indicate that headache is the most common symptom perceived by those who climb to high altitudes, it occurs in 25% of people who climb to 2000–3000 m.a.s.l., in 80% of those who climb to altitudes above 3000 m.a.s.l., and in almost all people at altitudes above 4500 m.a.s.l. The headache begins 8–24 h after reaching 2500 m.a.s.l. [5]. On the other hand, the results of Dekker et al. point out that the headache begins between 48 and 72 hours after beginning the ascent [7].

It is hypothesized that cerebral edema and increased intracranial pressure cause headache by compressing brain structures and causing stretching and displacement of unmyelinated pain-sensitive fibers within the trigemino-vascular system. Connections of afferent nerve fibers from the trigeminal nerve to vegetative centers in the brainstem may also explain accompanying symptoms such as nausea and vomiting [12].

The Headache Classification Committee of the International Headache Society (IHS) III edition of the International Classification of Headaches describes that altitude headache is frequently bilateral, worsens with exertion, is caused by ascent to altitude greater than 2500 m.a.s.l. and is resolved within 24 hours after the descent [13].

Said Committee points out the following criteria to identify altitude headache:

A. Headache meeting criterion C.
B. There has been an ascent to more than 2500 m.a.s.l.
C. Causation is demonstrated by at least two of the following characteristics:

1. The onset of the headache is temporally related to the ascent.
2. Any of the following characteristics:

    (a) The headache has significantly worsened simultaneously with the continued ascent.
    (b) The headache has resolved within 24 hours after descent to an altitude below 2500 m.a.s.l.

3. The headache has at least two of the following three characteristics:

    (a) Bilateral location.
    (b) Mild or moderate intensity.
    (c) Aggravated by exercise, movement, effort, coughing and/or trunk flexion.

D. Not attributable to another ICHD-III diagnosis.

Regarding its characteristics, Dekker et al. describe that in 30%–40% of cases this headache is dull and throbbing, develops during sleep and is perceived upon awakening [7]. For their part, Lafuente et al. describe that when the headache is part of the AMS, it is characterized by mild to moderate intensity, oppressive type, frontal reference, frontoparietal, bilateral, or holocranial, whose intensity is increased by exercise and movement of the head [5].

Lafuente et al [5] and Dekker *et al* [7], differentiate HACE headache from AMS headache by the following indicators: (1) affects 0, 5%–1.0% of people, (2) altitude greater than 4500 m.a.s.l., (3) generally between 24–36 hours after ascent to high altitude (late compared to AMS), (4) frequently associated with high altitude pulmonary edema [5, 7] commonly occurs with progressive ataxia, altered mental status, slurred speech, confusion, decreased consciousness, hallucinations Carod [14] notes that 32% of climbers experience hallucinations above 7500 m.a.s.l.], stupor, coma [5, 15], (5) also associated with intracranial hypertension (ICH), papilledema, retinal hemorrhages [with a frequency of 50% according to Carod [14], brain hernia [5], paralysis of the sixth nerve Dekker et al. point out that it is usually the first dysfunction of the cranial nerves [7].

The results of Dekker et al. show that the neurological signs of established HACE are papilledema (52%), incontinence (48%), extensor plantar reflexes (34%), abnormal tone/power (14%), and to a lesser extent, isolated visual field loss, paralysis of the sixth nerve, pupillary asymmetry and hearing loss [7]. The investigations of Joyce et al. [10], Davis [16], and Song et al. [15] report ataxia -for Joyce- in 40%–60% of cases [10], anorexia, nausea, for Davis vomiting and convulsions are rare [16]. Dekker et al. emphasize that hypoglycemia, dehydration, exhaustion, and hypothermia can make diagnosis difficult [7]. Who survive HACE recover in 3–14 days [17].

Diagnosis

Kanan et al. point out that the brain responds to hypoxia with increased blood flow, increased biochemical mediators induced by hypoxia, and increased permeability of the blood-brain barrier, causing mechanical stress [18]. The diagnosis of HACE involves, in part, identificate these phenomena. Davis adds the need to identify the environment and the symptoms, in addition, he points out that laboratory and imaging studies are useful -above all- to suppress alternative diagnoses. In this sense, the evidence shows that complete blood count electrolytes, glucose, ethanol level, carboxyhemoglobin and toxicological tests are useful to exclude other disorders. HACE can present with mild leukocytosis that requires clinical correlation to exclude an infectious process. When encephalitis or subarachnoid hemorrhage is suspected, lumbar puncture can be performed (provided there are no contraindications), taking into account that, in HACE, said puncture shows normal cell counts and high opening pressure [16].

Computed Tomography

Computed tomography of the brain exhibits white matter signal attenuation with flattening of gyri and effacement of sulci [16].

Magnetic Resonance

Joyce et al. explain that reductions in venous flow preceded by increased cerebral blood flow due to hypoxia probably cause an increase in the volume of the brain parenchyma [10].

Magnetic resonance imaging evidence 32 hours after high-altitude ascent showed that healthy people and those with AMS had larger brain volume in gray matter, possibly explained by compensatory increase in cortical cerebral blood flow [5].

Through this study, both the relaxation time (T2) and the apparent diffusion coefficient (ADC) allow us to distinguish between extracellular and intracellular edema. Low ADC (low diffusivity) corresponds to intracellular water and high ADC (high diffusivity) indicates extracellular water [5]. Lafuente *et al* teach that in people with AMS symptoms, hypoxia increased relaxation time (cerebral edema) but with a low ADC, indicating the existence of the intracellular component. They also show that, in the absence of brain inflammation, the decrease in ADC translates into "fluid redistribution" from the extracellular to the intracellular space rather than brain water gain. However, they observe that since the edema affects the corpus callosum, the symptoms of AMS would not be explained, but rather a disconnection syndrome [5].

In this same sense, Kanaan et al. state that reversible vasogenic cerebral edema is noted with increased T2 signal in the corpus callosum and subcortical white matter, indicative of the permeability of the blood brain barrier [16]. On the other hand, Burtscher et al. found Microhemorrhages in the cerebellar peduncles of a high-altitude climber, indicative of a correlation between the anatomical site of injury and ataxia [11].

Davis describes that autopsies showed microbleeds in the white matter and corpus callosum consistent with those seen in MRIs of HACE survivors [16]. Likewise, Burtscher et al. point out that magnetic resonance imaging can show hemosiderin deposits in the splenium of the corpus callosum after microbleeding even months after recovery from HACE [11]. Lafuente et al. explain that corpus callosum could be irrigated by short, small, perforating arterioles without adrenergic tone, predisposed to hypoxic vasodilation, autoregulatory failure and overperfusion, with subsequent microbleeding. They add that the microhemorrhages are due to the obstruction of the venous flow, this hypothesis is based on the presence of dilation of the retinal veins and retinal microhemorrhages present in people who ascend to high altitude [5].

Optic Nerve Sheath

Kanan et al. indicate that there is a correlation between the diameter of the optic nerve sheath and increased intracranial pressure, given that the intraorbital sub-arachnoid space expands due to increased intracranial pressure [17] and show that, while a large cross-sectional study positively associated severity of AMS with increased optic nerve sheath diameter seen on ultrasound, two other prospective studies concluded a weak/no relationship between optic nerve sheath diameter and high-altitude headache or AMS [18].

The Standard Approach to Management

Prophylaxis

Dekker et al. establish that they do not require pharmacological prophylaxis:

1. Those who ascend up to 2500 m.a.s.l.
2. Those who ascend gradually for 2 (two) or more days up to 3000 m.a.s.l. Davis points out that graduated ascent is the best prevention, pointing out that: (a) above 2500 m.a.s.l. one should not ascend more than 500 m/day and (b) after the 1500 m ascent an additional night is necessary for acclimatization [16].
3. Those who ascend 500 m/day.
4. Those who do not have a history of having suffered from AMS [7].

So also Dekker *et al* point out that drug prophylaxis should be considered for people who:

1. They have a history of having suffered from AMS.
2. They ascend to more than 2500 m.a.s.l. in one day.
3. They ascend 500 m/day or more above 3000 m.a.s.l.
4. They ascend to very high or extreme altitudes.
5. They ascend rapidly [7].

Prophylaxis Drugs

Acetazolamide (Az)

Recommended dose of Az for AMS prophylaxis is 125 [11] to 250 mg bid from the day before altitude exposure and low-dose pretreatment (125 mg bid) should be started 2 days before altitude exposure to altitude [2, 10] and continue for 48 hours once arrived at the destination altitude. Joyce et al. indicate that the 62.5 mg BID dose may be just as effective in preventing AMS [10].

Administration of acetazolamide as prophylaxis with recommendation grade (RG): 1A [19].

Dexamethasone (Dx)

4 mg every 12 hours intramuscularly (IM), or intravenously (IV), (RG: 1A) [19].

Acetaminophen/paracetamol

1 g 3 times daily (RG: 1C) [19].

Ibuprofen

600 mg 3 times daily (RG: 2B) [19].

The Treatment

Non-pharmacological Treatment

1. Ensure that the patient's head is elevated to 30° in the supine position.
2. Evidence indicates that people with AMS can remain at high altitude with symptomatic treatment [7]. However, the main treatment for AMS and HACE is descent [7, 16] or as far as symptoms cease [3].
3. Portable hyperbaric chambers (Gamov bags) [7]: Aksel *et al,* indicate that limited evidence demonstrates the usefulness of portable hyperbaric chambers when descent is impossible. The treatment lasts long hours, not without problems (nausea, claustrophobia, etc.) and the symptoms can reappear at its conclusion [3]. Davis reports that 0.9 kg/2.5 cm^2 (2 pound/inch^2) intra-chamber pressure simulates a descent of up to 1500 m (4,920 ft). Chamber depressurization should be gradual to avoid middle ear contraction and barotrauma [16]. The use of a portable hyperbaric chamber is useful for people who climb snowy peaks or mountains, while the descent is carried out safely until arrival at a hospital (RG: 1B) [19].
4. Other measures, we recommend not consuming alcoholic beverages when arriving in high-altitude cities, as well as notably reducing tobacco consumption (ideally avoiding it) until arriving in the country of origin.

Pharmacotherapy

1. Oxygen through nasal cannulas or mask, with saturation titrated at 90% for all patients with suspected HACE, even more so due to the frequent concomitance of HAPE and critical condition [16]. Evidence shows that low-flow O_2 (2L/min)

via nasal cannula during sleep alleviates the physiological stress of hypobaric hypoxia and effectively simulates sea level below 3000 m.a.s.l. [16] It recommends avoiding prolonged hyperoxia in critically ill patients due to increased mortality. Oxygen administration with RG: 1A [19].

2. Oxygen through the advanced airway in comatose patients [16] maintaining an O2 saturation of at least 90%, avoiding hyperventilation (at 3600 m.a.s.l. -La Paz Bolivia- normal $PaCO_2$ is 30 mmHg) and arterial hypotension, both factors can cause cerebral ischemia and hinder the neurological prognosis.
3. Evidence indicates that analgesics (acetaminophen/paracetamol 650-1000 mg) or non-steroidal anti-inflammatory drugs (ibuprofen 600 mg) can be used to relieve high altitude headache [3].
4. Given the need to administer parenteral solutions, isotonic solutions are used. Avoid overhydrating the patient and/or administer hypotonic solutions.

Carod indicates that pharmacological treatment seeks Increase ventilatory response, and decrease cytokine release and inflammation [14]:

Increase Ventilatory Response

Acetazolamide (Az)

Acetazolamide inhibits aquaporin, modulates reactive oxygen species (ROS), heat shock protein 70 (HSP-70), the IL-1 receptor agonist, HIF, regulates cyclic adenosine monophosphate (cAMP) [9] and inhibits renal carbonic anhydrase by stimulating the loss of bicarbonate (HCO3−) and sodium (Na^+) in the urine with retention of H^+ and chloride (Cl−) and effective reduction of serum pH plus subsequent metabolic acidosis that stimulates minute ventilation and increases PaO2 [14, 10].

HACE can be treated with Az 125–250 mg/8–12 h [17], however, due to adverse effects (e.g. paresthesia, polyuria, rash, dysgeusia, etc.) it is important to establish the dose minimum effective [10]. Davis discusses the importance of avoiding the use of Az in people with a history of anaphylaxis to sulfa antibiotics and keeping Stevens-Johnson syndrome in mind [2, 16].

Metazolamide (Mtz)

The administration of 150 mg of Mtz is as effective as that of Az with fewer adverse effects. Joyce et al. point out that Mtz, in vitro, activates the gene transcription factor related to nuclear factor 2 (Nrf-2) that positively regulates antioxidant proteins that eliminate reactive oxygen species (ROS), it is not clear if this effect would occur in vivo [10].

Benzolamide (Bz)

Bz has similar efficacy to Az with less psychomotor effect efficacy due to its lower penetration to the central nervous system [10].

Decrease Cytokine Release and Inflammation

1 Dexamethasone (Dx)

Joyce et al. show that Dx reduces ROS generation, positively regulates endogenous antioxidants/HSP-707/adrenomedullin, causes sympatholysis, improves O2 saturation and modifies aquaporin expression [10], Carod adds blockade of VEGF factor expression and reversal hypoxia-induced cerebral edema [14]. Aksel et al. [3] and Joyce et al. initially recommend 8–10 mg of Dx intramuscularly (IM), or intravenously (IV), followed by 4 mg every 6 hours [2, 10].

Controversial Aspects of Management

Pre-acclimatization through a tent, chamber or commercial hypoxia mask, showing that brief and intermittent exposure to hypoxia of less than 6 h/day does not seem to prevent AMS and remote ischemic preconditioning, the application of which lacks support in the literature [16].

Aksel et al. emphasize that there is no evidence authorizing the use of hypertonic saline, loop diuretics, or mannitol in patients with HACE. In addition, they advocate avoiding loop diuretics due to the danger of hypotension, cerebral hypoperfusion and ischemia. There is insufficient evidence to support the use of ginkgo biloba, and budesonide [3].

The group of Geng et al., conducted a study in adult male mice subjected to the combination of LPS (0.5 mg/kg, intraperitoneal injection) and exposure to hypobaric hypoxia in a hypobaric hypoxia chamber (mimicking 6000 m.a.s.l.) in order to create the HACE model. The mice received gipenoside-14 (GP-14), a bioactive fraction during the plant *Gynostemma pentaphyllum* 7 days and that would have antihypoxic activity in vitro and in vivo. The study emerged that GP-14 suppressed the NF-κB pathway, inhibited microglial activation and inflammatory cytokine production in a mouse HACE model, however further studies are still required for its administration in HACE [20].

On the other hand, Mehany et al., studied the effects of *quercetin* (a component of various vegetables, plants and fruits) with antioxidant and anti-inflammatory effect. The rats subjected to hypoxic chamber to simulate a decreased atmospheric pressure and an altitude of 5000 m.a.s.l. received 20 mg/Kg of quercetin. The results showed increased concentrations of biomarkers such as: glutathione, glutathione S-transferase, glutathione reductase, glutathione peroxidase, superoxide dismutase, catalase and a decrease in malondialdehyde levels, it would also have the ability to scavenge free radicals resulting from hypoxia [21].

In relation to the coca plant, it is native to South America, probably domesticated about 4000 years ago. The variety *Erythroxylum coca var. coca* is found in Bolivia and is made up of three alkaloids: cocaine, cis-cinamilcocafoa, trans-cinamilcocafoa indicated by a study by the Bolivian Institute of High-altitude Biology published in 1997 [22]. It is ingested as an infusion (coca tea) by most visitors to cities above 3000 m.a.s.l., in order to reduce the symptoms/signs of *"Sorojchi"* (Altitude Sickness/Mountain Sickness). Among the studies related to the coca leaf, Spielvogel et al. investigated the use of coca and its relationship with effort, they subjected 60 men from two communities of the Bolivian Altiplano (32 male coca leaf chewers and 23 non-consumers) to exercise tests using a stationary bicycle. It was evaluated oxygen consumption (VO2), carbon dioxide production (VCO2), the exchange ratio of these two gases (R = VCO2/VO2) called respiratory quotient, ventilation (VE) and respiratory equivalent (VE/VO2). There is also fever, heart rate (HR), blood oxygen saturation (SaO_2), glucose, free fatty acids, lactate, and the hormones epinephrine and norepinephrine flourish in blood samples. The respiratory quotient (R) was lower in the coca leaf users than in the non-users in the maximum effort, while the other variables were similar in both, the users showed a lower SaO_2 and a Higher HR in relation to non-users, epinephrine and norepinephrine was higher in the consumer group. In the group of non-consumers, VO2 was higher in relation to the duration of the test, while in the group of consumers it remained stable for 30 minutes with a late increase. The results indicate that chewed coca leaves could help to work for a longer time before exhaustion sets in [23]. To date there are no studies with scientific evidence to support the use of coca tea or chewed coca leaves to be used as part of the treatment or prevention of HACE.

References

1. Lawley JS, Levine BD, Williams MA, Malm J, Eklund A, Polaner DM, Subudhi AW, Hackett PH, Roach RC. Cerebral spinal fluid dynamics: effect of hypoxia and implications for high-altitude illness. J Appl Physiol. 2016;120:251–62.
2. Zelmanovich R, Pierre K, Felisma P, Cole D, Goldman M, Lucke-Wold B. High altitude cerebral Edema: improving treatment options. Biologics. 2022;2(1):81–91.
3. Aksel G, Çorbacıoğlu Şeref K, Özen C. High-altitude illness: management approach. Turkish J Emerg Med. 2019;19:121–6.
4. Imray C, Wright A, Subudhi A, Roach R. Acute Mountain sickness: pathophysiology, prevention, and treatment. Prog Cardiovasc Dis. 2010;52:467–84.
5. Lafuente JV, Bermudez G, Arce LC, Bulnes S. Blood-brain barrier changes in high altitude. CNS Neurol Disord Drug Targets. 2016;15:1188–97.

6. Luks AM. Physiology in medicine: a physiologic approach to prevention and treatment of acute high-altitude illnesses. J Appl Physiol. 2015;118:509–19.
7. Dekker MCJ, Wilson MH, Howlett WP. Mountain neurology. Pract Neurol. 2019:1–8.
8. Turner REF, Gatterer H, Falla M, Lawley JS. High-altitude cerebral edema: its own entity or end-stage acute mountain sickness? J Appl Physiol. 2021;131:313–25.
9. Britze J, Arngrim N, Schytz HW, Ashina M. Hypoxic mechanisms in primary headaches. Cephalalgia. 2016:1–13.
10. Joyce K, Lucas S, Imray C, Balanos G, Wright AD. Advances in the available non-biological pharmacotherapy prevention and treatment of acute mountain sickness and high altitude cerebral and pulmonary oedema. Expert Opin Pharmacother. 2018;19(17):1–12.
11. Burtscher M, Hefti U, Hefti JP. High-altitude illnesses: old stories and new insights into the pathophysiology, treatment and prevention. Sports Med Health Sci. 2021;3(2):59–69.
12. Berger M, Schiefer L, Treff G, Sareban M, Swenson E, Bärtsch P. Acute high-altitude illness: updated principles of pathophysiology, prevention, and treatment. German J Sports Med. 2020;71:267–74.
13. Sociedad Internacional de Cefaleas. III edición de la Clasificación internacional de las cefaleas. Cephalalgia. 2018;38(1):1–211.
14. Carod-Artal F. Cefalea de elevada altitud y mal de altura. Neurologia. 2014;29(9):533–40.
15. Song T-T, Bi Y-H, Gao Y-Q, Huang R, Hao K, Xu G, Tang J-W, Ma Z-Q, Kong F-P, Coote JH, Chen X-Q, Du J-Z. Systemic pro-inflammatory response facilitates the development of cerebral edema during short hypoxia. J Neuroinflammation. 2016;13(63):1–14.
16. Davis C, Hackett P. Advances in the prevention and treatment of high altitude illness. Emerg Med Clin North Am. 2017;35(2):241–60.
17. Srivastava S. High altitude brain swelling. Emerg Med Clin North Am. 2016;7(3):1–2.
18. Kanaan NC, Lipman GS, Constance BB, Holck PS, Preuss JF, Williams SR. Optic nerve sheath diameter increase on ascent to high altitude: correlation with acute mountain sickness. Emerg Med Clin North Am. 2015;34(9):1677–82.
19. Luks AM, Auerbach PS, Freer L, Grissom CK, Keyes LE, SE MI, Rodway GW, Schoene RB, Zafren K, Hackett PH. Wilderness medical society practice guidelines for the prevention and treatment of acute altitude illness: 2019 update. Wilderness Environ Med. 2019:1–16.
20. Geng Y, Yang J, Cheng X, Han Y, Yan F, Wang C, Jiang X, Meng X, Fan M, Zhao M, Zhu L. A bioactive gypenoside (GP-14) alleviates neuroinflammation and blood brain barrier (BBB) disruption by inhibiting the NF-κB signaling pathway in a mouse high-altitude cerebral edema (HACE) model. Int Immunopharmacol. 2022;107:1–10.
21. Mehany ABM, Belal A, Santali EY, Shaaban S, Abourehab MAS, El-Feky OA, Diab M, Abou Galala FMA, Elkaeed EB, Abdelhamid G. Biological effect of quercetin in repairing brain damage and cerebral changes in rats: molecular docking and in vivo studies. Biomed Res Int. 2022:1–12.
22. Sauvain M, Moretti C, Rerat C, Ruiz E, Bravo J, Muñoz V, Saravia E, Arrázola S, Gutierrez E, Bruckner A. Estudio químico y botánico de las diferentes formas de *Erythroxylum coca var. coca* cultivadas en Bolivia. Instituto Boliviano de Biología de Altura; 1997. p. 35–46.
23. Spielvogel H, Cáceres E, Favier R. Coca y esfuerzo físico. Instituto Boliviano de Biología de Altura; 1997. p. 51–61.

Chapter 14
High Altitude Cor Pulmonale

Gunjan Chanchalani, Kanwalpreet Sodhi, and Manender Kumar Singla

Case

A previously healthy, 36 year old male had been on vacation with his wife in Lahaul Spiti (India; 5000 m height) for 3 days. He presented to the emergency with progressively worsening clinical symptoms over the past 48 hours, with moderate headache and dizziness since landing, relieved by taking a paracetamol, and later followed by cough associated with progressively increasing dyspnea.

On physical examination, he appeared tachypneic with a respiratory rate of 32 breaths per minute, oxygen saturation of 84% on room air, rales in bilateral lung bases, elevated jugular venous pressure, loud second heart sound and pedal edema.

On further investigation, there was leukocytosis; Chest X-ray showed multiple bilateral alveolar opacities, predominantly in peri-bronchovascular region; ECG showed right axis deviation, QR wave in lead V1, and dominant R wave in leads V1 to V3 with no other abnormality.

Echocardiography showed dilated right ventricle (RV) with RVEDA of 18.7 cm^2/m^2; the right-to-left ventricular end-diastolic area ratio of 65% with the bowing of the interventricular septum into the left ventricle (LV) giving a characteristic D

G. Chanchalani
KJ Somaiya Hospital and Research Centre, Sion, Mumbai, Maharashtra, India

K. Sodhi (✉)
Critical Care, Deep Hospital, Ludhiana, Punjab, India

M. K. Singla
Cardiac Anesthesia, Fortis Hospital, Ludhiana, Punjab, India

J. Hidalgo et al. (eds.), *High Altitude Medicine*,
https://doi.org/10.1007/978-3-031-35092-4_14

configuration of the LV (consistent with volume and pressure overload of the RV), estimated pulmonary artery systolic pressure of 84 mm Hg (mean of 46 mmHg) and IVC diameter of 2.2 cm at expiration, non-collapsing during inspiration. The maximal velocity of the tricuspid regurgitant jet was increased, with a calculated trans tricuspid pressure gradient of 62 mmHg. The right atrium was dilated with the bulging of the inter auricular septum into the left atrium. On doppler imaging, the right heart showed a decreased ejection wave.

Standard Approach to Management

Clinical Presentation

The classical symptoms and signs of cor pulmonale include dyspnea, cough, cyanosis, sleep disturbance, irritability, and clinical signs of right heart failure. Signs of backward RV failure include features of systemic congestion with elevated jugular venous pressure with dilated jugular veins, facial and lower limb edema, congestive hepatomegaly, ascites, pericardial effusion and effort angina.

In severe forms, it can lead to compromised LV diastolic filling, due to interventricular dependence, causing forward failure with hypotension and organ hypoperfusion.

Chest Radiography

Chest X-ray shows cardiomegaly, prominence of central and peripheral pulmonary arteries (Fig. 14.1).

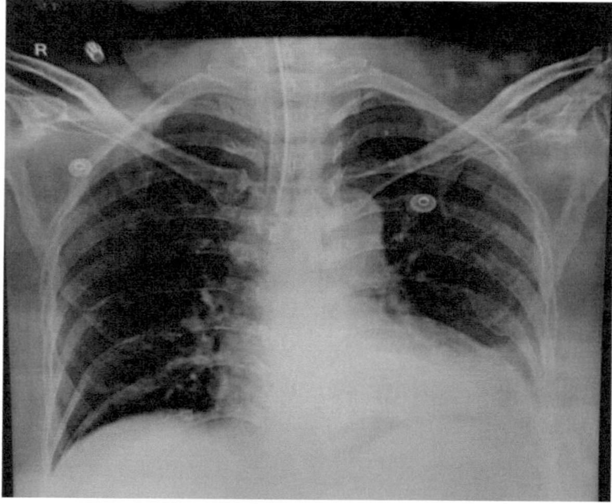

Fig. 14.1 CXR showing cardiomegaly, with relatively oligemic lung fields

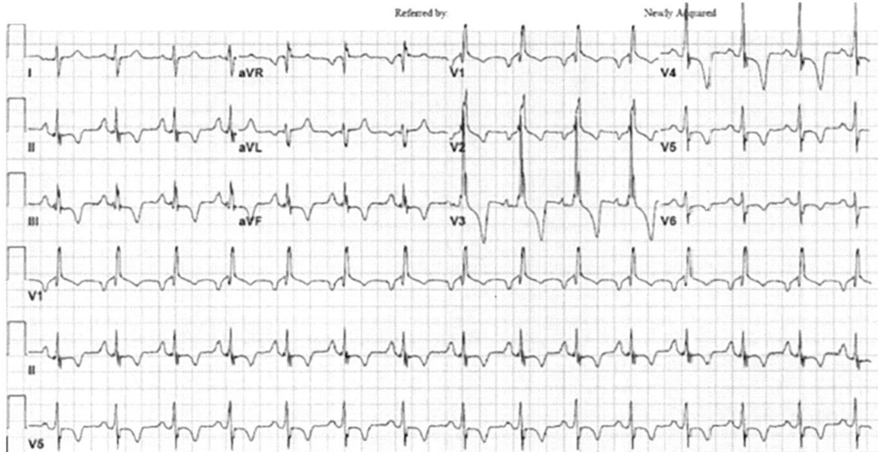

Fig. 14.2 ECG showing sinus tachycardia with incomplete right bundle branch block

Electrocardiogram

ECG shows right axis deviation and evidence of marked right ventricular hypertrophy. Other ECG criteria include RS-ratio in lead V5 or V6 $\leq$ 1, S in V5 or V 6 $\geq$ 7 mm, P-pulmonale or a combination of these. RV failure may often be associated with atrial flutter or atrial fibrillation (Fig. 14.2).

Echocardiography

2D echocardiography assists in diagnosis by evidence of features of right ventricular hypertrophy and/or right heart failure.

A transthoracic echocardiogram shows marked increase in mean and systolic pulmonary arterial pressure, with an increase in the tricuspid regurgitant jet and a increase in the trans-tricuspid pressure gradient. The right ventricle is dilated, with an increase in the right ventricle end-diastolic area (RVEDA), and a high right-to-left end-diastolic area ratio, leading to flattening of interventricular septum, and paradoxical motion of the interventricular septum. The right atrium appears dilated too, with the interatrial septum bulging towards the left side. The inferior vena cava is dilated with loss of inspiratory decrease in size. On tissue doppler a decreased ejection wave of the RV is seen (Fig. 14.3).

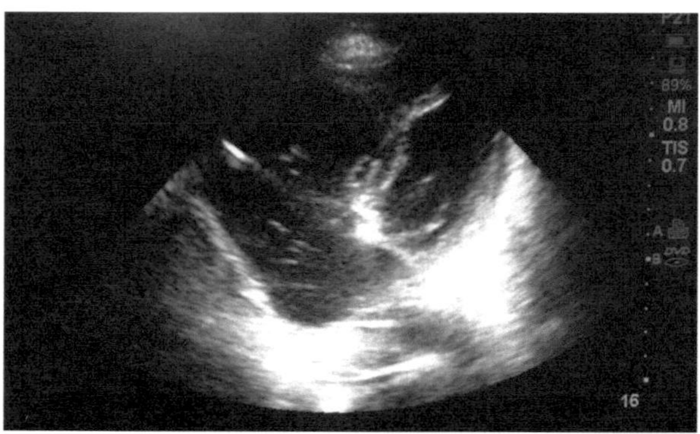

Fig. 14.3 Echocardiography showing dilated right atrium and right ventricle

Cardiac MRI

Cardiac MRI is now considered as the standard reference method to assess the cardiac chambers and function, when echocardiography findings may be limited due to poor visualization of the RV.

Treatment

The treatment for symptomatic high altitude cor pulmonale is moving to low altitude, which reverses the condition within few days to few weeks [1–3].

Oxygen supplementation may help temporarily.

Low level evidence exists for use of endothelin receptor blockers, phosphodiesterase-5 inhibitors, calcium channel blockers, or high-dose corticosteroids [3].

Treatment of RV failure involves volume optimization if preload dependent, or use of diuretics if evidence of congestion but usually diuretics are not helpful and may sometimes be harmful due to decrease in preload with worsening the cor pulmonale. Perfusion pressure can be maintained with use of Noradrenaline as vasopressor. A positive ionotropic drug (Dobutamine / Levosimendan) may be added to improve myocardial contractility. Use of Mechanical circulatory support may be considered. The role of pulmonary vasodilators is controversial.

Prognosis

The condition is reversible with descent to sea level and has a good prognosis [1].

Evidence Contour

(i) *The prevalence*

Congestive RV failure on exposure to high altitude was initially reported in the late nineteenth century in cattle transported to the high pastures of Utah and Colorado, named as "brisket" disease [4]. In adults, this syndrome was seen in 10–20% of soldiers, involved in strenuous activity at 5800–6700 m [5].

In humans, RV may be affected in long term inhabitants at high altitude known as "subacute mountain sickness"- rapidly progressing congestive heart failure [5].

A similar finding of acute right heart failure was objectified by echocardiography in a European tourist travelling to Bolivia [6].

(ii) *What is subacute mountain sickness (SMS)?*

Usually an insidious onset, with gradual worsening dyspnea and edema. The symptoms start becoming evident about 10.8 ± 5.9 weeks of stay at high altitude, usually presenting with gross anasarca with severe shortness of breath. The incidence is higher in children and in males [7].

(iii) *What is Chronic Mountain Sickness (CMS)?*

RV dysfunction is seen in some long-term residents at high altitude, with chronic pulmonary hypertension [8].

Chronic mountain sickness (CMS), or Monge's disease, affects about 5% to 10% of the population permanently living at high altitude, above 2500 m [1]. Progressive loss of ventilatory rate, and hypoxemia leads to polycythemia (Hb $\geq$19 g/dL for women and Hb $\geq$21 g/dL for men). This is also associated with pulmonary hypertension, which in advanced cases progresses to cor pulmonale [1].

(iv) *Susceptibility*

About 10% to 20% of the individuals stationed at high altitude were found to be affected in a study, however no clear-cut factors could be identified for this incidence [9].

Right heart failure induced by altitude, is usually seen at heights of 4000 m above sea level, and is secondary to hypoxic pulmonary hypertension. The incidence of pulmonary hypertension and thus cor pulmonale has shown to increase with higher altitude and with the longer duration of stay [10]. Few cases have been reported in children and adults at altitudes below 3000 m as well [7].

SMS occurs in adults usually at altitudes above 5500 m, whereas in infants it manifests at altitudes of 2500-3000 m. This is secondary to the fact that children develop greater pulmonary vasoconstrictor response and thus greater pulmonary hypertension to hypoxia. This response to hypoxia decreases with age [11].

Tibetans have a very low incidence of SMS [7], as they develop no or minimal pulmonary hypertension in response to hypoxia [12], and thus do not develop cor pulmonale. This natural selection to hypoxic atmosphere exposure makes Tibetans the best ethnicity to long-term adaptation to environmental hypoxia. These phenotypic, physiological, and genetic adaptations have been unchanged over the last generations, despite miscegenation [13].

(v) *Pathophysiology*

Pulmonary artery pressure inevitably rises on ascent to high altitude, along a parabolic curve [2], secondary to pulmonary artery vasoconstriction. Cor pulmonale usually manifests weeks to a few months of continuous exposure to hypoxia at high altitude. Exposure to alveolar hypoxia causes immediate and reversible pulmonary vasoconstriction, which is mediated by endothelin-1 and other mediators. Persistent and prolonged hypoxia leads to thickening and hypertrophy of the tunica media of the pulmonary vessels [9].

Due to increased afterload, the RV hypertrophies and dilates, and if this pulmonary hypertension is severe, it leads to cor pulmonale. Activation of the sympathetic nervous system, and adaptation of RV to hypovolemia may have an additive effect on the altered RV function. Other contributing factors may include polycythemia, remodeling of the pulmonary vasculature structure, the pulmonary vasoconstrictive effects of cold, and pulmonary thromboembolism [9].

In natives at high-altitude, similar findings in cardiac function were seen with both systolic and diastolic function indices being mildly depressed, an adaptation of the heart to relatively milder pulmonary hypertension. These differences on acclimatization may be secondary to different sympathetic nervous tone, hypovolemia and decreased preload, and possibly direct cardiac effects of prolonged chronic hypoxia [14, 15].

(vi) *Role of myocardial dysfunction*

Hypoxia at high altitude can cause myocardial depression [16, 17], however its contribution to the right heart failure at high altitude is not proven.

Exposure of healthy subjects to high altitude (over 6000 m) for 25 days, did not find an impairment of the cardiac function in the Everest II study [18, 19].

(vii) *Role of the kidney and neuro-endocrines*

Soldiers with adult subacute mountain sickness, were found to have a 20% increase in total body water and a increase in total body sodium of 23% [9].

In a study, Anand et al. measured body fluid compartments, renal blood flow, and plasma hormones in normal asymptomatic soldiers stationed for approximately 10 weeks at extreme altitude above 6000 m [20]. All the body fluid compartments - the total body water, plasma volume, blood volume, and total body exchangeable sodium were significantly increased. The effective renal plasma flow was reduced by 55%. The plasma hormonal response with rise in plasma norepinephrine and serum aldosterone levels, with unaffected plasma epinephrine and renin was seen [20].

Studies suggest a possibility that the salt and water retention seen in the normal subjects at extreme altitude and that seen in the soldiers with the subacute mountain sickness, could be secondary to mechanisms to reduce the renal blood flow, which is independent to the incidence of pulmonary arterial hypertension and myocardial dysfunction [21].

(viii) *Treatment and prevention*

Adults should avoid long stays at altitudes higher than 5500 m. Some adults improve temporarily with supplemental oxygen [22], as well as with nifedipine or sildenafil [23], although full remission of SMS (in children and adults) is only achieved by descending to low altitude [9].

Low level evidence exists for use endothelin receptor blockers, phosphodiesterase-5 inhibitors, calcium channel blockers, or high-dose corticosteroids [3].

(ix) *Reversibility*

Experimental data has proven that structural changes in the pulmonary vasculature occur with exposure to hypobaric hypoxia and are reversible over few months of exposure to euoxia [24].

On descent to sea level, there may be evidence of residual pulmonary hypertension, followed by the complete resolution of pulmonary arterial pressures over next 12 to 16 weeks, support the concept of structural remodeling of pulmonary vasculature in this group of patients [9].

References

1. Leon-Velarde F, Maggiorini M, Reeves JT, et al. Consensus statement on chronic and subacute high altitude diseases. High Alt Med Biol. 2005;6:147–57. https://doi.org/10.1089/ham.2005.6.147.
2. Penaloza D, Arias-Stella J. The heart and pulmonary circulation at high altitudes. Healthy highlanders and chronic mountain sickness. Circulation. 2007;115:1132–46. https://doi.org/10.1161/CIRCULATIONAHA.106.624544.
3. Bärtsch P, Gibbs S. Effect of altitude on the heart and the lungs. Circulation. 2007;116:2191–202.
4. Glover GH, Newsom IE. Brisket disease (dropsy of high altitude). Colo Agric Exp Station. 1915;204:3–24.
5. Anand IS, Malhotra RM, Chandrashekhar Y, Bali HK, Chauhan SS, Jindal SK, Bhandari RK, Wahi PL. Adult subacute mountain sickness: a syndrome of congestive heart failure in man at very high altitude. Lancet. 1990;335 561–5. https://doi.org/10.1016/0140-6736(90)90348-9.
6. Huez S, Faoro V, Vachiéry JL, Unger P, Martinot JB, Naeije R. Images in cardiovascular medicine. High-altitude-induced right-heart failure. Circulation. 2007;115(9):e308–9. https://doi.org/10.1161/CIRCULATIONAHA.106.650994.
7. Ge RL, Helun G. Current concept of chronic mountain sickness: pulmonary hypertension-related high-altitude heart disease. Wilderness Environ Med. 2001;12:190–4.
8. Maripov A, Mamazhakypov A, Karagulova G, Sydykov A, Sarybaev A. High altitude pulmonary hypertension with severe right ventricular dysfunction. Int J Cardiol. 2013;168(3):e89–90. https://doi.org/10.1016/j.ijcard.2013.07.129.
9. Anand IS, Wu T. Syndromes of Subacute Mountain sickness. High Alt Med Biol. 2004;5(2):156–70. https://doi.org/10.1089/1527029041352135.
10. Lockhart A, Saiag B. Altitude and the human pulmonary circulation. Clin Sci (London). 1981;1981(60):599–605.

11. Heath D, Williams DR. Infantile and adult subacute mountain sickness. In: Heath D, Williams DR, editors. High-altitude medicine and pathology. New York: Oxford University Press Inc; 1995. p. 213–21.

12. Groves BM, Droma T, Sutton JR, McCullough RG, McCullough RGE, Zhuang J, et al. Minimal hypoxic pulmonary hypertension in normal Tibetans at 3,658 m. J Appl Physiol. 1993;74:312–8.

13. Beall CM. Two routes to functional adaptation: Tibetan and Andean high-altitude natives. Proc Natl Acad Sci U S A. 2007;104:8655–60.

14. Naeije R. Physiological adaptation of the cardiovascular system to high altitude. Prog Cardiovasc Dis. 2010;52(6):456–66. https://doi.org/10.1016/j.pcad.2010.03.004.

15. Huez S, Faoro V, Guénard H, et al. Echocardiographic and tissue doppler imaging of cardiac adaptation to high altitude in native highlanders versus acclimatized lowlanders. Am J Cardiol. 2009;103:1605–9.

16. Hartley LH, Alexander JK, Modelski M, Grover RF. Subnormal cardiac output at rest and during exercise in residents at 3,100 m altitude. J Appl Physiol. 1967;23:839–48.

17. Tucker CE, James WE, Berry MA, Johnstone CJ, Grover RF. Depressed myocardial function in the goat at high altitude. J Appl Physiol. 1976;41:356–61.

18. Reeves JT, Groves BM, Sutton JR, Wagner PD, Cymerman A, Malconian MK, Rock PB, Young PM, Houston CS. Operation Everest II: preservation of cardiac function at extreme altitude. J Appl Physiol. 1987;63:531–9.

19. Suarez J, Alexander JK, Houston CS. Enhanced left ventricular systolic performance at high altitude during Operation Everest II. Am J Cardiol. 1987;60:137–42.

20. Anand IS, Chandrashekhar Y, Rao SK, Malhotra RM, Ferrari R, Chandana J, Ramesh B, Shetty KJ, Boparai MS. Body fluid compartments, renal blood flow, and hormones at 6,000 m in normal subjects. J Appl Physiol. 1993;74:1234–9.

21. Anand IS, Ferrari R, Kalra GS, Wahi PL, PooleWilson PA, Harris PC. Edema of cardiac origin. Studies of body water and sodium, renal function, hemodynamic indexes, and plasma hormones in untreated congestive cardiac failure. Circulation. 1989;80:299–305.

22. Poduval RG. Adult subacute mountain sickness a syndrome at extremes of high altitude. J Assoc Physicians India. 2000;48:511–3.

23. West JB, Schoene RB, Luks AM, Milledge JS. High altitude medicine and physiology. 5th ed. Boca Raton: CRC Press; 2013.

24. Fried R, Reid LM. Early recovery from hypoxic pulmonary hypertension: a structural and functional study. J Appl Physiol. 1984;57:1247–53.

Chapter 15
Nutritional Management of Critically Ill Patients in High Altitude Medicine

Víctor Manuel Sánchez Nava and Carlos Mauricio González Ponce

Initial Management of Nutrition in Air Transport

Case Presentation

A 32-year-old male patient with no significant pathological history, does not have a complete vaccination schedule for covid-19. He went to the emergency sequence service due to respiratory distress which has been exacerbating in recent days, the patient had severity criteria for intubation, so it is carried out quickly without complications and he is transferred to the intensive care unit. As there are no contraindications, it is decided to start enteral nutrition within the first 24 h, which is optimized in the following 48 h until 60% of their energy needs are achieved. During the first 72 h, he had a torpid respiratory evolution with severe ARDS criteria and PAFI less than 80 despite neuromuscular blockade and a prone cycle for 48 h, so it was decided to protocolize ECMO. Cannulation was performed by the ECMO team, and an international air transfer was decided by the multidisciplinary team to continue with ECMO support in another hospital unit.

V. M. S. Nava (✉)
Intensive Care Unit, Tec Salud, Monterrey, Nuevo León, Mexico

C. M. G. Ponce
Critical Care Medicine Fellowship, Tec Salud, Monterrey, Nuevo León, Mexico

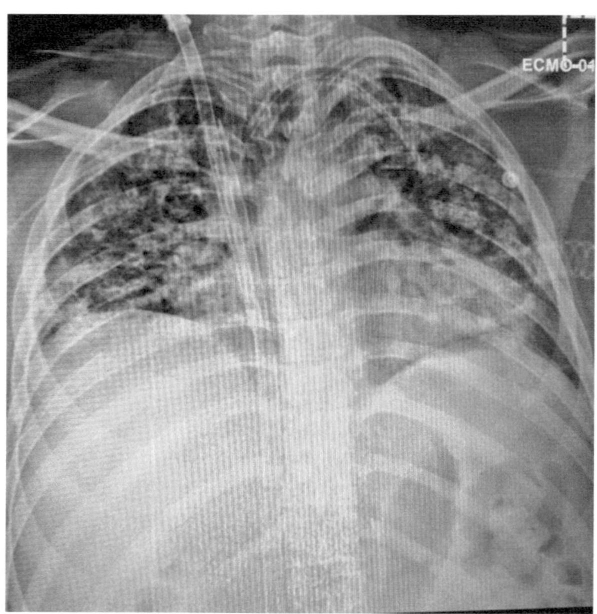

Question **What would be the best way to continue nutrition during the transfer?**

Answer
Considerations in altitude medicine and artificial enteral nutrition

In air transport, adverse effects may arise from the means of transport itself, as well as from the drop in atmospheric pressure.

The decrease in atmospheric pressure conditions the decrease in the partial pressure of oxygen in ambient air, in the alveolus and, therefore, produces a decrease in the conduction pressure of oxygen transported in the blood. Unpressurized helicopters do not fly at altitudes greater than 4000–5000 feet (1200–1500 m) above sea level. This assumes a barometric pressure greater than 632 mmHg, so the pAO2 will be greater than 80 mmHg. Under these conditions, the FIO2 required to maintain a pO2 of 100 mmHg will be less than 26%. In pressurized aircraft, the altitude reached in flight plays little part, generally maintaining pressures close to those obtained at sea level.

In critically ill patients, the slight hypoxia resulting from the decrease in the partial pressure of oxygen could determine its aggravation. The initiation or exacerbation of hyperventilation and increased cardiac output may be critical for the evolution of the process. Therefore, correct oxygenation must be guaranteed to patients evacuated by aircraft, supplying them with supplemental oxygen either in spontaneous or artificial ventilation, correcting the theoretically necessary FIO2 [1, 2].

The drop in atmospheric pressure also exerts effects on the gases enclosed in organic cavities. According to the Boyle-Mariotte law, volume is inversely proportional to pressure: $VK * T/P$; where V is the volume of gas, P is pressure, T is the temperature (which remains constant at around 37 $^\circ$ C) and K is a constant.

With the height of flight, an expansion of the gases is produced, which causes:

- Increased trapped volume in undrained pneumothorax
- Aggravation of mediastinal emphysema and expansion of non-reabsorbed residual air accumulations after thoracotomy.
- Increased intracranial pressure in patients with pneumocephalus.
- Increased intraocular pressure.
- Tympanic membrane rupture and barosinusitis.
- Distal ischemia after cast immobilization.
- **Gastrointestinal tract distension: worsening of intestinal ileus, dehiscence of sutures and abdominal anastomoses in post-surgical patients, reactivation of digestive bleeding and all the consequences in patients with previous intestinal pathology as far as mesenteric flow is concerned.**

All these effects become somewhat more significant at a height of 2000 m. where the volume of the gases can be increased by up to 30%.

Depending on the type of air transport used, there are some mechanical factors that can influence the patient's pathological state to a greater or lesser extent: acceleration-deceleration of the aircraft, vibrations, and noise; Despite this, none of these mechanical incident's conditions the indication of evacuation of patients on aircraft.

It is necessary to point out the possible impact on the distribution of blood volume caused by sudden changes in speed. The accelerations that occur in aerial media range between 0.5 g in aircraft takeoff and 0.3 g in helicopters, values below those achieved in ground vehicles. These accelerations may be more important in the transverse and vertical axis, so it is recommended that the patient be placed in the longitudinal axis of the aircraft, placed in decubitus, with the head backwards and the feet facing the direction of travel [3].

The vibrations that occur in the air are of high frequency and therefore exceed the most harmful range of amplitude 4–12 Hz, which is where resonance phenomena originate in organs and this clearly has repercussions on enzymatic secretion and mechanisms of internal sphincters, as well as the glandular functioning of bull the digestive tract. Helicopters with two blades produce vibrations of 18 Hz, reaching 28 Hz for those with three blades. The frequencies produced by airplanes are even higher [2].

It is important to consider all the pathophysiological aspects that the change in altitude may have as an impact on the different organs and pathologies of the patients who are going to be transferred to make the appropriate adjustments and, above all, consider transfer times to see the nutritional requirements during transport. There is no absolute contraindication to avoid feeding patients during transfers.

Principles of Management

Physiopathological Consequences and Metabolic Response to Stress

Under conditions of injury, as little as 16–24 h after fasting, liver glycogen stores are depleted; this results in protein degradation, which supplies amino acids to gluconeogenesis to maintain glucose production, and from there energy through glycolysis. However, the use of proteins during prolonged fasting is costly for the organism since their losses lead to a decrease in intracellular functions [4, 5] The metabolic response to stress (Fig. 15.1) is characterized by changes in hormones and inflammatory mediators. Hormonal changes (Fig. 15.2) are characterized by elevated adrenocorticotropic hormone (ACTH), cortisol, epinephrine, norepinephrine, vasopressin, glucagon, renin, aldosterone, and decreased thyroid-stimulating hormone (TSH), thyroxine (T.) free, total and free triiodothyronine (T4), which lead to hepatic proteolysis, lipolysis, gluconeogenesis and glycogenolysis.

The inflammatory response is characterized by complement activation, which generates the release of leukotrienes and prostaglandins, as well as complement fragments that can act as vasoactive kinins, which are the most important cellular factors of aggression. Both interleukin 1 (IL-1), the most active, as well as IL-2 and IL-6 and cachectic or tumor necrosis factor (TNF) have very harmful effects on the body (see Fig. 15.1). One of them is hypercatabolism, which is the increase in protein utilization without a proportional increase in synthesis, which leads to a negative nitrogen balance [6, 7].

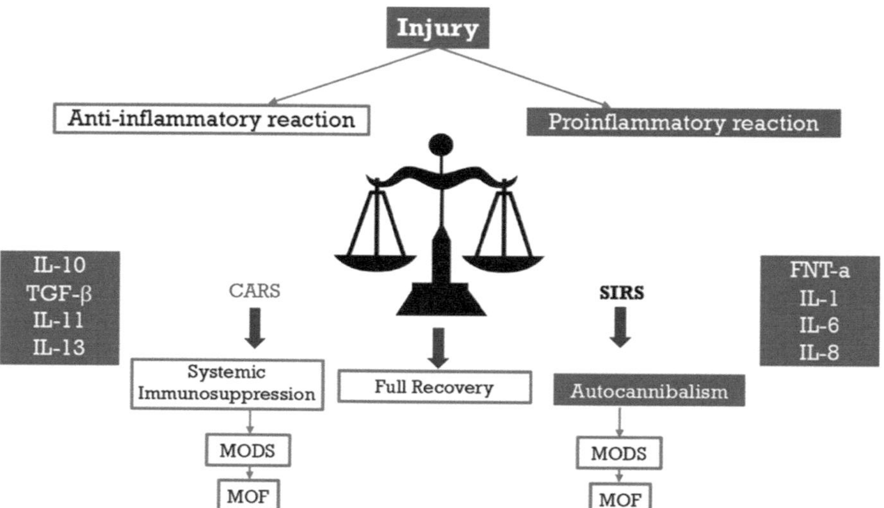

Fig. 15.1 Metabolic response to a serious aggression with systemic repercussion. Ugarte, S., Laca, M., Matos, A., & Sánchez, V. (2017). Fundamentos de Terapia Nutricional en Cuidados Críticos-FTNCC. Bogotá-Colombia: Grupo Distribuna (With the permission from Panamerican Nutrition Group)

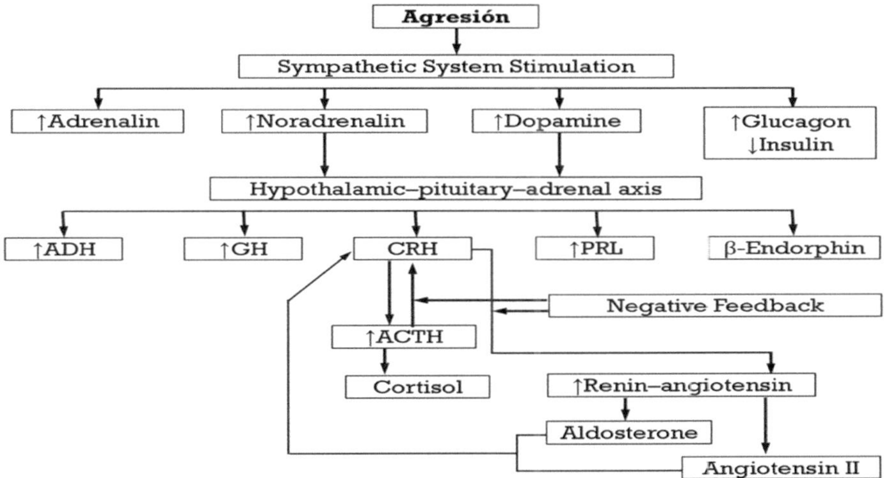

Fig. 15.2 Neuroendocrine response to the initial insult in critically ill patients. Ugarte, S., Laca, M., Matos, A., & Sánchez, V. (2017). Fundamentos de Terapia Nutricional en Cuidados Críticos-FTNCC. Bogotá-Colombia: Grupo Distribuna. (With the permission from Panamerican Nutrition Group)

The metabolic response to the combination of starvation and hypermetabolic stress generates an increase in the production of catecholamines, glucagon, insulin and growth hormone that favors lipolysis and gluconeogenesis. Liver glycogen is first used to further deplete muscle stores, contributing to the patient's cachexia.

Ketogenesis then occurs to save protein and amino acids, which worsens the patient's clinical picture.

In systemic inflammatory response syndrome (SIRS) there is increased IL with increased energy expenditure and protein catabolism. In the compensatory anti-inflammatory response syndrome (CARS) there is an increase in the release of TNF and IL-1 and 6 that inhibit the release of L-carnitine, which generates an increase in triglycerides and fatty acids; this generates immunoparalysis and facilitates infections (see Fig. 15.4).

There is a high metabolic rate with high amino acid and protein requirements. When the decrease in proteins reaches 30% or 40%, multiple organ failure occurs, which is incompatible with life.

The intestine, an organ that was traditionally considered exclusively related to the digestion and absorption of nutrients, we now know that it also intervenes in the regulation of endocrine, immunological, and metabolic processes, and acts as a barrier between the external and internal media. The presence of nutrients in the intestinal lumen, even in minimal amounts, stimulates the release of gastrointestinal hormones and improves intestinal motility and function, making it necessary to maintain its structural and functional integrity [8–10]. The loss of the barrier function of the intestine allows bacteria, endotoxins and antigenic macromolecules to pass into the portal and systemic circulation and, therefore, bacterial translocation.

This facilitates the release of mediators that trigger the systemic inflammatory response and thus establishes a relationship between barrier failure and multi-organ failure (MOF) [8, 11, 12].

These concepts related to the metabolic response to stress and the function of the intestine have opened new perspectives in the use of enteral nutrition (EN) in the search for specific substrates that can attenuate or counteract these effects [12, 13].

Figure 15.3 shows the stages of the response to stress, which must be known and managed properly to avoid increased morbidity and mortality. In the first moment (acute stage: ebb-flow) the goal is to maintain blood volume, hemodynamic functions, hydration, and acid-base balance.

In the flow stage, caloric intake is essential, with an adequate amount of protein, vitamins and minerals. In the second stage (maintenance) and in the third (anabolism, or recovery), nutritional management is essential, with an adequate caloric intake, with a balanced ratio of proteins and calories, and with adequate intake of vitamins and minerals.

In summary, we can say that the non-use of the digestive tract affects its subsequent functioning, as well as its structure and integrity, which decreases cell proliferation, mucosal mass and enzyme production. There is an increase in capillary permeability that increases the risk of bacterial translocation, with bacterial proliferation and less secretion of immunoglobulins. This makes it possible to create an environment conducive to bacterial translocation that worsens a pathology that is already highly fatal, such as sepsis and septic shock.

We must not overemphasize that wound healing will be slower, with a higher incidence of pressure ulcers.

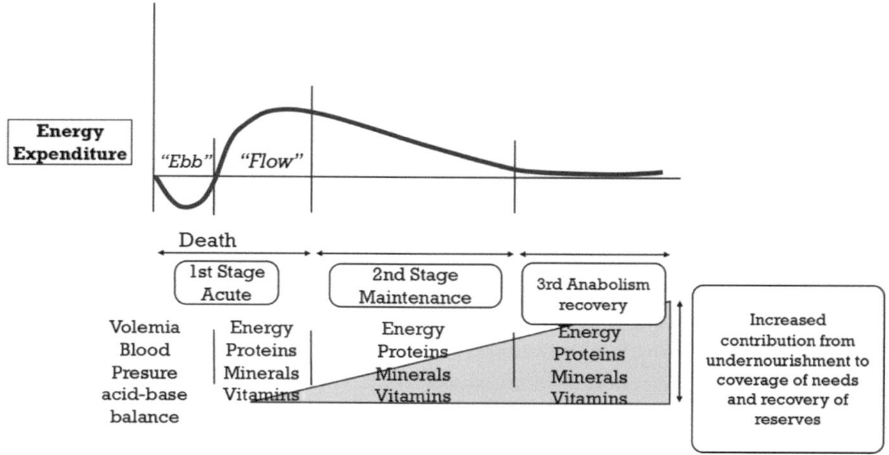

Fig. 15.3 Increased contribution from undernourishment to coverage of needs and recovery of reserves. Ugarte, S., Laca, M., Matos, A., & Sánchez, V. (2017). Fundamentos de Terapia Nutricional en Cuidados Críticos-FTNCC. Bogotá-Colombia: Grupo Distribuna (With the permission from Panamerican Nutrition Group)

An alteration of cellular immunity occurs, which leads to an increase in mortality, hospital stay (in 2–3 days) and hospital costs, which increase up to 67% [14–16]. It has been shown that the incidence of complications increases and reaches 27% in malnourished patients versus 16.8% in those with normal nutrition ($p < 0.05$) [17].

Nutritional Assessment

Every patient should have a nutritional evaluation upon admission, and no less than 30 tools are described in the literature. In hospitalized patients, the VGS, MUST and NRS-2002 scales have shown adequate sensitivity and specificity; In critically ill patients, the NUTRIC SCORE is used to identify patients who would benefit from the prescription of aggressive enteral nutrition, using variables such as age; APACHE II scale, SOFA; number of comorbidities and days prior to admission to the ICU [18], this being the best use for nutritional assessment due to its versatility. The use of this scale can be done together with the clinical examination looking for malnutrition data such as involuntary weight loss and muscle wasting, associated with inflammatory processes or decreased intake or assimilation of nutrients. Early enteral nutrition (<48 h upon admission) should be considered in all patients regardless of risk since patients with high risk or malnutrition could benefit from achieving caloric goals after the early acute phase (day 1 to 2) and those with low risk or without malnutrition assess hypocaloric intake the first 7 days [19].

The nutritional parameters to consider are:

Anthropometric: weight, height, skinfold, body mass index (BMI) and arm muscle circumference.

Biochemical: creatinine/height index. Serum albumin, 24-h urinary nitrogen, lymphocyte count, transferrin, prealbumin, and retinol-binding protein dosage.

Others: Sodium, potassium, calcium, zinc, iron, chromium, manganese, carotene, 25-hydroxyvitamin D, tocopherol, Vitamin B, folate and iron binding capacity.

These determinations and measurements have one exception in the critical patient, given the alteration of several parameters due to the high rate of volume transfer, edema, alterations in body weight and their response to stress, which affects the estimation nutritional status and sometimes underestimates the seriousness of its commitment [19].

One of the few assessments that has been well validated in intensive care units (ICUs) is the so-called subjective global assessment (SGA), since it facilitates the identification of patients at risk.

This subjective assessment involves questioning about the six points that we detail below:

Weight changes: Chronic loss (last 6 months) or acute loss in the last 2 weeks. Mild: 0–5% of the weight; moderate: 5–10% of the weight; and severe: >10% of previous weight. Changes in the diet eaten. Gastrointestinal symptoms (nausea, vomiting, diarrhea or anorexia).

Functional capacity: look for the existence of alterations in work capacity and/or activities of daily living.

Relationship between disease and nutritional need: for example, there is up to a 30% increase in need in cancer patients.

Directed physical exam: Loss of subcutaneous fat is sought. Loss of muscle tissue. Presence of malleolar edema, sacral edema and/or ascites. As well as stomatitis and glossitis.

Start of Therapeutic Nutrition

One way to estimate the energy requirement is through the Harris-Benedict equation: REE (resting energy expenditure):

$$\text{Men}: 66 + (13.7 \times \text{weight}) + (5 \times \text{height in cm}) - (6.76 \times \text{age})$$

$$\text{Women}: 65 + (9.6 \times \text{weight}) + (1.8 \times \text{height in cm}) - (4.7 \times \text{age})$$

The weight to use is the ideal—except in severely malnourished patients, in whom the REE is calculated with the actual weight, and in the obese patient, in whom the adjusted body weight (ideal weight + 0.4) is used.

The simplified formula can also be applied by calculating caloric requirements at 25 to 30 kcal/kg/day. Other methods include direct measurement by calorimetry or the use of the pulmonary artery catheter:

$$\text{REE} = \text{Cardiac output} \times \text{Hb} \times (\text{SaO}_2 - \text{SVO}_2) \times 95.18$$

Where Hb is hemoglobin and (SaO_2 − SVO_2) is the difference between arterial and venous oxyhemoglobin saturation.

The caloric need is then distributed in different percentages. Carbohydrates, 60%, and lipids, 30%. Protein needs are approximately 0.8–1 g/kg/day and in states of hypermetabolic stress, 1–2 g/kg/day. This last contribution must be adapted to renal function and controlled with nitrogen balances that allow estimating the loss of nitrogen in the urine.

In critically ill patients on mechanical ventilation with a BMI less than 30 kg/m², it is often preferred to estimate caloric requirements using the equation developed by researchers at Pennsylvania State University. In contrast, in mechanically ventilated patients with a BMI of 30 kg/m² or more, the Ireton-Jones equation modified in 2002 (or the Pennsylvania State University equation modified in 2011) is preferred, and for spontaneously breathing patients the 1992 Ireton-Jones formula (Table 15.1).

Table 15.1 Validated equations for calculating energy requirements in critically ill patients. Ugarte, S., Laca, M., Matos, A., & Sánchez, V. (2017). Fundamentos de Terapia Nutricional en Cuidados Críticos-FTNCC. Bogotá-Colombia: Grupo Distribuna (With the permission from Panamerican Nutrition Group)

Table 1. Validated equations for calculating energy requirements in critically ill patients

Author and year	Ecuation
Ireton-Jones 1992	GEE (s) = 629 – 11 (A) +25 (P) – 609 (O)
Ireton-Jones 2002	GEE (v) = 1784 / 11 (A) + 5 (P) + 244 (G) + 239 (TM) + 804 (Qdo)
Penn State 2003 / 2004	GER = Mifflin-St. Jeor (0,96) + Tmax (167) + VE (31) - 6212
Penn State 2011	GER = Mifflin-St. Jeor (0,71) + Tmax (85) + VE (64) - 3085
Mifflin St.Jeor 1990	Men: 10 (P) + 6,25 (H) – 5 (A) + 5 Women: 10 (P) + 6,25 (H) – 5 (A) - 161

Where EEE is estimated energy expenditure (kcal/24 hours); v is fan dependent; s is patient who is breathing spontaneously; E is the age (years); P is body weight (kg); H is height and is expressed in centimeters; G is the gender (masculine = 1; feminine = 0); TM is the diagnosis of trauma (current = 1; absent = 0); Qdo is the burn diagnosis (current = 1; absent = 0); Or it is obesity (>30% above ideal body weight [IBW] tables) from life insurance. Present = 1; absent = 0); REE is resting energy expenditure; Tmax is the maximum body temperature in the last 24 hours (expressed in degrees Celsius); VE is the ventilation volume exhaled in one minute (in liters per minute) at the time of

Routes of Administration of Nutrients

Oral/Enteral Nutrition

The different diets are started orally or enterally by tube if the gastrointestinal tract is intact. With this type of nutrition, the intestinal barrier is maintained, the metabolic response to injury or trauma is modulated and adequately stimulated system-associated lymphoid tissue (GALT; gut associated lymphoid tissue). This regulates the body's immunity. By starting EN early (within the first 24–48 h), infection rates, the formation of intestinal fistulas, days in intensive care, hospital stay and, therefore, costs are reduced [20].

Orally Administered

Clear liquid diets: to assess tolerance. Nutritionally inadequate [21].
Full liquid diet: thick liquids rich in lactose. Nutritionally inadequate [21].
Normal solid diet.
Low sodium diet: 4 g without additional salt or 2 g without salty foods or table salt [22].
Oral supplements: with better results in orthopedic surgery, when intake is less than 75% of what should be consumed. There is a lower rate of infections, shorter hospital stays and faster rehabilitation [23].

Nasogastric Tube Feeding (NGT)

It should be started when a patient does not have an adequate intake (defined as <60% of goal for >10 days). The tube can be nasogastric (NGS) or nasojejunal (NIS), installed blindly or under endoscopic guidance. It should be started as early as possible in critical patients, provided that their hemodynamic characteristics allow it, with progression to the objective caloric goal in the first 48–72 h; It should also be considered to supplement it if the objective is not reached in the first 10 days. In this way, bacterial translocation decreases, the immune system is stimulated with the release of lymphocytes and macrophages, and immunoglobulin A secretion increases.

Some of the more serious complications regarding enteral feeding should be considered, such as intestinal ischemia (4%), malabsorption disorders (20%), intestinal subocclusion (15%), constipation (15%), diarrhea (60%) and the presence of nausea, vomiting and regurgitation (20%). It should be taken into account that a contribution of only 25% of the calculated caloric goal already manages to significantly reduce bacterial translocation [24] thus maintaining enterocyte trophism.

Parenteral Nutrition (PN)

It is indicated when there is dysfunction of the gastrointestinal tract, in patients with moderate or severe malnutrition in whom oral intake is impossible or insufficient within 24–72 h of admission and in patients with adequate nutritional status but who a week after the start of enteral feeding cannot meet the caloric needs of the same. It should never be considered as the first option [25].

The components of PN are:

Dextrose (in different compositions; (25% or 50%), Lipids (10% or 20% soy or safflower), medium-chain and long-chain triglycerides Amino acids (5–10%)

Vitamins and minerals: vitamin and trace element packages

Electrolytes: They are added depending on the metabolic, hydroelectrolytic and acid-base status. Digestive losses are replaced, due to fistulas, ostomies, drains, skin, among others.

The subclavian puncture is preferred for central PN, for catheters that will be used for a short or medium period. Their placement should be carried out by an expert operator and under ultrasound guidance. The catheter should be used only for PN, and the bag exchange technique should be sterile and handled with care. Possible complications of their placement are pneumothorax, chylothorax, hemothorax, gas embolism, arterial puncture, and neurovascular injury.

There is also the possibility of using the placement of a peripheral catheter for the administration of PN.

Peripheral PN is simpler and helps to avoid delaying the start of feeding, being less expensive than central PN, it provides less than 20 kcal/day, less than 1.5 g/kg/day of protein and no more than 850 mOsm/L with high amount of lipids.

Care must be taken with the appearance of phlebitis and with the volumes administered and it should not be administered for more than 8–10 days. May supplement enteral feeding. The catheters used should preferably be made of polyurethane, of about 20–25 cm long. They should be rotated every 48 h preferably or at the slightest redness, swelling and/or pain. Healing can be done with transparent tegaderm-type barrier devices.

There must be strict interdisciplinary control between nursing, intensive care doctors, nutritionists and the laboratory to avoid complications. Long-term catheters (considered those dedicated to greater than 3 months) must be tunneled and with implantable subcutaneous ports, placed by experienced vascular surgeons. NP can cause hyperglycemia and metabolic acidosis, decreases chemotaxis, phagocytosis, and healing capacity with alterations in the complement cascade and an increase in inflammatory answer. A difference in mortality has not been demonstrated when selecting the enteral or parenteral route, but it was observed that enteral administration reduced the risk of infectious complications without a significant difference in the days of hospitalization [23].

Modulation of the Inflammatory and Metabolic Response to Stress

After the publications of Dudrick and Wilmore [24–26], total parenteral nutrition (TPN) became popular and became the most widely used form of nutritional therapy. However, this therapy was associated with significant metabolic complications, particularly in those years when patients were believed to require high calorie loads, especially carbohydrates. What was then called parenteral hypernutrition was used in which patients received up to 200% of their basal energy expenditure (GEB), which was associated with hyperglycemia, hyperosmolar states, and increased rates of infection.

In the 1980s, stress hyperglycemia was considered a physiological metabolic phenomenon [27], until new studies showed that severely ill patients benefited from lower nutrient loads and a trend toward decreased caloric intake began. At the same time, the first studies emerged on the feasibility and safety of using EN in many patients who until then had only been able to be fed intravenously.

Trauma, serious illnesses, and major surgeries are the origin of profound inflammatory and metabolic changes whose basic objective is to guarantee adequate defense of the body and prioritize metabolic pathways towards products for the acute phase of the disease. However, an exaggerated response on the part of the patient is associated with dysfunction and organ damage and systemic alterations and, therefore, the understanding and modulation of the metabolic response of our patients is a fundamental point to achieve adequate therapies and the best results of the interventions.

In 1992, Moore [28] showed that trauma patients had a significant reduction in the incidence of infections if they received EN instead of TPN. Multiple investigations confirmed these results and convinced the scientific community of the advantages of NE. In addition, there was a greater understanding of the mechanisms of this improvement: (a) maintaining the structure of the intestinal barrier, (b) modulating the metabolic response to injury and trauma, and (c) adequately stimulating GALT.

Although the maintenance of the structure of the intestinal barrier was the key to prevent bacterial translocation, it was later understood that the response of the intestinal lymphoid tissue had to be preserved intact, since it acts as a regulator of the general immunity of the organism. Thus, the intensity of the systemic inflammatory response is directly related to intestinal integrity, which is better preserved by using EN from very early on.

Recently, the Kudsk studies have shown better clinical results in critically ill patients (trauma and major abdominal surgery) using early EN [29, 30]. Experimental studies have also shown that the main mechanism of action is through stimulation of the intestinal lymphoid system and its role in the systemic inflammatory response [31, 32].

In recent years, numerous studies have been published comparing early EN supplemented with specific nutrients versus conventional EN or PN in different critical patient populations, including trauma, cancer, acute pancreatitis, and major burns. They have confirmed the advantage of using early EN with a lower rate of infection, intestinal fistulas, days in intensive care, days in the hospital and care costs [33, 34]. It is clear that the analysis of the current state of the evidence allows us to affirm that nutritional care must be an integral part of the care of all critically ill patients and that nutritional intervention must be early and

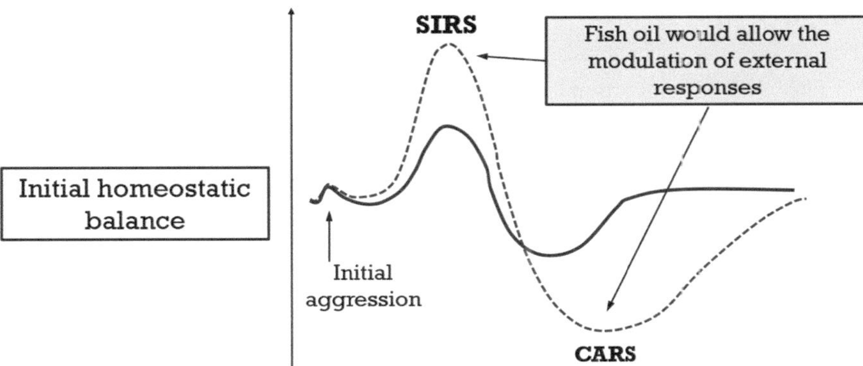

Hypothetical-didactic model of metabolic/inflammatory response
CARS: compensatory anti-inflammatory response syndrome
SIRS: systemic inflammatory response syndrome

Fig. 15.4 Suggested effects of modulators such as fish oil in a hypothetical-didactic model of metabolic/inflammatory response. Dotted line: baseline response; continuous line: response with action of fish oil. Ugarte, S., Laca, M., Matos, A., & Sánchez, V. (2017). Fundamentos de Terapia Nutricional en Cuidados Críticos-FTNCC. Bogotá-Colombia: Grupo Distribuna. (With the permission from Panamerican Nutrition Group)

adequate for each patient and involve the use of specific nutrients to achieve the best results by modulating the metabolic response to stress. In recent years, emphasis has been intensified on incorporating enriched enteral feeding that can help regulate the metabolic response (Fig. 15.4). Of all these new studies, it is worth mentioning two written by Pontes Arruda [35, 36] who have shown that early EN enriched with omega 3 fatty acids (fish oils) reduces mortality in septic patients by half.

No medical intervention has had such an impact on critically ill patients.

Immunonutrition

The different immunomodulatory nutrients are divided into the following categories:

(a) Immune system stimulators: arginine, iron, glutamine.
(b) Promoters of the integrity of the gastrointestinal tract (GIT): glutamine, probiotics, prebiotics.
(c) anti-inflammatories: eicosapentaenoic acids (EPA), gamma-linolenic acid (GLA).
(d) Antioxidants: vitamin E, A, C, selenium, and taurine. The composition of these diets must be appropriate according to the specific pathology of the patient, considering its pathophysiology.

Omega-3 Fatty Acids

w-3 fatty acids are incorporated into phospholipids in the cell wall and are a substrate for cyclooxygenases, lipoxygenases, and cytochrome P450. They influence the production of prostaglandins, thromboxanes, leukotrienes, and lipoxins and can reduce platelet aggregation and the production of proinflammatory cytokines.

They would attenuate lipid peroxidation in septic patients, improving the evolution of acute respiratory distress syndrome (ARDS) with increased survival and decreased stay in the intensive care unit (ICU) [36]. A meta-analysis of three studies in patients with acute lung injury (ALI) and/or ARDS on mechanical ventilation for 28 days showed a decreased risk of death ($p = 0.05$), time on assisted mechanical ventilation ($D < 0, 05$), ICU stay ($p < 0.05$) and risk of organ failure ($p < 0.05$). Currently, the evidence in its favor is grade A in postoperative head and neck, burn and polytraumatized patients, and grade B in patients on mechanical ventilation.

Glutamine

Glutamine is one of the 20 amino acids involved in protein formation. It is a non-essential amino acid, abundant in skeletal muscle that becomes conditionally essential in states of its deficiency (polytrauma, major burns, among others). Having 2 nitrogen atoms, it would act as a nitrogen donor in multiple enzymatic processes, thus being considered as an energy source to regulate the body's REDOX system.

It acts in different biochemical processes:

It participates as a primordial substrate in hepatic gluconeogenesis as well as being part of the urea cycle.

The generation of ammonium allows the synthesis of other amino acids, such as alanine and aspartate, through transamination reactions in the muscle, intestine, and liver.

Glutamate deamination generates reduced nicotinamide -adenine-dinucleotide-phosphate (NADPH), which is involved in glutathione regeneration.

Along with alanine, it is the nitrogen transporter to the kidney.

Plasma glutamine concentration decreases after surgery, sepsis, major trauma, or severe burn. This decrease in plasma levels has been correlated with an increase in mortality [37]. Glutamine is a basic energy substrate for lymphocytes and macrophages and is a precursor to nucleotides. Phagocytic activity increases in a dose-dependent manner upon glutamine administration and enhances apoptosis. This dose-dependent effect also appears when heat shock protein (HSP) expression is measured.

Glutamine has similar activity in the intestinal mucosa and associated lymphoid tissue (Fig. 15.5). Experimental studies have shown that low glutamine levels are associated with increased intestinal permeability and impaired the microscopic structure of the mucosa and with an increase in bacterial translocation.

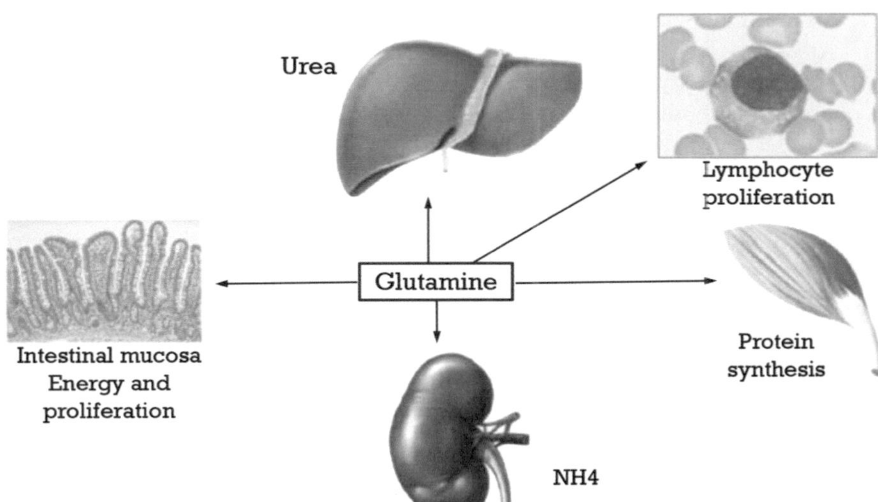

Fig. 15.5 Tissue interrelationships in glutamine metabolism. Ugarte, S., Laca, M., Matos, A., & Sánchez, V. (2017). Fundamentos de Terapia Nutricional en Cuidados Críticos-FTNCC. Bogotá-Colombia: Grupo Distribuna (With the permission from Panamerican Nutrition Group)

The metabolic response to stress, particularly severe infection, can lead to disruption of glutamine homeostasis (Fig. 15.5). This is favored by the existence of a previous poor nutritional status and the use of corticosteroids; also by the fast to which the critical patient is subjected. Glutamine is one of the glutathione precursors found in high concentrations in mammalian cells and is the most important endogenous oxygen free radical scavenger known powerful. Glutamine depletion is associated with a decrease in intracellular glutathione levels, the replacement of which is achieved by providing exogenous glutamine.

Glutamine administration can improve the ability to chelate free oxygen radicals and even inhibit the expression of inducible nitric oxide synthetase (iNOS), although experimental studies have revealed contradictory data [38].

Glutamine administration has also been associated with better insulin-mediated glycemic control. Glutamines are the primary substrate for gluconeogenesis in the liver, intestine, and kidney. Glutamine administration appears to improve insulin sensitivity and suppress gluconeogenesis. Intestinal. These findings are limited at the moment and do not allow to determine the real efficacy of glutamine on insulin resistance.

Evidence Contour Some specific situations of Artificial Nutrition have been found with suboptimal evidence or with differences in the consensus of the experts. That is why those topics that generate misinterpretation and therefore the application to the clinic in a heterogeneous way are exemplified below.

1. **Suboptimal Nutrition**—In a large observational study conducted in 167 ICUs, Alberda et al. [39] demonstrated a strong association between the reduced provision of energy and protein and worse outcomes. Weijs et al. [40] demonstrated that optimal nutritional therapy (calories and protein) in mechanically ventilated critically ill patients was associated with a 50% decrease in 28-day mortality.

   The energy deficit accumulated by underfeeding patients during their ICU stay has been shown to be an important factor in increasing the risk of adverse outcomes [41–43].

   The Society of Critical Care Medicine (SCCM) and American Society of Parenteral and Enteral Nutrition (ASPEN) guidelines [44], as well as the Canadian [45, 46] and European guidelines [47] all recommend that EN be initiated within 48 h in the critically ill patient who is unable to maintain volitional intake. It is important to emphasize that there is no known illness or disease that has been demonstrated to benefit from starvation.

   In the absence of a proven benefit of permissive underfeeding, critically ill patients should receive 12–30 kcal/kg/day and 0.6 g/kg/day – 1.2 g/kg/day protein [48]. The benefits of higher quantities of protein are controversial, with the SCCM/ASPEN guidelines recommending 1.2–2.0 g/kg/day [44]. However, increased provision of protein has not been demonstrated to limit muscle wasting, loss of lean body mass, or improve clinical outcomes.

   Catabolism is an important event to consider since the loss of up to 1 kg/day of muscle, therefore, considering the protein intake in the enteral diet is essential. Consider that even a reduced intake of up to 0.6 g/kg was associated with early weaning from mechanical ventilation and longer survival [48], but do not forget its increase to the target: 1.3 g/kg/day. Don't forget to mobilize your patient and prevent Acquired Weakness Syndrome [19].

2. **Parenteral nutrition is safe**

   It is now widely accepted that the GI tract is the preferred route of delivering nutritional support [49]. Furthermore, consensus guidelines strongly recommend "enteral over parenteral nutrition" (PN) in critically ill patients [44]. The institution of early EN in critically ill medical and postoperative patients has been demonstrated to improve outcome [50].

   The adverse sequela associated with PN results from the "double hit" of not directly feeding the bowel, as well as the metabolic, immunologic, endocrine, and infective complications associated with infusing a solution with a high glucose concentration and fat globules into a patient's systemic venous system [51]. PN bypasses the gut and liver. EN stimulates the release of a wide variety of enterohormones that play a crucial role in regulating gut function and metabolic pathways.

   Lack of enteral feeding results in GI mucosal atrophy, bacterial overgrowth, increased intestinal permeability, and translocation of bacteria and/or bacterial products. In a large cohort of critically ill patients, Grau et al. [52] demonstrated that PN was strongly associated with the development of liver dysfunction, whereas early EN was protective. EN has a major effect on the gut-associated lymphoid tissue (GALT), which is the source of most mucosal immunity in humans. PN results in rapid and severe atrophy of this tissue.

Heyland et al. [53] performed a metaanalysis of PN (compared with no nutritional support) in critically ill patients. These authors demonstrated that PN almost doubled the risk of dying (relative risk [RR], 1.78; 95% CI, 1.11–2.85). The SCCM/ASPEN guidelines state that "Enteral nutrition is the preferred route of feeding over parenteral nutrition (PN) for the critically ill patient who requires nutrition support therapy (Grade: B)" and that "if early EN is not feasible or available the first 7 days following admission to the ICU, no nutrition support therapy should be provided" However, if there is evidence of protein-calorie malnutrition at admission and all attempts at providing EN fail, the guidelines suggest that "it is appropriate to initiate PN as soon as possible following admission and adequate resuscitation" [44].

3. **Enteral nutrition contraindicated with vasopressors**—Many critically ill patients are hemodynamically unstable require vasopressors/inotropes to maintain adequate blood pressure and cardiac output. Vasopressors improve hemodynamics by shunting blood from the gut and other peripheral organs (i.e., bone marrow, skin, and kidneys) to the central circulation. These "nonessential" organs are more sensitive to vasoconstriction than are central "essential" organs (i.e., heart and brain). Thus, the effect of vasoconstrictor medications and hypotension is a decrease in gut blood flow. It has, therefore, been postulated that because these patients have limited oxygen delivery and that by increasing GI oxygen demand with enteral feeding, intestinal ischemia will develop. However, these propositions are based on evidence from animal models where the mesenteric artery was occluded and in patients with atherosclerotic occlusion of the mesenteric arteries [54]. Based on this information, many clinicians believe that EN will cause bowel ischemia and is contraindicated in patients receiving pressors. Anecdotal cases report of mesenteric ischemia in trauma patients receiving vasopressor agents are often cited to support this belief [55]. However, this theory is incorrect. Indeed, both experimental and clinical studies demonstrate that EN increases gut blood flow and protects against bowel ischemia. In the experimental and clinical setting, enteral infusion of nutrients prevents adverse structural and functional alterations of the gut barrier, increases epithelial proliferation, maintains mucosal integrity, decreases gut permeability, improves gut blood flow, and improves local and systemic immune responsiveness. These effects are mediated via both direct and indirect (i.e., hormonal, and neuronal) effects [56]

   The benefits of early EN in critically ill patients treated with vasopressors are supported by a multicenter study, which demonstrated a lower hospital mortality in patients fed within 48 h (34% vs 44%, $p < 0.001$) [57].

4. **Continuous or intermittent infusion?**
   Although there is no evidence that places one superiority over the other, in meta-analyses benefits have been discovered in continuous administration [58] such as greater tolerance to feeding and less risk of aspiration [58]. The administration of enteral formula without interruption for 24 h is associated with a

greater caloric debt when the infusion is interrupted throughout the day for various reasons (administration of enteral drugs, mobilization for studies), proposing the infusion at 20 h [59]. Therefore, it has been suggested to adjust the infusion based on total volume, modifying the infusion rate according to the volume remaining for the day. The use of intermittent infusion has been proposed as a more physiological measure which could have the benefit of promoting protein synthesis [60, 61] (avoiding the "full muscle" effect), this has not been clearly demonstrated, although current evidence indicates that said infusion has a benefit in achieving nutritional goals [62, 63]. The measurement of gastric residue has not been routinely recommended since it could generate a decrease in nutritional intake without achieving greater benefit in risk reduction [64–66].

5. **Enteral nutrition contraindicated with high volumes of gastric residue**

   Many clinicians monitor gastric residual volumes (GRV). The presumption is that GRV measurements are accurate and useful markers for the risk of aspiration and pneumonia. Enteral feeding is then interrupted when the GRV exceeds 150 mL. There is, however, no data to support this practice. High GRVs (i.e., >400 mL) do not necessarily predict aspiration, and low GRVs (i.e., <100 mL) are no guarantee that aspiration will not occur. Interrupting EN when the GRV exceeds 100–200 mL has not been shown to decrease the prevalence of aspiration. McClave et al. [67] randomized critically ill ventilated patients to two management strategies using a GRV more than 200 mL or GRV more than 400 mL for interrupting gastric feeding. In this study, the prevalence of aspiration was similar between groups. Similarly in a prospective multicenter study, Montejo et al. [68] randomized patients to a control group (GVR > 200 mL) or an intervention group in which tube feeds were held when the GRV exceeds 500 mL. In this study, there was no difference in the risk of pneumonia, ventilator-free days, organ failure, or mortality between groups. More recently, Reignier et al. [65] randomized mechanically ventilated patients to a group in which the GVR was not monitored and a group in whom tube feeds were held when the GRV exceeded 250 mL. These investigators demonstrated no difference in the risk of pneumonia between groups; however, the proportion of patients receiving their caloric goal was higher in the no-GRV group. It should, however, be noted that in this study, patients with abdominal surgery within the past month; a history of esophageal, duodenal, pancreatic, or gastric surgery; a history of GI bleeding; and contraindications to prokinetic agents were excluded. These data suggest that there is poor relationship between GVR and the risk of aspiration. Monitoring GVR may not be necessary in patients at low risk for aspiration and may only serve to reduce the amount of nutrition provided.

6. **Post-pyloric feeding and risk of aspiration**

   As an extension of the myth that the GRV is associated with the risk of aspiration pneumonia, many clinicians believe that all critically ill patients should receive postpyloric feeding. Cleary, there are some critically ill patients who have impaired gastric motility (especially patients with diabetes) who cannot tolerate early gastric feeds in whom EN is tolerated if delivered beyond the pylorus [69]. However, there is little consensus regarding the issue as to whether the routine use of postpyloric feeding decreases the risk of aspiration pneumonia. We performed a metanalysis comparing the risk of pneumonia in patients fed gastrically versus postpylorically [70]. In this meta-analysis, the risk of pneumonia was unrelated to the route of feeding. Ho et al. [71] reported similar findings. However, a meta-analysis by Alhazzani et al. [57] demonstrated a small reduction in the risk of pneumonia with small bowel feeding without affecting mortality, ICU length of stay, or duration of mechanical ventilation. We suggest placement of an orogastric tube and early (within 12 h of ICU admission) initiation of EN in all mechanically ventilated patients. In those patients who demonstrate intolerance to gastric feeding (abdominal distension, regurgitation), we suggest the use of prokinetic agents [72, 73]. Should this approach fail, we would then place a postpyloric feeding tube. In patients with known gastric dysmotility and those who are nursed supine (e.g., extracorporeal membrane oxygenation patients), we would suggest early placement of a postpyloric feeding tube.

7. **Enteral nutrition contraindicated in a patient without bowel sounds or paralytic ileus**—In 1905, Cannon [74] was the first clinician to formally suggest a relationship between abdominal auscultation and bowel function. Remarkably, abdominal auscultation has become part of the standard physical examination of patients, and yet, no studies have validated the value of this maneuver. Historically, ICU nurses have been trained to auscultate each of the four abdominal quadrants for the presence of bowel sounds, with the presence of bowel sounds indicating that it is safe to feed patients. Similarly, the return of bowel sounds after abdominal surgery has been regarded as an indicator of the resolution of postoperative ileus and an indicator that it is safe to commence EN. However, the absence of bowel sounds does not mean that the bowel is not working. Bowel sounds result from air moving through the small intestine. The presence of bowel sounds requires swallowing of air and gastric emptying. Many seriously ill patients have little movement of air from the stomach to the small intestine and therefore have decreased bowel sounds. The absence of bowel sounds after operation seems to result from "the emptiness of the gut." When fluid and air is injected into the duodenum, sounds can be heard immediately [75].

   Waldhausen et al. [76] measured GI myoelectric and clinical patterns of recovery after laparotomy. Small bowel myoelectric activity returned immediately after surgery, whereas it took on average 2.4 days for the return of bowel sounds and 5 days for the passage of flatus. These authors were unable to find any correlation between bowel myoelectric activity and bowel sounds. These data suggest that ausculting for bowel sound has limited clinical utility and should not be used to guide the initiation of EN. Indeed, multiple clinical trial have shown improved outcome with the early initiation of tube feeds following abdominal surgery in spite of the absence of bowel sounds or the passage of flatus. Current guidelines recommend that "in the ICU patient population, neither the presence nor the absence of bowel sounds nor evidence of the passage of flatus or stool is required for the initiation of enteral feeding" [44].

8. **EN contraindicated in post-operative intestinal surgery patients**
   Classic surgical teaching suggests that due to reflex inhibition, the alimentary tract becomes inactive after abdominal surgery [75]. The period of inactivity or postoperative ileus is thought to last for 3–5 days during which time the patient is tided over by gastric aspiration and parenteral fluids [75]. It has been assumed that the postoperative ileus precludes enteral feeding. Furthermore, it has been suggested that bowel distention following enteral feeding would disrupt the anastomoses. Consequently, EN is frequently withheld from postoperative abdominal surgery patients, particularly those with fresh GI tract anastomoses. This approach is detrimental to patients and without scientific evidence. Motility studies demonstrate return of small bowel peristalsis within hours after laparotomy providing support for early postoperative EN [76, 77]. Over 30 years ago, Moss [78] demonstrated the benefits of immediate EN following laparotomy and colorectal excision. In this study, a full-strength elemental diet was delivered into the duodenum immediately postoperatively. Using radiolabeled albumin, he demonstrated that 94% ± 4% of the albumin was absorbed with achievement of a positive protein balance by 5 h postoperatively. The GI tract produces approximately 6 L of fluid per day, and it is illogical to propose that an additional liter or so of tube feeds will cause excessive distention of the bowel with anastomotic dehiscence. Furthermore, wound healing is critically dependent on an adequate supply of protein; starvation with protein catabolism is likely to increase the risk of wound dehisce. In an animal model, Moss et al. [79] demonstrated that early enteral feeding doubled the bursting pressure of the colorectal anastomosis, with the anastomoses containing significantly higher concentration of collagen and collagen precursors than those of the unfed controls. Multiple experimental studies have demonstrated that early EN following bowel surgery is associated with improved wound healing, greater wound strength, and higher wound hydroxyproline and collagen accumulation [80–85]. This may explain the lower risk of anatomic leaks and fistulas in bowel surgery patients who receive early enteral as opposed to delayed feeding or PN [86].

   The experimental data demonstrating the benefit of early EN are supported by many studies which have demonstrated the safety and improved outcomes associated with early EN in patients who have undergone both small and large bowel surgery.

   Concern has been raised that early enteral feeding may cause bowel ischemia following abdominal surgery [44]. This is a very rare complication that was reported predominantly between 1986 and 2000 with isolated cases reported subsequently [87–92]. Most of these patients had sustained traumatic injuries, and almost all had undergone a laparotomy with surgical placement of a jejunostomy tube. Small bowel necrosis is very rare in postoperative patients who are initiated on early enteral feeding. Nevertheless, enteral feeding should be advanced slowly in patients at risk (severe abdominal trauma, large burns), and they should be discontinued in patients who developed abdominal complaints, such as pain, distention, and vomiting, until the status of bowel integrity can be evaluated. A semielemental formula may be advantageous in these patients.

9. **EN contraindicated in patients with open abdomen**

   Decompressive celiotomy has reduced the mortality of patients with abdominal compartment syndrome [93]. The management of these patients is challenging with the approach to the route and timing of nutritional support being controversial. Many patients are kept "nil per os" or receive PN on the assumption that these patients cannot be fed enterally due to bowel wall edema and bowel dysfunction. However, clinical studies have demonstrated that early EN is feasible in patients with an open abdomen and that this approach is associated with improved outcomes [94–96]. Collier et al. [95] demonstrated that early enteral feeding (within 4 day of celiotomy) was associated with earlier closure of the abdominal cavity and less fistula formation when compared with the delayed initiation of EN.

10. **EN contraindicated in patients with pancreatitis**

    In patients with acute severe pancreatitis, classic teaching suggested that "total parenteral nutrition should be initiated promptly and should judiciously replace nutrient deficits and provide the extra energy imposed on the patient by the inflammatory process" [97]. It was claimed that this approach was essential to "rest the pancreas" and that PN reduced mortality [98]. EN was considered an absolute contraindication as it would stimulate the pancreas and worsen pancreatic inflammation. Randomized clinical trials comparing EN versus PN in patients with moderate and severe pancreatitis have, however, proven these recommendations to be wrong. Meta-analyses have demonstrated that EN as compared with PN reduces infectious complications (particularly pancreatic abscesses), organ failure, length of hospital stay, and mortality [99, 100]. Nutritional support should be viewed as an active therapeutic intervention that improves the outcome of patients with acute pancreatitis. EN should begin within 24 h after admission and following the initial period of volume resuscitation and control of nausea and pain. Patients with mild acute pancreatitis should be started on a low-fat oral diet. In patients with severe acute pancreatitis, EN may be provided by the gastric or jejunal route [99].

11. **Patients should be fed in a 45° position**

    In an article published in 1999, Drakulovic et al. [101] demonstrated a lower frequency of clinically suspected ventilator associated pneumonia (VAP) in 39 intubated patients randomized to the semirecumbent (45°) as opposed to the supine body position (47 patients). In this study, the risk of pneumonia was highest for patients receiving EN in the supine body position. Based on this small single center study, it became standard of care to nurse all ICU patients in a semirecumbent 45° position particularly when receiving tube feeds. Indeed, the Centers for Disease Control and Prevention [102], the Agency for Healthcare Research and Quality [103], and the Institute for Healthcare Improvement [104] suggest elevating the head of the bed to 45° above horizontal to reduce gastroesophageal reflux and the prevalence of nosocomial pneumonia. The results of the study by Drakulovic et al. [101] have, however, not been reproduced. Van Nieuwenhoven et al. [105] randomized 112 intubated patients to the semirecumbent position with a target backrest elevation of 45° and 109 patients to a supine position with a backrest elevation of 10°. Average elevations were 9.8° and 16.1° at day 1 and day 7, respectively, for the supine group and 28.1° and 22.6° at day 1 and day 7, respectively, for the semirecumbent group. The target semirecumbent position of 45° was not achieved for 85% of the study time, and these patients more frequently changed position than supine-positioned patients. There was no difference in the risk VAP or any other outcome variable between groups. In an observational study of 66 ventilated patients, Grap et al. [106] reported a mean backrest elevation of 21.7° with no association between backrest elevation and the Clinical Pulmonary Infection Score. Rose et al. [107] performed 2112 backrest elevation measurements in 371 patients in 32 ICUs. Backrest elevation more than or equal to 45° was recorded in 5.3% of instances and elevation of between 30° and 45° in 22.3% of instances [107]. In this study, the mean backrest elevation was 23.8°. These studies suggest that nursing a patient semirecumbent at 45° is not feasible and attempts to do so may not reduce the risk of VAP. When the head of the bed is inclined at 45°, the patient often slides down; most of the weight of the upper body is applied on the sacral area, and this position becomes uncomfortable for the patient. Furthermore, experimental models suggest that the semirecumbent position may enhance the flow of mucous into the lungs with an increased risk of bacterial colonization and pneumonia [98]. Although maintaining a patient supine (0°) probably increases the risk of pneumonia, there is no strong evidence that elevation of the head of the bed between 10° and 30° is associated with a greater risk of pneumonia than a semirecumbent 45° position.

12. **What do we know about indirect calorimetry?**
It is the measurement of O_2 consumption (VO_2) and CO_2 production representing energy metabolism in real time. Its use in connection with the use of equations that calculate energy demand shows that it can prevent underfeeding and overfeeding. In addition, a meta-analysis has shown a reduction in mortality at 28 days using indirect calorimetry with isocaloric nutrition. Despite these benefits, its cost and investment in devices, consumables, calibration gas and service make it a method that is not very reproducible in our hospital units [108].

The ESPEN recommendation [19], the use of 25 kcal/kg has good accuracy for the use of nutrition; consider that the start of the enteral diet of the critically ill patient should not be delayed for more than 24–48 h, as well as the examination of eating habits prior to admission. Many patients have fasted for more than 24 h prior to hospital admission, or failing that, their nutritional assessment may show a certain degree of malnutrition. Therefore, it is recommended to use diets of ≈500 kcal/day or 10 kcal/kg and gradually increase the caloric intake up to a maximum of 25 kcal/day in a period of 3–7 days, considering the production of endogenous energy that it reaches up to 500–1400 kcal/day [109] and avoids overfeeding syndrome.

13. **Liquefied, handmade or polymeric?**

The use of terminology in the hospital setting is often heterogeneous, but blended and traditional diets share the same concept: preparation of mixed foods (liquefied) poured into a bag for administration to critical patients who do not have the orally available, they are prepared in order to administer them by naso or orogastric, naso-jejunal or gastrostomy tubes [110]. Ideally it is recommended to use a software [111] for the calculation of portions, consider contacting your Nutrition and Diet service to determine how they perform the calculation.

On the other hand, the polymeric diet in its standard isocaloric formulation 1 kcal/mL provides the micronutrients in their intact form in quantities very similar to that of a conventional diet. Consider that, for their administration, they require a normal production of pancreatic enzymes for their digestion and absorption.

14. **Hyperglycemia in enteral feeding?**

It is a common alteration, often associated with systemic inflammatory response/trauma or the use of corticosteroids, but the great association between nutrition and excess caloric intake is often the main alteration. Provide management of hyperglycemia and treat the cause [111]; monitor glucose closely. Avoid the use of hydrolyzed formulas due to their high carbohydrate content [112].

Not only the medications that we administer as corticosteroids can increase hyperglycemia levels, but if you do not consider the infusions in your patient from Propofol, dextrose solutions or administration of citrate, they can condition contributions of up to ≈400 kcal due to the use of Propofol. Consider that the 1 ml Propofol emulsion provides 1.1 kcal. So, count your intake and adjust the enteral diet to meet your nutritional goal [113].

15. **What is refeeding syndrome?**

It is the full manifestation in patients who undergo prolonged fasting, due to medical indication or course of critical illness and the abrupt onset with administration of the total nutritional requirements, which presents with hydroelectrolytic alterations secondary to the abrupt increase in insulin levels, as well as metabolic after the resumption of feeding. It usually occurs within 2–5 days of feeding [114]. Clinical detections in critical patients are a challenge because in this population the alterations observed can be multifactorial and not only due to the refeeding syndrome, such as rhabdomyolysis, arrhythmias, edema, confusion or encephalopathy. It is recommended to detect those patients at high risk and start the administration of thiamine (200–300 mg/day for 3–10 days), as well as the gradual increase in calories with monitoring of serum electrolytes, the presence of hypophosphatemia being an indicator of said syndrome. Consider the cut-off value for hypophosphatemia of relevance as the decrease greater than 0.5 mg/dL, achieving optimization of serum levels <2.0 mg/dL within the first 72 h of starting feeding [115].

References

1. Chaves JV. Cuadernos de Emergencia. 1994;2:61–71.
2. Perez HY. Preparación del paciente para evacuaciones aéreas. Emergencias. 1997;9:35–43.
3. Chuliá VC, Ortiz P. Transporte Sanitario. Fisiopatología. Las norias de evacuación. En: Alvarez Leiva C, Chuliá Campos V, Hernando Lorenzo A; Manual de Asistencia Sanitaria en las Catástrofes. Ed. ELA, Madrid, 1992, 123.
4. Cox J. Nutrition. En: Siberry G, Lannone R. Handbook. 15th. The Johns Hopkins Hospital: Mosby; 2000. p. 481-518.
5. García Roig C. Soporte nutricional en el paciente pediátrico critico. En: Montemerlo H, Menéndez AM, Slobdianik NH (editors). Nutrición enteral y parenteral. Argentina: Abbott Laboratorios; 1999. p. 225-233.
6. Brooks S, Kearns P. Nutrición enteral y parenteral. En: Ekhard E, Ziegler EE, Filer L. Conocimientos actuales sobre nutrición. 7. edición. Washington DC: OPS/OMS ILSI Press: 1997. D. 567-76.
7. Patino JF, de Pimiento SE, Vergara A, Sabino P, Rodriguez M, Escollan J. Hipocaloric support in the critically ill. World J Surg. 1999;6:553–99.
8. Ruza F, Alvarado F, Delgado MA, Garcia S, Hernández A. Soporte nutricional en situaciones especiales. En: Borrajo E, López M, Pajarón M.Nuevas perspectivas en nutrición infantil. Madrid: Ediciones Ergon;1995. p. 339-341.
9. Mena Miranda VR, Riverón Corteguera RL, Pérez Cruz JA. Nuevas consideraciones fisiopatológicas sobre el sindrome de respuesta inflamatoria sistémica relacionada con la sepsis. Rev Cuba Pediatr. 1996;68(1):57–70.
10. Mena Miranda VR, Riverón Corteguera RL, Pérez Cruz JA. Translocación bacteriana: un problema para reflexionar. Rev Cuba Pediatr. 1996;68(1):50–6.
11. Van Eys J. Benefits of nutritional intervention on nutritional status, quality of live and survival. Int J Cancer Suppl. 1998;11:66–8.
12. Mejia-Aranguren JM. Malnutrition in childhood lymphoblastic leukaemia: a predictor of early mortality during the induction to remission phase of the treatment. Unidad de Investigaciones Hospital Pediátricode México. Arch Med Res. 1999;30(2):150–3.
13. Ami LA, Moss RL. Nutritional support of the pediatric surgical patient. Curr Opin Pediatr. 1999;11/3:237–40.
14. Roediger WE. Famine, fiber, fatty acids, and failed colonic absorption: dos fiber fermentation ameliorate diarrhea? JPEN. 1994;18(1):4–8.
15. Green R, Miller JW. Folate deficiency beyond megaloblastic anemia: hyprehomoysteinemia and other manifestations of dysfunctional folate status. Semin Haematol. 1999;36(1):47–64.
16. Correia MI, Waitzberg DL. The impact of malnutrition on morbidity, mortality, length of hospital stay and costs evaluated through a multivariate model analysis. Clin Nutr. 2003;22(3):235–9.
17. Waitzberg DL, Caiaffa WT, Correia MI. Hospital malnutrition: the Brazilian national survey (IBRANUTRI): a study of 4,000 patients. Nutrition. 2001;17:573–80.
18. Kyle UG, Kossovsky MP, Karsegard VL, Pichard C. Comparison of tolls for nutritional assessment and screening at hospital admission: a population study. Clin Nutr. 2006;25:409–17.
19. ESPEN guideline on clinical nutrition in the intensive care unit. Clin Nutr. 2019;38:48–79.
20. Marik P. Immunonutrition in critically ill patients; a systematic review and analvsis of the literature. Int Care Med. 2008;34:1980–90.
21. Toulson MI, Costa P, Machado GA. Perioperative nutritional management of patients undergoing laparotomy. Nutr Hosp. 2009;24(4):479–84.
22. Niedert KC, Position of the American Dietetic Association. Liberalization for the diet prescription improves quality of life for older adults in long-term care. J Am Diet Assoc. 2005;105:1955–65.
23. Heyland DK. Nutritional support in the critically ill patient: a critical review of the evidence. Crit Care Clin. 1998;14:423–40.

24. Wilmore DW, Dudrick SJ. Growth and development of an infant receiving all nutrients exclusively by vein. JAMA. 1968;203:860–4.
25. Dudrick SJ, Wilmore DW, Vars HM, Rhoads JE. Long-term total parenteral nutrition with growth, development, and positive nitrogen balance. Surgery. 1968;64:134–42.
26. Wilmore DW, Dudrick SJ. Effects of nutrition on intestinal adaptation following massive small bowel resection. Surg Forum. 1969;20:398–400.
27. Vary TC, Siegel JH, Nakatani T, Sato T, Aoyama H. Regulation of glucosa metabolism by altered pyruvate dehydrogenase activity. I. Potential site of insulin resistance in sepsis. JPEN. 1986;10:351–5.
28. Moore FA, Feliciano DV, Andrassy RJ. Early enteral feeding, compared with parenteral, reduces postoperative septic complications. The results of a meta-analysis. Ann Surg. 1992;216:172–83.
29. Kudsk K, Jonathan E. Rhoads lecture: of mice and men... And a few hundred rats. JPEN. 2008;32:460–73.
30. Kudsk KA. Beneficial effect of enteral feeding. Gastrointest Endosc Clin N Am. 2007;17:647–62.
31. Hermsen JL, Gómez FE, Maeshima Y, Sano Y, Kang W, Kudsk KA. Decreased enteral stimulation alters mucosal immune chemokines. JPEN. 2008;32:36–44.
32. Hermsen JL, Gómez FE, Sano Y, Kang W, Maeshima Y, Kudsk KA. Parenteral feeding depletes pulmonary lymphocyte populations. JPEN. 2009;33:535–40.
33. Marik P, Zaloga G. Immunonutrition in critically ill patients: a systematic review and analysis of the literature. Int Care Med. 2008;34:1980–90.
34. Mazaki T, Ebisawa K. Enteral versus parenteral nutrition after gastrointestinal surgery: a systematic review and meta-analysis of randomized controlled trials in the English literature. J Gastrointest Surg. 2008;12:739–55.
35. Pontes-Arruda A, Aragão AM, Albuquerque JD. Effects of enteral feeding with eicosapentaenoic acid, gamma-linolenic acid, and antioxidants in mechanically ventilated patients with severe sepsis and septic shock. Crit Care Med. 2006;34:2325–33.
36. Pontes-Arruda A, Demichele S, Seth A, Singer P. The use of an inflammation-modulating diet in patients with acute lung injury or acute respiratory distress syndrome: a meta-analysis of outcome data. JPEN. 2008;32:596–605.
37. Lacey JM, Wilmore DW. Is glutamine a conditional essential amino acid? Nutr Rev. 1990;48:297–309.
38. Fukatsu K, Ueno C, Hashiguchi Y, Hara E, Kinoshita M, Mochizuki H, et al. Glutamine infusion during ischemia is detrimental in a murine gut ischemia/ reperfusion model. JPEN. 2003;27:187–92.
39. Alberda C, Gramlich L, Jones N, et al. The relationship between nutritional intake and clinical outcomes in critically ill patients: results of an international multicenter observational study. Intensive Care Med. 2009;35:1728–37.
40. Weijs PJ, Stapel SN, de Groot SD, et al. Optimal protein and energy nutrition decreases mortality in mechanically ventilated, critically ill patients: a prospective observational cohort study. JPEN J Parenter Enteral Nutr. 2012;36:60–8.
41. Singer P, Pichard C, Heidegger CP, et al. Considering energy deficit in the intensive care unit. Curr Opin Clin Nutr Metab Care. 2010;13:170–6.
42. Faisy C, Candela Llerena M, Savalle M, et al. Early ICU energy deficit is a risk factor for Staphylococcus aureus ventilator-associated pneumonia. Chest. 2011;140:1254–60.
43. Faisy C, Lerolle N, Dachraoui F, et al. Impact of energy deficit calculated by a predictive method on outcome in medical patients requiring prolonged acute mechanical ventilation. Br J Nutr. 2009;101:1079–87.
44. McClave SA, Martindale RG, Vanek VW, et al. A.S.P.E.N: Board of Directors; American College of Critical Care Medicine; Society of Critical Care Medicine: Guidelines for the provision and assessment of nutrition support therapy in the adult critically ill patient: Society of Critical Care Medicine (SCCM) and American Society for Parenteral and Enteral Nutrition (A.S.P.E.N.). JPEN J Parenter Enteral Nutr. 2009;33:277–316.

45. Heyland DK, Dhaliwal R, Drover JW, et al; Canadian Critical Care Clinical Practice Guidelines Committee: Canadian Clinical Practice.
46. 2013 Canadian Clinical Practice Guidelinee. Available at: http://www.criticalcarenutrition. com/. Accessed July 5, 2022.
47. Kreymann KG, Berger MM, Deutz NE, et al. DGEM (German Society for Nutritional Medicine); ESPEN (European Society for Parenteral and Enteral Nutrition): ESPEN guidelines on enteral Nutrition: intensive care. Clin Nutr. 2006;25:210–23.
48. Matejovic M, Huet O, Dams K, et al. Medical nutrition therapy and clinical outcomes in critically ill adults: a European multinational, prospective observational cohort study (EuroPN). Crit Care. 2022;26:143.
49. Zaloga GP. Parenteral nutrition in adult inpatients with functioning gastrointestinal tracts: assessment of outcomes. Lancet. 2006;367:1101–11.
50. Marik PE, Zaloga GP. Early enteral nutrition in acutely ill patients: a systematic review. Crit Care Med. 2001;29:2264–70.
51. Marik PE, Pinsky M. Death by parenteral nutrition. Intensive Care Med. 2003;29:867–9.
52. Grau T, Bonet A, Rubio M, et al. Working Group on Nutrition and Metabolism of the Spanish Society of Critical Care: liver dysfunction associated with artificial nutrition in critically ill patients. Crit Care. 2007;11:R10.
53. Heyland DK, MacDonald S, Keefe L, et al. Total parenteral nutrition in the critically ill patient: a meta-analysis. JAMA. 1998;280:2013–9.
54. Kles KA, Wallig MA, Tappenden KA. Luminal nutrients exacerbate intestinal hypoxia in the hypoperfused jejunum. JPEN J Parenter Enteral Nutr. 2001;25:246–53.
55. McClave SA, Chang WK. Feeding the hypotensive patient: does enteral feeding precipitate or protect against ischemic bowel? Nutr Clin Pract. 2003;18:279–84.
56. Siregar H, Chou CC. Relative contribution of fat, protein, carbohydrate, and ethanol to intestinal hyperemia. Am J Phys. 1982;242:G27–31.
57. Alhazzani W, Almasoud A, Jaeschke R, et al. Small bowel feeding and risk of pneumonia in adult critically ill patients: a systematic review and meta-analysis of randomized trials. Crit Care. 2013;17:R127.
58. Ma Y, Cheng J, Liu, Chen K. Intermittent versus continuous enteral nutrition on feeding intolerance in critically ill adults: a meta-analysis of randomized controlled trials. Int J Nurs Stud. 113:103783.
59. Lichtenberg K, Guay-Berry P, Pipitone A, Bondy A, Rotello L. Compensatory increased enteral feeding goal rates: a way to achieve optimal nutrition. Nutr Clin Pract. 2010;25(6):653–7.
60. Bharal M, Morgan S, Husain T, Hilari K, Morawiec C, Harrison K, Bassett P, Culkin A. Volume based feeding versus rate based feeding in the critically ill: a UK study. J Intensive Care Soc. 2019;20(4):299–308.
61. Flower L, Haines R, McNelly A, Bear D, Koelfat K, Damink S, et al. Effect of intermittent or continuous feeding and amino acid concentration on urea-to-creatinine ratio in critical illness. J Parenter Enter Nutr. 2021;46(4):789–97.
62. McNelly A, Bear D, Connolly B, Arbane G, Allum L, Tarbhai A, et al. Effect of intermittent or continuous feed on muscle wasting in critical illness. Chest. 2020;158(1):183–94.
63. Bear D, Hart N, Puthucheary Z. Continuous or intermittent feeding. Curr Opin Crit Care. 2018;24(4):256–61.
64. Wang Z, Ding W, Fang Q, Zhang L, Liu X, Tang Z. Effects of not monitoring gastric residual volume in intensive care patients: a meta-analysis. Int J Nurs Stud. 2019;91:86–93.
65. Reignier J, Mercier E, Le Gouge A, et al. Effect of not monitoring residual gastric volume on risk of ventilator-associated pneumonia in adults receiving mechanical ventilation and early enteral feeding: a randomized controlled trial. JAMA. 2013;309(3):249–56.
66. Galindo Martín C, Mandujano González J, Pérez Félix M, Mora Cruz M. Síndrome de realimentación en el paciente críticamente enfermo: del metabolismo al pie de cama. Revista Mexicana De Patología Clínica. 2019:154–9.

67. McClave SA, Lukan JK, Stefater JA, et al. Poor validity of residual volumes as a marker for risk of aspiration in critically ill patients. Crit Care Med. 2005;33:324–30.
68. Montejo JC, MinÃÉambres E, BordejeÃÅ L, et al. Gastric residual volume during enteral nutrition in ICU patients: the REGANE study. Intensive Care Med. 2010;36:1386–93.
69. Chapman MJ, Nguyen NQ, Fraser RJ. Gastrointestinal motility and prokinetics in the critically ill. Curr Opin Crit Care. 2007;13:187–94.
70. Marik PE, Zaloga GP. Gastric versus post-pyloric feeding: a systematic review. Crit Care. 2003;7:R46–51.
71. Ho KM, Dobb GJ, Webb SA. A comparison of early gastric and postpyloric feeding in critically ill patients: a meta-analysis. Intensive Care Med. 2006;32:639–49.
72. Ritz MA, Chapman MJ, Fraser RJ, et al. Erythromycin dose of 70mg accelerates gastric emptying as effectively as 200 mg in the critically ill. Intensive Care Med. 2005;31:949–54.
73. Zaloga GP, Marik P. Promotility agents in the intensive care unit. Crit Care Med. 2000;28:2657–9.
74. Cannon WB. Auscultation of the rhythmic sounds produced by the stomach and intestines. Am J Phys. 1905;14:339–53.
75. Rothnie NG, Harper RA, Catchpole BN. Early postoperative gastrointestinal activity. Lancet. 1963;2:64–7.
76. Waldhausen JH, Shaffrey ME, Skenderis BS 2nd, et al. Gastrointestinal myoelectric and clinical patterns of recovery after laparotomy. Ann Surg. 1990;211:777–84. discussion 785
77. Nachlas MM, Younis MT, Roda CP, et al. Gastrointestinal motility studies as a guide to postoperative management. Ann Surg. 1972;175:510–22.
78. Moss G. Maintenance of gastrointestinal function after bowel surgery and immediate enteral full nutrition. II. Clinical experience, with objective demonstration of intestinal absorption and motility. JPEN J Parenter Enteral Nutr. 1981;5:215–20.
79. Moss G, Greenstein A, Levy S, et al. Maintenance of GI function after bowel surgery and immediate enteral full nutrition. I. Doubling of canine colorectal anastomotic bursting pressure and intestinal wound mature collagen content. JPEN J Parenter Enteral Nutr. 1980;4:535–8.
80. Kiyama T, Efron DT, Tantry U, et al. Effect of nutritional route on colonic anastomotic healing in the rat. J Gastrointest Surg. 1999;3:441–6.
81. YurtcÃßu M, Toy H, Arbag H, et al. The effects of early and late feeding on healing of esophageal anastomoses: an experimental study. Int J Pediatr Otorhinolaryngol. 2011;75:1289–91.
82. Tadano S, Terashima H, Fukuzawa J, et al. Early postoperative oral intake accelerates upper gastrointestinal anastomotic healing in the rat model. J Surg Res. 2011;169:202–8.
83. Fukuzawa J, Terashima H, Ohkohchi N. Early postoperative oral feeding accelerates upper gastrointestinal anastomotic healing in the rat model. World J Surg. 2007;31:1234–9.
84. Cihan A, Oguz M, Acun Z, et al. Comparison of early postoperative enteral nutrients versus chow on colonic anastomotic healing in normal animals. Eur Surg Res. 2004;36:112–5.
85. Khalili TM, Navarro RA, Middleton Y, et al. Early postoperative enteral feeding increases anastomotic strength in a peritonitis model. Am J Surg. 2001;182:621–4.
86. Collier B, Guillamondegui O, Cotton B, et al. Feeding the open abdomen. JPEN J Parenter Enteral Nutr. 2007;31:410–5.
87. Schunn CD, Daly JM. Small bowel necrosis associated with postoperative jejunal tube feeding. J Am Coll Surg. 1995;180:410–6. 103
88. Lawlor DK, Inculet RI, Malthaner RA. Small-bowel necrosis associated with jejunal tube feeding. Can J Surg. 1998;41:459–62.
89. Marvin RG, McKinley BA, McQuiggan M, et al. Nonocclusive bowel necrosis occurring in critically ill trauma patients receiving enteral nutrition manifests no reliable clinical signs for early detection. Am J Surg. 2000;179:7–12.
90. Melis M, Fichera A, Ferguson MK. Bowel necrosis associated with early jejunal tube feeding: a complication of postoperative enteral nutrition. Arch Surg. 2006;141:701–4.

91. Sarap AN, Sarap MD, Childers J. Small bowel necrosis in association with jejunal tube feeding. JAAPA. 2010;23:28–32.
92. Gwon JG, Lee YJ, Kyoung KH, et al. Enteral nutrition associated non-occlusive bowel ischemia. J Korean Surg Soc. 2012;83:171–4.
93. Asensio JA, Petrone P, RoldaÃÅn G, et al. Has evolution in awareness of guidelines for institution of damage control improved outcome in the management of the posttraumatic open abdomen? Arch Surg. 2004;139:209–14.
94. Moore EE, Jones TN. Benefits of immediate jejunostomy feeding after major abdominal trauma—a prospective, randomized study. J Trauma. 1986;26:874–81.
95. Tsuei BJ, Magnuson B, Swintosky M, et al. Enteral nutrition in patients with an open peritoneal cavity. Nutr Clin Pract. 2003;18:253–8.
96. Cothren CC, Moore EE, Ciesla DJ, et al. Postinjury abdominal compartment syndrome does not preclude early enteral feeding after definitive closure. Am J Surg. 2004;188:653–8.
97. Latifi R, McIntosh JK, Dudrick SJ. Nutritional management of acute and chronic pancreatitis. Surg Clin North Am. 1991;71:579–95.
98. Li Bassi G, Zanella A, Cressoni M, et al. Following tracheal intubation, mucus flow is reversed in the semirecumbent position: possible role in the pathogenesis of ventilator-associated pneumonia. Crit Care Med. 2008;36:518–25.
99. Marik PE. What is the best way to feed patients with pancreatitis? Curr Opin Crit Care. 2009;15:131–8.
100. Petrov MS, van Santvoort HC, Besselink MG, et al. Enteral nutrition and the risk of mortality and infectious complications in patients with severe acute pancreatitis: a meta-analysis of randomized trials. Arch Surg. 2008;143:1111–7.
101. Drakulovic MB, Torres A, Bauer TT, et al. Supine body position as a risk factor for nosocomial pneumonia in mechanically ventilated patients: a randomised trial. Lancet. 1999;354:1851–8.
102. Tablan OC, Anderson LJ, Besser R, et al. CDC; Healthcare Infection Control Practices Advisory Committee: Guidelines for preventing health-care–associated pneumonia, 2003: Recommendations of CDC and the Healthcare Infection Control Practices Advisory Committee. MMWR Recomm Rep. 2004;53:1–36.
103. Strategies to Prevent Ventilator-Associated Pneumonia in Acute Care Hospitals. Rockville, MD, Agency for Healthcare Research and Quality, 2008. Available at: http://www.guideline.gov/content.aspx?id=13396NGC-6807. Accessed June 25, 2012.
104. Institute for Healthcare Improvement: Implement the IHI Ventilator Bundle, 2012. Available at: http://www.ihi.org/knowledge/pages/changes/implementtheventilatorbundle.aspx. Accessed June 25, 2012.
105. van Nieuwenhoven CA, Vandenbroucke-Grauls C, van Tiel FH, et al. Feasibility and effects of the semirecumbent position to prevent ventilator-associated pneumonia: a randomized study. Crit Care Med. 2006;34:396–402.
106. Grap MJ, Munro CL, Hummel RS 3rd, et al. Effect of backrest elevation on the development of ventilator-associated pneumonia. Am J Crit Care. 2005;14:325–32. quiz 333
107. Rose L, Baldwin I, Crawford T, et al. Semirecumbent positioning in ventilator-dependent patients: a multicenter, observational study. Am J Crit Care. 2010;19:e100–8.
108. Waele D, van Zanten. Routine use of indirect calorimetry in critically ill patients: pros and cons. Crit Care. 2022;26:123.
109. Tappy L, Schwatrz JM, Schneiter P, Cayeux C, Revelly JP, Fagerquist CKL. Effects of isoenergetic glucose. Based or lipid based parenteral nutrition on glucose metabolism, de novo lipogenesis and respiratory gas exchanges in critically ill patients. Crit Care Med. 1998;26:860–7.
110. Borghi R, Araujo TD, Airoldi-Vieira RI, et al. ILSI Task Force on enteral nutrition: estimated composition and cost of blenderized diets. Nutr Hosp. 2013;28(6):2033–8.
111. Gosmanov AR, Umpierrez GE. Management of hyperglycemia during enteral and parenteral nutrition therapy. Curr Diab Rep. 2013;13(1):155–62.

112. Escuro AA, Humell AC. Enteral formulas in nutrition support practice: is there a better choice for your patient? Nutr Clin Pract. 2016;31(6):709–22.
113. Huang Y. An analysis of non-nutritive calories from propofol, dextrose, and citrate among critically ill patients receiving continuous renal replacement therapy. J Parenter Enter Nutr. 2022;
114. Skipper A. Refeeding syndrome or refeeding hypophosphatemia: a systematic review of cases. Nutr Clin Pract. 2012;27(1):34–40.
115. Galindo Martín C, Mandujano González J, Pérez Félix M, Mora Cruz M. Síndrome de realimentación en el paciente críticamente enfermo: del metabolismo al pie de cama. Revista Mexicana De Patología Clínica. 2019:154–7.

Chapter 16
Energy Balance and Nutrition in High Altitude

Prakash Deb, Prithwis Bhattacharyya, and Debasis Pradhan

Case Presentation

A multinational expedition team of ten members are climbing and planning to camp at a height of 5000 (m) metres on Mount Kilimanjaro (5895 m). Total duration of this adventure trip is 3 weeks. At the end of tenth days, the ration in-charge raises concern regarding unused rations which were meant to be finished 3 days earlier. Then, the team physio realised a decrease in the body weight among seven of them and per person there was a loss of around 4 kilogram (kg). Then, the team plans to increase the dietary intake to avoid further weight loss which may compromise the expedition outcome.

P. Deb
Department of Anaesthesiology, Critical care & Pain medicine, AIIMS, Guwahati, India

P. Bhattacharyya (✉)
Departments of Critical Care Medicine & Trauma & Emergency Medicine, Pacific Medical College, Udaipur, Rajasthan, India

D. Pradhan
Anaesthesia, NHS Derby and Burton, Derby, UK

© The Author(s), under exclusive license to Springer Nature Switzerland AG 2023
J. Hidalgo et al. (eds.), *High Altitude Medicine*,
https://doi.org/10.1007/978-3-031-35092-4_16

What Are the Effects of High Altitude (HA) on Energy Balance?

If the nutrition aspect is not addressed during a HA expedition, then one can have negative energy balance, negative nitrogen balance, weight loss, loss of fat free mass (includes muscle) and fat.

What Physiological Changes Might Be Responsible for Such Altitude Effects on Nutrition?

HA increases basal metabolic rate (BMR), resting energy expenditure (REE), decreases maximum oxygen consumption capacity (VO2 max). At the same time, it reduces appetite, substrate utilisation, and alters dietary composition. All these changes lead to weight loss and loss of both fat and fat free mass (FFM) (FFM shares a major portion).

What Dietary Modifications Possibly May Impede or Minimise Such HA Impact on Energy Balance?

Successful increase in dietary intake to support the basal requirement by providing special high caloric, nutrient dense, branched chain amino acids (Leucine) rich, balanced (Protein 0.8 g/kg for sedentary and 1.2–1.5 g/kg for strenuous activities, complex carbohydrates and fat providing 60% and 25–28% of total energy requirement) and palatable product. Fluid intake should be sufficient to cover insensible water loss and diuresis (usually amounts to 4 litres a day).

Introduction

Exposure to High altitude (HA) poses multiple challenges for the mountaineer like low barometric pressure, low oxygen concentration, extreme cold, radiation, sleep irregularities, acute mountain sickness in addition to the fluid and calorie imbalance, the severity of which varies with the rate of ascent, altitude climbed, fluid and energy intake, physical built and degree of physical activity.

When climbing high altitude or doing physical activities, daily energy requirements are not achieved and finally ends up with weight loss which includes both fat and fat free mass [1]. So, exposure to high altitude causes decrease in body mass leading to loss of around 5 kilogram during a normal civilian expedition. Causes of negative energy balance include decreased input, increased energy output and altered homeostasis. Interventions which may prevent or slow down such changes include but not limited to, increased dietary intake with appropriate composition and palatability, supplementation with branched chain amino acid such as leucine and antioxidants, appropriate acclimatization and proper hydration.

Impact of High Altitude on Metabolism and Weight

The impact of high altitude on metabolic processes is evident from the weight loss, which is almost inevitable and can reach up to 15% depending upon multiple factors [2]. The fundamental reason being an imbalance between energy, fluid intake and expenditure. The intake may reduce due to anorexia, inadequate supply and the palatability of food [3].

Anorexia can be a part of acute Mountain sickness or may occur alone. Food intake can drop by 25–50% at high altitude. Increased rate of ventilation, exposure to dry, cold air and cold induced diuresis lead to negative fluid balance and add to the weight loss. There is a reduced digestive capacity, motility and enzyme secretion in hypoxic conditions of high altitude, which in addition to the anorexia and malabsorption lead to extreme reduction of energy intake and weight loss [4].

Decreased Energy Intake

Leptin is released from the adipose tissue and enterocytes of the small intestine and by acting on hypothalamus plays a major role in appetite regulation, alters body metabolism and energy homeostasis. Acute short-term high-altitude exposure increases the level of hypoxia inducible factor 1 (HIF 1) which in turn stimulates production of leptin. Blood leptin level increases during the first two weeks of climbing and correlates with the duration of high-altitude exposure and contributes to anorexia [5, 6]. Study of isolated human adipocytes has shown time dose-response curve between leptin and GLUT1. HIF 1 is responsible for up and downregulation of GLUT1 leading to reduced and increased appetite for fat contributing towards loss and gain of weight at high altitude. Ghrelin, produced by the enteroendocrine cells of the intestine, is responsible for maintenance of hunger. Its level decreases following acute exposure to high altitude hypoxia contributing to anorexia [7]. At high altitude, early satiety and decreased hunger is attributed to the alteration in leptin-ghrelin balance secondary to hypoxia.

Increased Energy Expenditure

At high altitude, there is increased energy requirement in healthy individuals which is more than two times that of sea level individuals at rest. Inadequate energy intake along-with an increase in expenditure leads to rapid weight loss. With increasing hypoxia associated with high altitude, there is a sympathetic stimulation and an increase in BMR by 30% which may not come down easily even after weeks of acclimatization.

Decrease in VO2 max at high altitude partially explains the increase in exercise effort for the same physical activity. With 10% fall in VO2 max for every 1000 m increase in altitude above 2000 m, equivalent work will require a greater proportion of available maximal effort at HA and VO2 max falls. Even a low-level activity can become a high intensity activity, increasing metabolic demands, at high altitude [8].

Digestive Function at High Altitude

Food digestion and assimilation is very effective in a healthy person at sea level and only 4–7% of energy is lost in the faeces [9]. Hypoxia has been linked to malabsorption both at the sea level and high altitude. There is no definite evidence of malabsorption at high altitude causing energy deficit, weight loss and negative protein balance, however it has been hypothesized by some that a decrease in splanchnic circulation secondary to hypobaric hypoxia leads to enterocyte malfunction and altered absorption [7, 10, 11].

The Energy Gap at High Altitude

The energy gap (difference between intake and expenditure) at high altitude is one of the common reasons behind the alteration in body composition and weight loss. Daily energy expenditure in the range of 3250–7871 kcal per day has been reported during Mt. Everest expedition which is significantly higher than sea-level expenditure. Factors other than physical activity which determine the energy expenditure include but are not limited to diet-induced thermogenesis, body size (which influences BMR) and genetic make-up [12–14].

Energy deficit at high altitude mimics chronic starvation. On an average, 480 kcal per day of calorie deficit has been calculated which results in a weekly weight loss of ~0.5 kg which is also dependant on many other factors like duration of stay at high altitude, rate of ascent and ultimate altitude achieved. It is necessary to correct the energy gap in the form of increased intake or reducing physical activity, later would be unavoidable in most of the circumstances. Attempts should be made to improve intake by providing food of individual choice, increasing palatability along with proper motivation and education about the beneficial effects of increased intake. Even with all the necessary measures the energy gap is never mitigated completely [15–17].

Macronutrients at High Altitude

Protein Intake

Relative calorie deficit results in weight loss, of which loss of muscle mass is the major concern which reduces physical endurance, aerobic capacity, induces fatigue, depresses immune system, increases vulnerability to infection and other illnesses. There is a decrease in fluid, fat, Fat free Mass (FFM) or lean body mass in case of negative energy balance at high altitude. Hypoxia in a calorie deficit individual causes more loss of FFM compared to a normoxic condition in addition to other influencing factors like age, gender or physical fitness.

Numerous studies have been done to measure the changes in body composition using some of the available tools like dual-energy x-ray absorptiometry (DXA), ultrasound guided skinfold measurement, bioelectrical impedance analysis (BIA), hydrostatic weighing. They reported a large loss of FFM (60–70%) compared to fat mass at high altitude though there are differences in methods of measurement, altitude achieved, age, gender and the duration of stay at high altitude [14, 18–24].

Skeletal muscle mass constitutes more than 55% of FFM and the muscle protein synthesis is greatly influenced by hypoxia which is a dominant force at high altitude. Muscle protein synthesis is centred around rapamycin pathway (mTOR) which is downregulated under hypoxic conditions at high altitude contrary to that at sea level.

Increased muscle proteolysis and reduced synthesis in response to hypobaric hypoxia at high altitude suggests that replacing nutrition alone may not prevent muscle wasting however an energy-protein deficient state can magnify the complication. Low calorie intake in addition to hypoxia increased REDD1 gene expression which would lead mTOR downregulation and reduced Muscle protein synthesis [25].

Adequate protein intake is protective along with diet rich in carbohydrate however increased protein intake may be even harmful considering its action on satiety promoting anorexia and more oxygen requirement for utilisation. Branched chain amino acids like leucine can stimulate muscle protein synthesis by stimulating mTOR pathway and preventing proteolysis.

So, a protein intake of 1.2–1.5 gm/kg body weight along with addition of Leucine should be able to prevent FFM loss if given with adequate carbohydrate, which is discussed in details later in this chapter.

Carbohydrate and Fat

Glucose is the most efficient fuel consuming less oxygen per unit of energy produced than either fat or protein. In hypobaric hypoxia at HA, glucose metabolism helps by increasing the alveolar partial pressure of oxygen. Fat is a larger source of energy when compared to carbohydrate but requires more oxygen to breakdown energy making it less energy efficient macronutrient at high altitude.

Let us consider Respiratory Quotient to understand the fact;

Respiratory quotient is the ratio of CO_2 release and O_2 consumed

$$RQ = vol\, CO_2\ released\ /\ vol\, O_2\ absorbed$$

Under normal conditions, *vol CO_2 released is 200 ml/min and vol O_2 absorbed is* 250 ml/min resulting in a RQ of 0.8 however the value varies with the type of macronutrients consumed. Fat has a RQ of 0.7, as it produces less CO_2 for each oxygen utilised to break the substrate and release energy. Carbohydrate on the other hand has a RQ of 1, implying less oxygen consumption per unit of substrate which is very cost effective in the hypoxic conditions at high altitude.

Glucose being the most oxygen efficient source of energy, at sea level, exercise intensities above 50% of VO2 max needs more carbohydrates than lipids.

Diet modification at high altitude should consider not only the proportion of macronutrients but also the timing and form in which it is taken. Carbohydrate intake before a planned physical exertion may reduce the high-altitude symptoms like anorexia, improve oxygen saturation, tissue oxygenation and prevent muscle protein breakdown. Carbohydrate intake before exercise prevents chances of hypoglycaemia during exercise and adequate intake post training replenishes glycogen store and help recovery of injured muscle. Before starting a physical training or exertional activity, a carbohydrate diet with high glycaemic index like glucose drink, sugar bar, energy drink etc. is helpful to compensate for high expenditure of energy during training, however normal diet with low glycaemic index like fruit, vegetables, bread etc. is preferable to replenish the glycogen store [26–29]. Carbohydrate should constitute 60% of the total energy intake at high altitude however it should be increase (even up to 65%) in case of higher physical activity.

A daily requirement of fat as 22–25% of total dietary intake is essential to preserve the energy store, maintain insulation, maintain cellular integrity, absorption of fat-soluble vitamins, providing essential fatty acids, for hormone synthesis and many other vital functions of the body. Diet high in fat is rather detrimental in hypoxic condition and may precipitate acute mountain sickness symptoms. If fatty diet is to be taken for some reason, it should be accompanied with carbohydrate so that total dependence on fat for energy generation can be avoided.

From the above discussions, it is clear that increased energy requirement associated with reduced uptake is the usual pattern at high altitude. So, a higher calorie intake than normal becomes essential especially in athletes, military trainees. Carbohydrates requires 8–10% of less oxygen is the main macronutrient in such hypoxic environment both at rest and during physical exertion making it a major contributor of total calorie intake at high-altitude.

Hydration

Dehydration at high altitude occurs when water loss from respiratory system, kidney, skin etc. are not replaced adequately. Dry and cold air predisposes to loss of water from respiratory tract. Increased minute ventilation in response to many metabolic adjustments at high altitude also increases respiratory loss of water. Cold induced diuresis is another protective response to hypothermia where the blood is shunted from periphery to vital organs including kidney for preserving the core temperature. The increased renal blood flow and mean arterial pressure leads to increased diuresis. Dehydration causes fatigue, mental confusion, decreased physical endurance, inversely related to symptoms of acute mountain sickness and decreased cardiovascular performance.

One practical way of assessment of dehydration status is by regularly observing urine osmolality and specific gravity. How much fluid is adequate is difficult to prescribe and rather than focussing on a fixed amount, it should be guided by the level of activity and the humidity. There are reports of fluid intake up to 10 L a day by cyclist in the mountain zone. Adequate fluid requirement may be replenished through fruits, vegetables, energy rich drink devoid of caffein (has diuretic property). This would also provide essential micronutrients and anti-oxidants along with water.

Replacement of Other Micronutrients

It is essential to provide essential micronutrients like copper, selenium, manganese, iron, zinc etc. to continue many of the vital cellular processes where they act co-factor.

Iron

The role of increasing oxygen delivery to the exercising muscle by increasing red cell mass is important in hypoxic locations. Erythropoiesis occurs in response to high altitude hypoxia to improve red cell mass and oxygen carrying capacity but at the expense of iron reserve of the body. It is therefore essential to measure the ferritin and iron level before planned high altitude expedition starts in order to replenish the iron reserve weeks before the planned trip. Iron available in food may not alone be sufficient in some individuals with low iron stores and those involved in heavy physical training. So, a supplementation with 100 mg/day may be required in them [30].

Vitamins and Anti-Oxidants

Studies done on athletes at high-altitude have demonstrated protective role of anti-oxidants from free radial induced injury of exercising muscle while others deny the same and claim that antioxidants themselves may be a source of injury [31–33].

A large number of reactive oxygen and nitrogen species (RONS) are generated during physical activity under hypoxic conditions at high altitude causing widespread damage to the cellular structures. Superoxide dismutase, glutathione peroxidase or reductase are the main endogenous scavengers which act on the reactive oxygen species and protects the muscle from injury and inflammation. The role of vitamin E, A and C are well known.

There are differences in the dose and combinations of vitamins prescribed for the purpose. Some considered vitamin E 400 IU/day as effective dose while others considered Vitamin C 1 gm combination with vitamin E 200 IU as superior. Rather than supplementing with individual antioxidants, it is a better choice to include different types of fruits, vegetables in diet which would provide hydration, carbohydrate along with beneficial antioxidants like, vitamin C, E, carotenoids, glutathione and phytochemicals in adequate quantity.

Vitamin D is known to have cardiovascular effect and influence on skeletal muscle health by improving oxygenation and strength. Vitamin D deficiency is common as such in general population which is more common after long stay at mountains, though there is a hypothetical advantage of UV radiations promoting endogenous vitamin D synthesis. For a longer stay at high altitude, a daily supplementation of vitamin D with 4000 IU may be considered.

Conclusion

Nutritional requirement at high altitude cannot be generalised because energy expenditure varies among different groups of athletes, military personals and mountaineers depending upon the age, gender, body mass, level of activity, altitude achieved, environmental conditions like temperature, humidity and genetic influences. Studies are also not sufficient on these aspects of high-altitude medicine and the results are not comparable because of the above differences. However, one thing is clear that there is an increased energy expenditure and reduced intake in high altitude climbers making an energy deficient state which should be considered in all mountaineers and replaced with increased carbohydrate intake owing to its ability to deliver instant energy at the cost of low oxygen consumption which is beneficial in hypoxic conditions of high altitude. Dehydration is also common and has to be taken care of especially during extreme physical activity. Vitamins, minerals and anti-oxidants should preferably be supplied through diet in the form of varieties of fruits, vegetables, legumes, cereals etc. and supplementation should be considered in individuals with limited baseline stores and those susceptible for deficiencies.

References

1. Westerterp KR, Kayser B. Body mass regulation at altitude. Eur J Gastroenterol Hepatol. 2006;18:1–3.
2. Reynolds RD, Lickteig JA, Deuster PA, Howard MP, Conway JM, Pietersma A, de Stoppelaar J, Deurenberg P. Energy metabolism increases and regional body fat decreases while regional muscle mass is spared in humans climbing Mt. Everest. J Nutr. 1999;129:1307–14.
3. Cymerman A. The physiology of high-altitude exposure. In: Marriot BM, Carlson SJ, editors. Nutritional needs in cold and in high-altitude environments: applications for military personnel in field operations. Washington, D.C.: National Academy Press; 1996. Ch 16.
4. Westerterp KR. Energy and water balance at high altitude. Physiology. 2001;16(3):134–7.
5. Netzer NC, Chytra R, Küpper T. Low intense physical exercise in normobaric hypoxia leads to more weight loss in obese people than low intense physical exercise in normobaric sham hypoxia. Sleep Breath. 2008;12:129–34.
6. Debevec T. Hypoxia-related hormonal appetite modulation in humans during rest and exercise: mini review. Front Physiol. 2017;8:366.
7. Hamad N, Travis SPL. Weight loss at high altitude: pathophysiology and practical implications. Eur J Gastroenterol Hepatol. 2006;18:5–10.
8. Brooks GA, Butterfield GE, Wolfe RR, et al. Increased dependence on blood glucose after acclimatization to 4,300 m. J Appl Physiol. 1991;70:919–27.
9. Milledge JS. Arterial oxygen saturation and intestinal absorption of xylose. Br Med J. 1972;3:557–8.
10. Westerterp KP, Meijer EP, Rubbens M, Robach P, Richalet J-P. Operation Everest III: energy and water balance. Eur J Appl Physiol. 2000;439:483–8.
11. Travis SPL, Edwards JSA, Westerterp K, Menzies IS. Carbohydrate intake, hydrolysis and permeation at high altitude (5600m) [abstract]. Gastroenterology. 1996;110:A845.
12. Hill NE, Stacey MJ, Woods DR. Energy at high altitude. J R Army Med Corps. 2011;157:43–8.
13. Maggiorini M, Bühler B, Walter M, Oelz O. Prevalence of acute mountain sickness in the Swiss Alps. BMJ. 1990;301:853–5.
14. Rose MS, Houston CS, Fulco CS, Coates G, Sutton JR, Cymerman A. Operation Everest. II: nutrition and body composition. J Appl Physiol. 1988;65:2545–51.
15. Butterfield GE, Gates J, Fleming S, Brooks GA, Sutton JR, Reeves JT. Increased energy intake minimizes weight loss in men at high altitude. J Appl Physiol. 1992;72:1741–8.
16. Roberts AC, Reeves JT, Butterfield GE, et al. Altitude and beta-blockade augment glucose utilization during submaximal exercise. J Appl Physiol. 1996;80:605–15.
17. Todd KS, Butterfield GE, Calloway DH. Nitrogen balance in men with adequate and deficient energy intake at three levels of work. J Nutr. 1984;114:2107–18.
18. Westerterp KR, Kayser B, Brouns F, Herry JP, Saris WH. Energy expenditure climbing Mt. Everest. J Appl Physiol. 1992;73:1815–9.
19. Westerterp KR, Kayser B, Wouters L, Le Trong JL, Richalet JP. Energy balance at high altitude of 6542 m. J Appl Physiol. 1994;77:862–6.
20. Tanner DA, Stager JM. Partitioned weight loss and body composition changes during a mountaineering expedition: a field study. Wilderness Environ Med. 1998;9:143–52.
21. Armellini F, Zamboni M, Robbi R, Todesco T, Bissoli L, Mino A, Angelini G, Micciolo R, Bosello O. The effects of high altitude trekking on body composition and resting metabolic rate. Horm Metab Res. 1997;29:458–61.
22. Pulfrey SM, Jones PJ. Energy expenditure and requirement while climbing above 6000 m. J Appl Physiol. 1996;81:1306–11.
23. Wing-Gaia SL, Gershenoff DC, Drummond MJ, Askew EW. Effect of leucine supplementation on fat free mass with prolonged hypoxic exposure during a 13-day trek to Everest Base Camp: a double-blind randomized study. Appl Physiol Nutr Metab. 2014;39 https://doi.org/10.1139/apnm-2013-0319.

24. Boyer SJ, Blume FD. Weight loss and changes in body composition at high altitude. J Appl Physiol. 1984;57:1580–5.
25. Favier FB, Costes F, Defour A, Bonnefoy R, Lefai E, Bauge S, Peinnequin A, Benoit H, Freyssenet D. Downregulation of Akt/mammalian target of rapamycin pathway in skeletal muscle is associated with increased REDD1 expression in response to chronic hypoxia. Am J Physiol Regul Integr Comp Physiol. 2010;298:R1659–66.
26. Golja P, Flander P, Klemenc M, Maver J, Princi T. Carbohydrate ingestion improves oxygen delivery in acute hypoxia. High Alt Med Biol. 2008;9:53–62.
27. Burke LM, Hawley JA, Wong SH, Jeukendrup AE. Carbohydrates for training and competition. J Sports Sci. 2011;29:17–27.
28. Jeukendrup AE, McLaughlin J. Carbohydrate ingestion during exercise: effects on performance, training adaptations and trainability of the gut. In: Maughan RJ, Burke LM, editors. Sports nutrition: more than just calories—triggers for adaptation, vol. 69. Basel, Switzerland: Karger AG; 2011. p. 1–17.
29. Jeukendrup A. A step towards personalized sports nutrition: carbohydrate intake during exercise. Sports Med. 2014;44:25–33.
30. Lukaski HC. Vitamin and mineral status: effects on physical performance. Nutrition. 2004;20:632–44.
31. Tauler P, Aguiló A, Gimeno I, Fuentespina E, Tur JA, Pons A. Response of blood cell antioxidant enzyme defences to antioxidant diet supplementation and to intense exercise. Eur J Nutr. 2006;45:187–95.
32. Gomez-Cabrera MC, Domenech E, Romagnoli M, Arduini A, Borras C, Pallardo FV, Sastre J, Viña J. Oral administration of vitamin C decreases muscle mitochondrial biogenesis and hampers training-induced adaptations in endurance performance. Am J Clin Nutr. 2008;87:142–9.
33. Teixeira VH, Valente HF, Casal SI, Marques AF, Moreira PA. Antioxidants do not prevent postexercise peroxidation and may delay muscle recovery. Med Sci Sports Exerc. 2009;41:1752–60.

Chapter 17
Exercise at High-Altitude

Antonio Gandra d´Almeida

Clinical Case

Male, 38 years old, no medical history, no medication, Arrived to Tibete on the 22nd of April and started climbing the Himalaias on the next day. When he was at 3000 m high he started feeling headache, náusea and fatigue. When he started to descend he started feeling better.

Introduction

Due to the lower availability of oxygen, the intensity of the exercise is reduced in altitude, and the adaptations generated by this exposure are the main factors to be evaluated when a competition at high altitude is programmed.

An adequate stay at altitude develops a series of physiological changes, which aim at better oxygen transport. Seeking to improve the delivery of oxygen to tissues, many elite athletes use training at altitude to improve physical fitness and improve performance at sea level. Exposure time and altitude level are the main factors that can lead to an optimized performance or damage to the athlete's health.

A. G. d´Almeida (✉)
North Delegation, National Institute Emergency Medicine, Porto, Portugal

J. Hidalgo et al. (eds.), *High Altitude Medicine*,
https://doi.org/10.1007/978-3-031-35092-4_17

Acclimatization

The main adjustments that occur in response to acute exposure to altitude are hyper-ventilation and increased cardiac output (at rest and at submaximal exercise). Prolonged exposure to altitude provides adjustments that occur more slowly, to improve tolerance to hypoxia, such as an acid-base balance of body fluids, an increase in the number of red blood cells and a higher concentration of hemoglobin.

The major cause of altitude illnesses is going too high too fast. Given time, the body can adapt to the decrease in oxygen molecules at a specific altitude. A number of changes take place in the body to allow it to operate with decreased oxygen.

- The depth of respiration increases.
- This ventilatory response to hypoxia induced, essentially, by stimulation of chemo-peripheral receptors sensitive to variations in the arterial oxygen content, allows the increase of ventilation by 2 to 5 times in relation to the values obtained at sea level and, thus, the increase in partial alveolar pressure of alveolar oxygen
- Pressure in pulmonary arteries is increased, "forcing" blood into portions of the lung which are normally not used during sea level breathing.
- The body produces more red blood cells to carry oxygen,
- Myoglobin, a protein similar to a subunit of hemoglobin, is found in large amounts in muscle, functioning as an additional reservoir of oxygen. As it has a greater affinity for oxygen in relation to hemoglobin, in any pO2, myoglobin receives the O2 transported by hemoglobin and releases it in very low pO2 conditions, to be used by muscle cell mitochondria.
- The low partial pressure of oxygen, associated with the effects of altitude, stimulates an increase in the production of erythropoietin by the kidneys, in response to an arterial hypoxia. With the synthesis of elevated erythropoietin, it increases the production of red blood cells, and consequently the number of available hemoglobin, improving the oxygen binding capacity.
- Regarding cardiovascular adaptations, acute exposure to hypobaric hypoxia triggers an increase in sympathetic autonomic nervous system activity, which promotes increased heart rate and cardiac output at rest and under-mage and changes in blood flow by selective vasoconstriction
- The body produces more of a particular enzyme that facilitates the release of oxygen from hemoglobin to the body tissues.

The ideal time required for acclimatization, on a general average, is around 15 days for an altitude of 2500 m, from then on, each 610 m increase requires an additional week for full acclimatization. The adaptations produced by acclimatization dissipate in about 20 days after returning to sea level.

Physical Performance at Altitude

Exercises with a predominantly anaerobic characteristic, of short duration, do not show a decrease in performance or difficulty in performing as a result of the effects of altitude. During exercise at altitude, the main energetic substrate used is glycogen, as it is the substrate that generates the most ATP per liter of oxygen consumed. The use of fatty acids for energy production during physical exercises at altitude would not be interesting, as in addition to having a slower rate of oxidation, the production of energy through these sources would use a greater volume of oxygen, which would lead to a reduction in exercise intensity. The reduced oxygen concentration, exercises performed above the lactate threshold and a high degradation of glycogen can lead to an early state of fatigue.

The main interest in performing altitude training is the improvement in the oxygen transport capacity in the blood, through an increase in the hemoglobin content.

The improvement in the movement economy occurs regardless of the training environment, but in this case, the improvement in the performance at sea level after a period of training at altitude, in relation to the movement economy, happens by an increase in the production of ATP per mol oxygen and by decreasing the cost of ATP for muscle contraction.

Training and Altitude

Trained people when exposed to altitude show a greater reduction in VO2max than untrained people. Elite athletes have been using altitude training for a long time, although the efficiency of this practice, in relation to improved performance at sea level, is still questioned by studies.

Live and Train at Altitude (Live High + Train High)

The original model of altitude training was to live and train at medium altitudes (live high + train high, LH + TH) that even though it has been used for several decades, its benefits in improving physical performance at sea level remain uncertain. A potential limitation of training in hypoxic conditions is the fact that many athletes are unable to reach the level of intensity necessary to generate the physiological changes that would improve performance, and in many cases, return to sea level in an untrained state, with 3–8% reductions in physical performance.

Live Low and Train at Altitude (Live Low + Train High)

Although the name indicates training in altitude, in the model LL + TH (live low + train high), the athlete lives and trains at sea level, with short periods of hypoxia (5–180 min) where he breathes through a gas mask with the percentage of oxygen reduced during the recovery interval or during the training session. The method is mainly indicated as a means of pre-acclimatization before ascending to altitude for athletes who intend to compete or train in high regions.

Live at Altitude and Train at Low (Live High + Train Low)

In this model, the athlete lives at altitude to obtain the benefits of acclimatization (increase in the production of erythropoietin, resulting in an increase in red blood cells) and trains at a lower location to achieve a training intensity similar to that of sea level. Athletes who use the LH + TL method live and/or sleep at a moderate altitude (2000–3000 m) and train at a low elevation (<1500 m).

Only for athletes with a very high level of conditioning does altitude training become significant as an additional stimulus, since the improvement in performance occurs in a minimal percentage. Living and training at altitude can be a viable alternative for athletes who are in the regenerative period, where the intensity of the training is mild to moderate.

Intermittent exposure to hypoxia can be used by athletes or teams whose competition calendars do not allow adequate acclimatization time, thus minimizing the appearance of possible complications during acute exposure to altitude. Staying at altitude and training at a lower altitude seems to be the ideal model to be adopted as an alternative to optimize the results obtained with training. According to the adaptations generated to improve oxygen transport, the pre-competition period would be the best time to apply this method, since its effects dissipate in a short period of time.

Thus, different individuals seem to respond differently to the same hypoxic stimulus of altitude, calling into question the generalization of the effectiveness of this new model of altitude training.

Sports Activities at Moderate and High Altitudes

There are 3 groups of individuals classified according to their way of responding to hypobaric hypoxia. The groups are the following: (1) healthy people living at sea level or at low altitudes; (2) those who were born and live at moderate and high altitudes; (3) those with heart diseases, pulmonary diseases and hemoglobinopathies. The first group can be subdivided into sedentary, active and athletic individuals.

The acclimatization process has no direct correlation with the previous level of physical conditioning. An athlete with high aerobic conditioning is equally exposed to the diseases of altitude as a sedentary individual. In absolute values, however, especially after the acclimatization period, the differences in the cardiopulmonary capacities are kept as at sea level. Physical training and the intensity of the exercises should be differentiated and adequate to each subgroup. Patients with pulmonar hypertension, decompensated heart failure, unstable angina, recent acute myocardial infarction, noncontrolled severe atrial hypertension, severe pulmonary disease, homozygote sickle cell anemia, recurrent thromboembolic episodes, and patients with a severe anemia or reduction in SaO2 can be at high risk. On the other hand, some individuals with the sickle cell trait have their first crisis of vascular occlusion during exercise at these altitudes. In competitions, they have the tolerance to exercise reduced, which until then had not been observed at sea level. Several sports activities are particularly dependent on high altitudes and have their peculiarities. A typical example is mountaineering.

Mountaineering As a general rule, in long ascents at altitudes higher than 3000 m, the positive difference of the altitudes between two consecutive nights should not exceed 300 m, and there should be two nights at the same altitude at every 3 days. To reduce the risks of dehydration caused by inspiration in a cold and dry environment, an abundant hydration with 3–5 L of liquids per day is fundamental, as well as a diet rich in carbohydrates, which release more energy (5.0 kcal/L O2) than lipids (4.7 kcal/L O2).

Athletic Training Acclimatization usually takes 2 weeks at moderate altitudes up to 2300 m. Beyond this altitude, to each additional ascent of 610 m, 1 week should be added, up to the altitude of 4572 m, characterizing a gradual acclimatization considered more physiological and safer. One characteristic of the low threshold of sensitivity to hypobaric hypoxia that we observed was the elevation of the HR at rest, when waking up, 24 h after the arrival at the altitude, in relation to the HR obtained at the wake up time at sea level. An 80% increase would indicate clinical complications at that altitude, requiring an individualized training.

It is believed that in prolonged sports competitions involving races and successive stops, such as soccer and basketball, the players may suffer little influence of the hypobaric hypoxia as a result of a reduced intensity training. This reduction in the intensity of the physical training does not imply reduction in the tactical training, which should be maintained. This is especially important so that the players can get used to a change in the dynamics of the displacement of the ball consequent to the smaller atmospheric pressure. A training carried out correctly, at the ideal level of altitude respecting the acclimatization periods, with a nutritional monitoring and reaching the appropriate training intensity, will certainly be a differential for the performance of endurance athletes. The risks exist, but they can be controlled and eliminated if the necessary precautions are taken.

What Causes Altitude Illnesses?

The concentration of oxygen at sea level is about 21% and the barometric pressure averages 760 mmHg. In order to properly oxygenate the body, your breathing rate (even while at rest) has to increase. This extra ventilation increases the oxygen content in the blood, but not to sea level concentrations. Since the amount of oxygen required for activity is the same, the body must adjust to having less oxygen. In addition, for reasons not entirely understood, high altitude and lower air pressure causes fluid to leak from the capillaries which can cause fluid build-up in both the lungs and the brain. Continuing to higher altitudes without proper acclimatization can lead to potentially serious, even life-threatening illnesses.

Risk Factors

It is not possible to know in advance if someone will become ill when traveling to a high altitude. In addition, being physically fit does not decrease the chances of developing a high altitude illness. However, certain groups are at increased risk, including people who:

- Have a prior history of high altitude illness
- Overexert themselves or drink alcohol before adjusting to the change in altitude
- Ascend rapidly from low elevation to sleeping altitudes above 8000 feet (2400 m).
- Ascend rapidly (>500 to 1000 m/day in sleeping altitude), when over 9000 feet (2700 m).
- Pre-existing cardiopulmonary disease
- Have not been to altitude in the previous few weeks

Preexisting Medical Problems

Travelers with medical conditions such as heart failure, myocardial ischemia (angina), sickle cell disease, any form of pulmonary insufficiency or preexisting hypoxemia, or obstructive sleep apnea (OSA) should consult a physician familiar with high-altitude medical issues before undertaking such travel.

Travel to high elevations does not appear to increase the risk for new events due to ischemic heart disease in previously healthy persons. Patients with well-controlled asthma, hypertension, atrial arrhythmia, and seizure disorders at low elevations generally do well at high elevations. All patients with OSA should receive acetazolamide; those with mild to moderate OSA may do well without their CPAP machines, while those with severe OSA should avoid high elevation travel unless given supplemental oxygen in addition to their CPAP. People with diabetes can travel safely to high elevations, but they must be accustomed to exercise and carefully monitor their blood glucose. Altitude illness can trigger diabetic ketoacidosis, which may be more difficult to treat in those taking acetazolamide. Not all glucose meters read accurately at high elevations.

Most people do not have visual problems at high elevations. However, at very high elevations some people who have had radial keratotomy may develop acute farsightedness and be unable to care for themselves. LASIK and other newer procedures may produce only minor visual disturbances at high elevations.

Travel to high elevations during pregnancy warrants confirmation of good maternal health and verification of a low-risk gestation. A discussion with the traveler of the dangers of having a pregnancy complication in remote, mountainous terrain is also appropriate. That said, there are no studies or case reports of harm to a fetus if the mother travels briefly to high elevations during her pregnancy. It may nevertheless be prudent to recommend that pregnant women do not stay at sleeping elevations above 10,000 ft. (3048 m).

Acute Mountain Sickness

Acute mountain sickness (**AMS**) is the most common of the altitude diseases; it occurs in approximately 40 to 50 percent of people who live at a low altitude and sleep at an altitude above 10,000 feet (3000 m), and in approximately 25 percent of those sleeping above 8000 feet (2400 m). Some people can develop AMS as low as 6500 feet (2000 m).

Symptoms usually occur within 6 to 12 hours of arrival at altitudes above 8000 feet (2400 m). Symptoms can begin as soon as 1 h or as long as 24 h after arriving. AMS does not occur after adjusting to a given altitude for three or more days.

AMS is common at high altitudes. At elevations over 10,000 feet (3048 meters), 75% of people will have mild symptoms. The occurrence of AMS is dependent upon the elevation, the rate of ascent, and individual susceptibility. Many people will experience mild AMS during the acclimatization process. Symptoms usually start 12–24 hours after arrival at altitude and begin to decrease in severity about the third day. The symptoms of Mild AMS are headache, dizziness, fatigue, shortness of breath, loss of appetite, nausea, disturbed sleep, and a general feeling of malaise. Symptoms tend to be worse at night and when respiratory drive is decreased. Mild AMS does not interfere with normal activity and symptoms generally subside within 2–4 days as the body acclimatizes. As long as symptoms are mild, and only a nuisance, ascent can continue at a moderate rate. When hiking, it is essential that you communicate any symptoms of illness immediately to others on your trip.

There are no clinical signs for AMS and the diagnosis is made in the history, The difficulty in identifying AMS is the non-specific nature of symptoms, which climbers may assign to fatigue or sleep deprivation. The scoring system for symptom severity is subjective and relies on self-reporting. In the context of field diagnosis, it is wise to assume that such non-specific symptoms are AMS unless strong evidence is available implicating an alternative cause. It is also important not to overlook conditions with similar non-specific presentations, for example hypothermia, dehydration, hypoglycaemia and hyponatraemia.

Moderate AMS

Moderate AMS includes severe headache that is not relieved by medication, nausea and vomiting, increasing weakness and fatigue, shortness of breath, and decreased coordination (ataxia). Normal activity is difficult, although the person may still be able to walk on their own. At this stage, only advanced medications or descent can reverse the problem.

Severe AMS

Severe AMS presents as an increase in the severity of the mentioned symptoms, including shortness of breath at rest, inability to walk, decreasing mental status, and fluid buildup in the lungs.

High Altitude Cerebral Edema

High altitude cerebral edema **(HACE)** is a rare life-threatening altitude disease, and is a severe form of acute mountain sickness (AMS). It is caused by leaky capillaries in the brain, which causes fluid accumulation and brain swelling. it is most often associated with HAPE. In addition to AMS symptoms, lethargy becomes profound, with drowsiness, confusion, and ataxia on tandem gait test, similar to alcohol intoxication. A person with HACE requires immediate descent; if the person fails to descend, death can occur within 24 h of developing ataxia. It usually happens at altitudes higher than 4500 m. The victim is usually tired, with no conditions to objectively evaluate his/her own status.

The fine movements of the hands, fingers and eyes are affected. Edema and petechial hemorrhages are typically found in the brain at autopsy. Prevention can be done through a slow ascent, good hydration and avoidance of strenuous exercises.

Descent is the treatment and it should be started immediately because evolution to death can be rapid. Oxygen improves the symptoms, but when interrupted, the situation aggravates even more. Dexamethasone does not affect cerebral edema, but reduces the symptoms and, therefore, makes the descent easier.

The mechanism for HACE is better understood than for AMS. Cerebral edema develops following cerebral vasodilation secondary to hypoxia. Hypoxaemia results in overperfusion of microvasculature, an increase in hydrostatic pressure and leakage from capillaries. Autopsies reveal edema and magnetic resonance imaging (MRI) studies demonstrate white matter changes in keeping with oedema in the splenium of the corpus callosum.

High Altitude Pulmonar Edema (HAPE)

HAPE is a noncardiogenic pulmonar edema. It is accompanied by pulmonary hypertension, an increase in the pulmonar capillary permeability and hypoxemia. Hypoxic pulmonary vasoconstriction has been proposed as being non-uniform throughout the pulmonary circulation, causing regional overperfusion. Endothelial dysfunction may also be instigated. Endothelial nitric oxide synthase gene polymorphisms confer genetic suspectibility, and therefore impaired nitric oxide synthesis may be an underlying mechanism in HAPE.

There are several hypotheses to explain this increase in permeability and some of them are listed below:

1. pulmonary arterial hypertension;
2. hypoxia inducing the release of inflammatory mediators, such as cytokines, ET-1, and intercellular adhesion molecule (ICAM-1)
3. hyperperfusion of the pulmonary vessels not undergoing vasoconstriction (hypoxic pulmonar vasoconstriction is extensive but not uniform) leading to dilation and high flow in the capillaries and consequente capillary lesion.

HAPE typically occurs in young and healthy mountaineers and is precipitated by rapid ascents at altitudes above 2500–3000 m. There is an individual susceptibility and it tends to recur. HAPE clinically manifests 2–5 days after acute exposure to hypobaric hypoxia, 78% of the cases appear until the tenth day, with the following symptoms: abnormal dyspnea on effort and, later, even at rest, cyanosis, dry cough that evolves to a mucous-sanguinolent cough, and tachycardia. Teleradiography shows diffuse alveolar images unevenly distributed. The alveolar fluid is rich in proteins and inflammatory mediators. An electrocardiogram demonstrates sinus tachycardia, right axis deviation, right bundle branch block or right strain. It is important to consider other causes of this clinical presentation, for example respiratory infection or cardiac conditions. HAPE is a severe and potentially fatal condition and immediate descent is mandatory.

The Differential Diagnosis

The differential diagnosis of is broad and includes: dehydration, exhaustion, hypoglycemia, hypothermia, hyponatremia, asthma, acute bronchitis, heart failure, mucus plugging, myocardial infarction, pneumonia, pulmonary embolus. Infections, drug effects, neurologic problems. Focal neurologic symptoms and seizures are rare in HACE and should lead to suspicion of an intracranial lesion or seizure disorder.

Encephalopathy from any cause may mimic HACE. Acute psychosis, intracranial vascular malformation, intracranial mass lesions, carbon monoxide poisoning, infection of the central nervous system, migraine, seizure, stroke, and transient ischemic attacks are all potential confounding disorders and must be considered in the differential diagnosis.

Diagnosis

Patients suffering from more severe forms of altitude-related illness, such as HAPE or HACE, are frequently in austere environments where access to diagnostic studies is limited. In these cases, a diagnosis of altitude-related illness must be made on clinical grounds and treatment initiated without the benefit of confirmatory laboratory testing or diagnostic imaging.

Currently, no widely accepted confirmatory laboratory studies exist for the diagnosis of AMS, HACE, or HAPE. Laboratory abnormalities may be secondary to accompanying dehydration and stress. Arterial blood gases, particularly in HAPE, may demonstrate marked hypoxia.

When imaging modalities are available, patchy, peripheral infiltrates representing pulmonary edema are seen on chest radiographs or CTs in the early stages of HAPE. As the disorder progresses, the edema becomes homogenous and diffuse.

In AMS, MRI studies may show a mild increase in cerebral volume, possibly reflecting minor cerebral edema. Brain MRI findings in HACE are more consistent and characterized by increased T2 signal intensity in the corpus callosum and centrum semiovale, as well as micro hemorrhages in the corpus callosum.

Prevention of Altitude Illnesses

Prevention of altitude illnesses falls into two categories, proper acclimatization and preventive medications. Below are a few basic guidelines for proper acclimatization.

- If possible, don't fly or drive to high altitude. Start below 10,000 feet (3048 m) and walk up.
- If you do fly or drive, do not over-exert yourself or move higher for the first 24 hours.
- If you go above 10,000 feet (3048 m), only increase your altitude by 1000 feet (305 m) per day and for every 3000 feet (915 m) of elevation gained, take a rest day.
- "Climb High and sleep low." This is the maxim used by climbers. You can climb more than 1000 feet (305 m) in a day as long as you come back down and sleep at a lower altitude.
- If you begin to show symptoms of moderate altitude illness, don't go higher until symptoms decrease
- If symptoms increase, go down!
- Keep in mind that different people will acclimatize at different rates. Make sure all of your party is properly acclimatized before going higher.
- Stay properly hydrated. Acclimatization is often accompanied by fluid loss, so you need to drink lots of fluids to remain properly hydrated (at least 3–4 quarts per day). Urine output should be copious and clear.
- Take it easy; don't over-exert yourself when you first get up to altitude. Light activity during the day is better than sleeping because respiration decreases during sleep, exacerbating the symptoms.
- Avoid tobacco and alcohol and other depressant drugs including, barbiturates, tranquilizers, and sleeping pills. These depressants further decrease the respiratory drive during sleep resulting in a worsening of the symptoms.
- Eat a high carbohydrate diet (more than 70% of your calories from carbohydrates) while at altitude.
- The acclimatization process is inhibited by dehydration, over-exertion, and alcohol and other depressant drugs.

Pharmacological Prophylaxis

For those at moderate or high risk of developing AMS, pharmacological prophylaxis may be considered:

- Acetazolamide is effective with a low risk of side effects. Prophylactic doses of acetazolamide are 125 mg twice daily for adults and 2.5 mg/kg twice daily in the pediatric population.
- Although acetazolamide is the preferred agent, dexamethasone is effective in preventing AMS at a dose of 2 mg every 6 h or 4 mg every 12 h.
- In rare circumstances that dictate the need for rapid ascent to very high altitude (over 3500 meters) with exertion, consideration may be given to concomitant use of both acetazolamide and dexamethasone.
- Prophylaxis should be started one day prior to ascent and may be stopped after 2–3 days at maximum elevation or upon initiation of descent.

Treatment

AMS treatment AMS treatment includes rest, descent, and may also include medicines to relieve symptoms. You should not exercise or proceed higher until your symptoms have resolved. You should also know when and if you need to seek help.

- The best and most effective treatment for HACE, HAPE, or severe AMS is descent.
- Since exertion may exacerbate altitude-related illness, individuals should minimize exertion during descent. The descent should be at least 1000 m or should be continued until symptoms improve. If available, supplemental oxygen may be titrated to achieve an oxygen saturation of >90 percent.
- Portable hyperbaric chambers, such as the Gamow bag, may be used for treatment of HACE or HAPE. Although effective, these devices require knowledgeable personnel for operation, and caution must be used with patients who are claustrophobic or vomiting.
- Portable hyperbaric chambers are inflatable pressure bags used in remote settings that can treat people with HACE when immediate descent is not feasible.
- While use of acetazolamide at higher doses than those used for prophylaxis has been employed in treatment of severe AMS, the agent is used primarily in mild or moderate AMS. In adults, the treatment dose for acetazolamide is 250 mg twice daily.
- Acetazolamide inhibits carbonic anhydrase, and thus reduces the conversion of carbon dioxide to bicarbonate and protons. It causes a bicarbonate diuresis and a metabolic acidosis through its inhibition in the renal system. It increases poikilo-

capnic HVR, accelerating a mechanism that occurs usually with acclimati¬sation. Other potential beneficial effects include increasing carbon dioxide retention through inhibition of vascular carbonic anhydrase, and the decrease of CSF production.

- A randomised controlled trial comparing higher doses showed no improved AMS prophylactic efficacy and an increase in the side-effect of paraesthesia, typically experienced in the extremities. Possible side effects include tingling of the lips and finger tips, blurring of vision, and alteration of taste. These side effects may be reduced with the 125 mg. dose. Side effects subside when the drug is stopped.
- Dexamethasone is used for moderate or severe AMS or HACE and may be administered orally, intramuscularly, or intravenously. The initial dose is 8 mg, followed by 4 mg every 6 h until symptoms abate.
- Dexamethasone is comparable to acetazolamide in terms of prophylactic efficacy in reducing AMS symptom scores when rapidly ascending to altitude in a randomised controlled trial, but should be reserved for the emergency treatment of AMS and HACO. The mechanism of prevention is unknown but is likely to be related to vessel permeability and cytokine regulation. You should take it immediately if you develop signs of HACE, with the recommended dose being 8 to 10 mg by mouth. You should take 4 mg every 6 h thereafter until you have descended. You should take dexamethasone before entering a hyperbaric chamber.
- While the literature is replete with reports of other pharmacological adjuncts in the treatment of HAPE, descent and supplemental oxygen remain the mainstays of management. Nifedipine has demonstrated some efficacy in the treatment of acute HAPE with a recommended dose of 60 mg of the sustained release preparation daily. Reports exist for combination therapy with pulmonary vasodilators, acetazolamide and inhaled beta-2 agonists. Utilization of positive pressure ventilation and oxygen supplementation has also been described with beneficial effects. The use of sildenafil for HAPO is appealing because of its primary vasodilator action on pulmonary rather than systemic vessels, perceivably decreasing the risk of systemic hypotension and cerebral hypoperfusion when compared with nifedipine. No robust studies of phosphodiesterase inhibitors in HAPO treatment have yet been conducted and there is some clinical experience that it increases AMS severity, so its use is not currently recommended. Current guidelines focus on descent in the remote setting with supplementary oxygen or nifedipine adjuncts. Hyperbaric therapy should not delay descent but can be used whilst awaiting evacuation. There is no role for diuretics in HAPO treatment.

In general, for those without previous history of AHAI, pharmacological prophylaxis should not be required and an appropriately controlled ascent rate should be employed to prevent AMS and HACO. In high-risk situations, where (a) the individual is susceptible, (b) an altitude greater than 3500 m is attained in 1 day or (c) ascent must be faster than 300 m/day, acetazolamide 125 mg twice daily is considered first line.

Oxygen supplementation can be used as an alternative to descent in selected patients, or as an adjunct to descent in severe AMS or HACO. Oxygen saturations greater than 90% should be achieved. Portable hyperbaric chambers can also be used, but this should not delay descent and, practically, their use in patients with severe nausea, vomiting or decreased conscious level can be challenging.

- Headache – non-prescription medicines for headache, such as aspirin, acetaminophen, or ibuprofen
- Nausea or vomiting – a prescription medicine such as ondansetron may be helpful, if it is available.

Prognosis

With adequate rest and adherence to treatment guidelines, individuals with mild or moderate AMS generally recover within a few days. HACE and HAPE are often fatal if left untreated. Clinical features of HAPE often improve after several days at a lower altitude. Neurological symptoms from HACE may take weeks or longer to resolve.

After an episode of AMS, ascent can be re-attempted once symptoms have completely resolved. Non-pharmacological prophylactic measures such as slow rate of ascent and pharmacological prophylaxis should be undertaken. In the case of HAPE and HACE, it is more controversial but there are no guidelines contraindicating re-ascent. Once again, prophylactic measures must be strongly considered.

What Other Considerations Exist for Patients Travelling to High Altitudes?

Retinal hemorrhages are relatively common at altitude, with reported incidences up to 56%. Most hemorrhages are asymptomatic and transient. Their development does not mandate descent unless the macula is involved and visual acuity is compromised. Acute exposure to the hypobaric hypoxia of altitude may exacerbate underlying chronic illness. Travel to high altitude is contraindicated in patients with pulmonary hypertension and uncompensated congestive heart failure, as the hypoxic environment increases mean pulmonary artery pressure. Patients with sickle-cell disease are prone to development of splenic infarcts and sickle-cell crises at high altitude and should avoid such environments.

Patients with severe COPD should not travel to altitude. Those with milder COPD may travel, but they should have access to pulse oximetry and supplemental oxygen.

Cardiac arrhythmias are more common at high altitude than at lower altitudes. Patients with a history of arrhythmias should have ready access to supplemental oxygen and should limit physical exertion at altitude. Patients with a history of coronary artery disease should be evaluated by a cardiologist prior to ascent to altitude; a cardiac stress test may be warranted. Asthma is not exacerbated by ascent to high altitude; usual asthma management should be continued. Although mild increases in blood pressure accompany ascent to altitude, the patient's sea-level antihypertensive regimen does not usually require modification.

Recommendations

The following recommendations can be given from these considerations related to the preparation of an endurance competition at altitude in terms of psychological aspects:

- Firstly, an early arrival (at least 42–52 h prior to the competition) is preferable to avoid possible riskier decision making, mood disturbances and the related detrimental effects on endurance performance. An early arrival is also recommended on the basis of physiological aspects.
- Secondly, a preexposure of the athlete to moderate altitude to study the athlete's individual reaction in terms of cognitive functions and mood states is advised. Ideally, the pre-exposure takes place in the same or a similar environment and altitude as the competition. In cases, where this is not possible, a pre-exposure to normobaric hypoxia corresponding to the competition altitude might be used. A preexposure might also be used for imagery training.
- Thirdly, CHO and/or cafeine supplementation might support to decrease the perceived effort during competition.

HAPE is one of most dangerous conditions related to increased altitude exposure among unacclimatized athletes. Athletes should be aware that the acclimatization process does not correlate with the level of physical conditioning. However, after acclimatization, cardiopulmonary capacity is the same as it is at sea level.

- Within the first days of acclimatization, athletes are at high risk of dehydration due to increased respiratory water loss by enhanced ventilation, increased urinary water loss, and an increase in basal metabolic rate. Thus, athletes should be encouraged to drink sufficient fluids while at altitude.
- Overall, authors recommend regular monitoring of body mass and urine osmolality during altitude training to ensure proper hydration and to prevent overdrinking since both hypohydration and hyperhydration impair performance and present a risk to health. At altitude, the stress response to exercise is enhanced, and thus CHO requirements are higher than at sea level. CHO consumption before exercise in hypoxia can mitigate some of the negative symptoms of high altitude, like less oxygen saturation and ventilation.

Conclusion

The optimum for achieving better results in endurance competitions at altitudes is to be born or at least live permanently and train at such altitudes or to move to altitude at any time over the course of the sporting carrier. If for logistical and/or socio-economic reasons athletes cannot move permanently to a higher altitude, it seems optimal to undergo an at least 2- to 4-week training camp before a important competition. The specific preparation cannot be done successfully without prior repeated testing in training camps at altitude to learn the course of acclimatization of the individual athlete.

From the presented findings of various aspects of an optimal preparation for endurance competition at altitude, it may be concluded that the acclimatization process and performance recovery nearly reach a plateau after about 2 weeks at altitudes up to 4500 m. Individual psychological conditions and appropriate diet and training are important modifiers of the preparation progress and related competition success. However, in reality preparation regimens may largely deviate.

Bibliography

1. Bartsch P, Swenson ER. Acute high-altitude illnesses. N Engl J Med. 2013;369(17):1666–7.
2. Hackett P. High altitude and common medical conditions. In: Hornbein TF, Schoene RB, editors. High altitude: an exploration of human adaptation. New York: Marcel Dekker; 2001. p. 839–85.
3. Hackett PH, Roach RC. High altitude cerebral edema. High Alt Med Biol. 2004;5(2):136–46.
4. Hackett PH, Roach RC. High-altitude medicine and physiology. In: Auerbach PS, editor. Wilderness medicine. 6th ed. Philadelphia: Mosby Elsevier; 2012. p. 2–32.
5. Johnson TS, Rock PB, Fulco CS, Trad LA, Spark RF, Maher JT. Prevention of acute mountain sickness by dexamethasone. N Engl J Med. 1984;310(11):683–6.
6. Luks AM, McIntosh SE, Grissom CK, Auerbach PS, Rodway GW, Schoene RB, et al. Wilderness Medical Society consensus guidelines for the prevention and treatment of acute altitude illness. Wilderness Environ Med. 2010;21(2):146–55.
7. Luks AM, Swenson ER. Medication and dosage considerations in the prophylaxis and treatment of high-altitude illness. Chest. 2008;133(3):744–55.
8. Maggiorini M, Brunner-La Rocca HP, Peth S, Fischler M, Bohm T, Bernheim A, et al. Both tadalafil and dexamethasone may reduce the incidence of high-altitude pulmonary edema: a randomized trial. Ann Intern Med. 2006;145(7):497–506.
9. Pollard AJ, Murdoch DR. The high altitude medicine handbook. 3rd ed. Abingdon, UK: Radcliffe Medical Press; 2003.
10. Pollard AJ, Niermeyer S, Barry P, Bartsch P, Berghold F, Bishop RA, et al. Children at high altitude: an international consensus statement by an ad hoc committee of the International Society for Mountain Medicine, March 12, 2001. High Alt Med Biol. 2001;2(3):389–403.
11. Bärtsch P, Swenson ER. Acute high-altitude illnesses. N Engl J Med. 2013;369:1666.
12. Luks AM, Auerbach PS, Freer L, et al. Wilderness Medical Society Clinical Practice Guidelines for the prevention and treatment of acute altitude illness: 2019 update. Wilderness Environ Med. 2019;30:S3.

13. Gore CJ, Clark SA, Saunders PU. Nonhematological mechanisms of improve sea-level performance after hypoxic exposure. Med Sci Sports Exerc. 2007;39(9):1600–9.
14. Gore CJ, Hopkins WG. Counterpoint: positive effects of intermittent hypoxic (live high – train low) on exercise performance are not mediated primarily by augmented red cell volume. J Appl Physiol. 2005;99(5):2055–7.
15. Kohin S, et al. Preconditioning improves function and recovery of single muscle fibers during severe hypoxic and reoxygenation. Am J Physiol Cell Physiol. 2001;281:142–6.
16. Levine BD, Stray-Gundersen J. Point: positive effects of intermittent hypoxia (live high – train low) on exercise performance are mediated primarily by augmented red cell volume. J Appl Physiol. 2005;99(5):2053–5.
17. Lorenz KA, et al. Effects of hypoxic on the onset of muscle deoxygenation and the lactate threshold. J Physiol Sci. 2006;56(4):321–3.
18. Mazzeo RS. Physiological responses to exercise at altitude. Sports Med. 2008;38(1):01–8.
19. Mcardle W, Katch FI, Katch VL. Fisiologia do Exercício: Energia, Nutrição e Desempenho Humano. 5th ed. Rio de Janeiro: Guanabara Koogan; 2003. p. 1175.
20. Muza SR. Military applications of hypoxic training for high-altitude operations. Med Sci Sports Exerc. 2007;39(9):1625–31.
21. Ogura Y, et al. Sprint- interval training-induced alterations of myosin heavy chain isoforms and enzymes activities in rat diaphragm: effects of normobaric hypoxia. Jpn J Physiol. 2005;55(6):309–16.
22. Robach P, et al. Strong iron demand during hypoxia-induced erythropoiesis is associated with down-regulation of iron-related proteins an myoglobin in human skeletal muscle. Blood. 2007;109(11):4724–31.
23. Szubski C, Burtscher M, Löscher WN. Neuromuscular fatigue during sustained contractions performed in short-term hypoxic. Med Sci Sports Exerc. 2007;39(6):948–54.
24. West JB. The physiologic basis of high-altitude diseases. Ann Intern Med. 2004;141(10):789–800.
25. Wilber RL. Application of altitude/hypoxic training by elite athletes. Med Sci Sports Exerc. 2007;39(9):1610–24.
26. Wilber RL, Stray-Gundersen J, Levine BD. Effect of hypoxic "dose" on physiological responses and sea-level performance. Med Sci Sports Exerc. 2007;39(9):1590–9.

Chapter 18
Importance of the Diagnosis of Patent Foramen Ovale to Prevent Ischemic Stroke in Height Altitude and Diving

Ignacio Previgliano

The Case

A 28 years old male arrives to the emergency room at 1 a.m. with a left hemiparesis and a National Institute of Health Stroke Scale (NIHSS) scale of 12 points. His wife said that it presented suddenly after parking the car 30 minutes ago and he was a healthy person, and put as an example they just arrived 12 h ago from a diving holiday in Cozumel, México. His vital signs were: Blood Pressure (BP) 160/100 mmHg, Heart Rate (HR) 68 per minute, Respiratory Rate 18 per minute. He has a normal electrocardiogram. Twenty minutes after admission he was sent to the radiology department for a CT scan. The study was informed as normal without early warning signs of middle cerebral artery infarction. With this CT findings, according to the protocol [1], recombinant Tissue Plaminogen Activator (rTPA) was started at a dose of 0.9 mg/kg, 10% in bolus and 90% in one hour infusion. Cerebrolysin, a

I. Previgliano (✉)
Hospital General de Agudos J. A. Fernandez, Ciudad Autonoma de Buenos Aires, Argentina

© The Author(s), under exclusive license to Springer Nature Switzerland AG 2023
J. Hidalgo et al. (eds.), *High Altitude Medicine*,
https://doi.org/10.1007/978-3-031-35092-4_18

neurotrophic factors preparation with neuroprotective and neuroregenerative action, was also started at a dose of 30 ml/day for 10 days [2, 3]. After treatment the patient was moved to the Intensive Care Unit. Transcranial doppler (TCD) ultrasound showed a 30% difference in blood flow velocities (BFV) in mean cerebral arteries (MCA) due to the decrease in the right velocities. Neck vessels ultrasound and transthoracic echocardiography were normal.

After 12 hours from admission his NIHISS worsened to 20 points, a new CT scan was performed and showed a right middle cerebral artery infarction. After the scan the patient deteriorated with a NHISS of 22 points, due to coma. Neurosurgical consultation was performed and decompressive craniectomy with dural expansion was decided [1]. A fiberoptic catheter was placed in the left hemisphere. After surgery the patient was mechanically ventilated, adapted with midazolam and fentanyl. Intracranial (ICP) and mean arterial pressure (MAP) monitoring was performed and the treatment objective was to maintain a cerebral perfusion pressure (CPP) above 70 mmHg. Meanwhile a transesophageal echocardiogram (TEE) with hydro-air contrast was performed and ruled out Patent Foramen Ovale (PFO).

After 5 days of neurointensive management the patient was weaned from ventilator, drugs and monitoring devices. His NIHSS returned to initial values (11 points). A new TCD showed symmetric BFV in both MCAs and microembolic signals (MES). As the patient was lucid and collaborative a TCD with hydro-air contrast was performed. The first examination revealed "drop passage" (6 bubbles) while the second with the Valsalva maneuver showed "curtain passage" (more than 30 bubbles). All these findings were compatible with right to left shunt, probably due to PFO in spite of negative TEE results [4, 5].

According to the best evidence-based treatment [6] PFO closure with an AMPLATZER device was decided.

The patient was derived to a rehabilitation facility and his NHISS at 90 day was 3 (very mild facial and left leg paresis, mild dysarthriaslurring but can be understood). Magnetic Resonance Imaging diffusion tensor imaging and tractography.

The Standard Approach to Management

This patient received the standard approach to diagnosis and treatment according to stroke guidelines. Mechanical thrombectomy was not possible to perform due to logistic troubles, so decompressive craniectomy was chosen.

Beyond these clinical considerations, this case motivated us to consider aspects that would have passed by without adequate critical reflection:

1. Is there any relationship between PFO and diving, decompression sickness or high-altitude pulmonaryedema, or stroke onset?
2. Which is the best diagnostic maneuver for PFO identification?
3. Is any indication for PFO screening or closure in divers or heigh altitude climbers?

Is there any Relationship Between PFO and Diving, Decompression Sickness or High-Altitude Pulmonaryedema, or Stroke Onset?

During embryogenesis, tissue oxygenation of the fetus takes place through exchange with maternal blood through the placenta. Because the fetal lungs are obviously inactive, the atria are widely communicated through the foramen ovale in order to provide a fast circulation.

At the time of birth, with the first breath, there is a decrease in pulmonary vascular resistance and pressures in the right atrium, with which the foramen ovale, part of the septum primun, adheres to the septum secundum, closing the atrial communication. This process of independence of the right and left circulations remains active during the first two years of life.

Nevertheless in 20–25% of the population this foramen remains patent. In these PFO population some physiological conditions as deep breathing, coughing, sneezing, or physical activities that involve a Valsalva maneuver can lead to a transient right-to-left shunt. Atrial septum aneurysm is another septal defect that it is associated with 15% to 18% of POF, mainly with the larger ones.

The respiratory system is crucial in the hemostatic homeostasis. The fine pulmonary vessels fulfill a filter function for venous blood, retaining mechanically or by specific adherence, aged blood cells, micro clots, adipose cells, placental cells, etc., elements that are normally forming in or entering the bloodstream. It is logical to hypothesize that many of these detritus could pass through PFO during transient right-to-left shunting. This situation could explain white matter hyperintensities, formally ischemic lesions [7], seen in young patients with asymptomatic PFO. It goes without saying that in the presence of a larger emboli source, such as deep vein thrombosis, a larger clot can cause a paradoxical embolism in a larger cerebral artery.

The relationship between stroke and PFO was established in two studies [8, 9] in patients from 40 to 55 years old with cryptogenic stroke in which PFO was present 40–50% and absent in 10–15%, using contrast echocardiography. Further studies confirmed these findings [10].

Decompression sickness is caused by the generation of bubbles produced as a consequence of the nitrogen saturation in the tissues that occurred during the descent. As the diver returns to the surface, the sum of the gas stresses in the tissue can exceed the ambient pressure and cause the release of free gas from the tissues in the form of bubbles.

They can alter organ function by occluding blood vessels, compressing tissues and / or causing endothelial damage with subsequent activation of the coagulation and inflammation cascades.

Gas bubbles are generally present in the venous circulation due to the low pressure and high tension of the gas. The presence of bubbles alone does not necessarily mean that DCS will develop.

Nevertheless, several studies demonstrate that the presence of a PFO is associated with a two- to fivefold increase in the risk for developing severe DCS, and that the risk is greater PFO size and septal mobility.

Although skydiving has a similar physic than diving, there are no articles relating the activity to stroke, except for one that attribute it to carotid artery dissection.

Acute Mountain Sickness [11] (AMS)is characterized by headache, gastrointestinal upset, fatigue, difficulty sleeping, and lightheadedness of sudden onset while there is a rapidly ascend to significant altitudes. AMS can progress to life threatening conditions such as High-Altitude Pulmonary Edema (HAPE) and High-Altitude Cerebral Edema (HACE) [10].

A prospective study [12] studied PFO prevalence in 137 hikers and AMS developing. PFO search was performed by contrast TCD, identifying it in 43% of the study population.

There was a higher prevalence of PFO in hikers with AMS 15/24 (63%) compared to hikers without AMS 44/113 (39%); $p = 0.034$. In the multivariate model, the presence of a PFO significantly increased the risk for developing AMS: OR 4.15. In a previous research Allemand [13] found that a PFO was 4 to 5 times more likely to be identified in professional mountain climbers who were HAPE-susceptible compared to those who were HAPE-resistant.

A very illustrative study from Lovering et al. [14] state that effects on physiological processes are likely dependent on both the presence and size of the PFO. The involved pathophysiologic mechanism could be worsened pulmonary gas exchange and blunted ventilatory acclimatization.

Exaggerated pulmonary hypertension and right ventricular dysfunction have been found in patients with PFO living at high altitude. This was associated with enlargement of the right ventricle at rest and an exaggerated increase in the pressure gradient and dysfunction of the right ventricle and a moderate increase in the fractional area change of the ventricle right ventricle during light exercise [15].

Individuals who undergo successful closure of their PFO can travel or live at high altitudes without difficulty [77].

Which Is the Best Diagnostic Maneuver for PFO Identification?

As we have analyzed above PFO's presence, size and associated septal defects are related to diving and heigh altitude complications. So, it diagnostic is mainfull.

Although TEE is considered "the gold standard" for PFO diagnosis, meta-analyzes seem to indicate that this is not the case.

Our first warning that DTC could become a more important tool than echocardiographic techniques for the diagnosis of PFO came from the study performed by Gonzalez-Alujas et al. [16]. They prospectively analyzed 134 patients performing simultaneously transthoracic ecocardiogram (TTE) with TCD and TEE with TCD, using agitated saline solution to detect right to left shunt. TTE and TCD showed higher sensitivity (100% vs 97%; non-significant difference) than TEE in the diagnosis of PFO (86%; $p < .001$). TEE underestimated shunt severity.

For the purposes of this chapter, we review the related literature, finding three important meta-analyzes [17–19] that supported Gonzalez-Aluja study.

Regarding the TCD's accuracy for intracardiac right-to-left shunt diagnosis [15], the meta-analysis examined data from 27 studies with 1968 patients and concluded that "TCD is a reliable, noninvasive test with excellent diagnostic accuracies, making it a proficient test for detecting RLS. TCD can be used as a part of the stroke workup and for patients being considered for PFO closure. If knowledge of the precise anatomy is required, then TEE can be obtained before scheduling a patient for transcatheter PFO closure".

Reviewing the diagnostic value of TTE for PFO diagnosis [16], the meta-analysis surveyed 16 studies with 1831 patients and revealed a sensitivity of 88% and specificity of 97%. Data suggested "that TTE is a test with high sensitivity and specificity in detection of PFO, but it may not be appropriate for screening for PFO in all patients, especially patients with a small right-left shunt".

With only 164 patients included, meta-analysis of TEE diagnostic value [17] showed a weighted sensitivity of 89.2% and specificity of 91.4% to detect PFO, but it's still considered for many investigators as the gold standard for PFO diagnosis.

According the American Academy of Neurology [20], compared with TEE, TCD has a sensitivity of 100% and a specificity greater than 95%.

It's important to bear in mind the operator dependence of all ultrasound studies. In our experience with 55 patients studied with TCD for PFO diagnosis, we found a 96% of positive predictive value and a 100% negative predictive value for TCD compared with right heart catheterization, the real gold standard. In these case series TTE reached the same values but after repeating the study with an experienced operator in 10 patients. This fact highlights the operator dependence as in all US proceedings.

A proper bubble TCD examination should be performed with the following technique: (a) patient at 45 °, (b) placement of a peripheral venous line in the right or left upper limb (ulnar vein) and placement of a 3-way stopcock, (c) continuous isonation of at least one middle cerebral artery, (d) contrast preparation: a syringe with 9 ml of isotonic saline solution and another syringe with 1 ml of air, (e) contrast stirring and bolus injection through the 3-way stopcock, and (f) repetition of the procedure with the performance of the Valsalva maneuver with a resistance of 40 mmHg [21]. The correct Valsalva maneuver is crucial to PFO opening and shunt demonstration.

The passage of bubbles is categorized into 4 groups: (a) negative result (without passage), (b) from 1 to 10 bubbles ("in drop"), (c) from 10 to 20 ("in rain") and (d) more than 20 ("In curtain"), where the large number of bubbles does not allow their counting (Fig. 18.1).

With a similar technique, in Figs. 18.2 and 18.3, are examples of contrast TTE and TEE findings in PFO diagnosis.

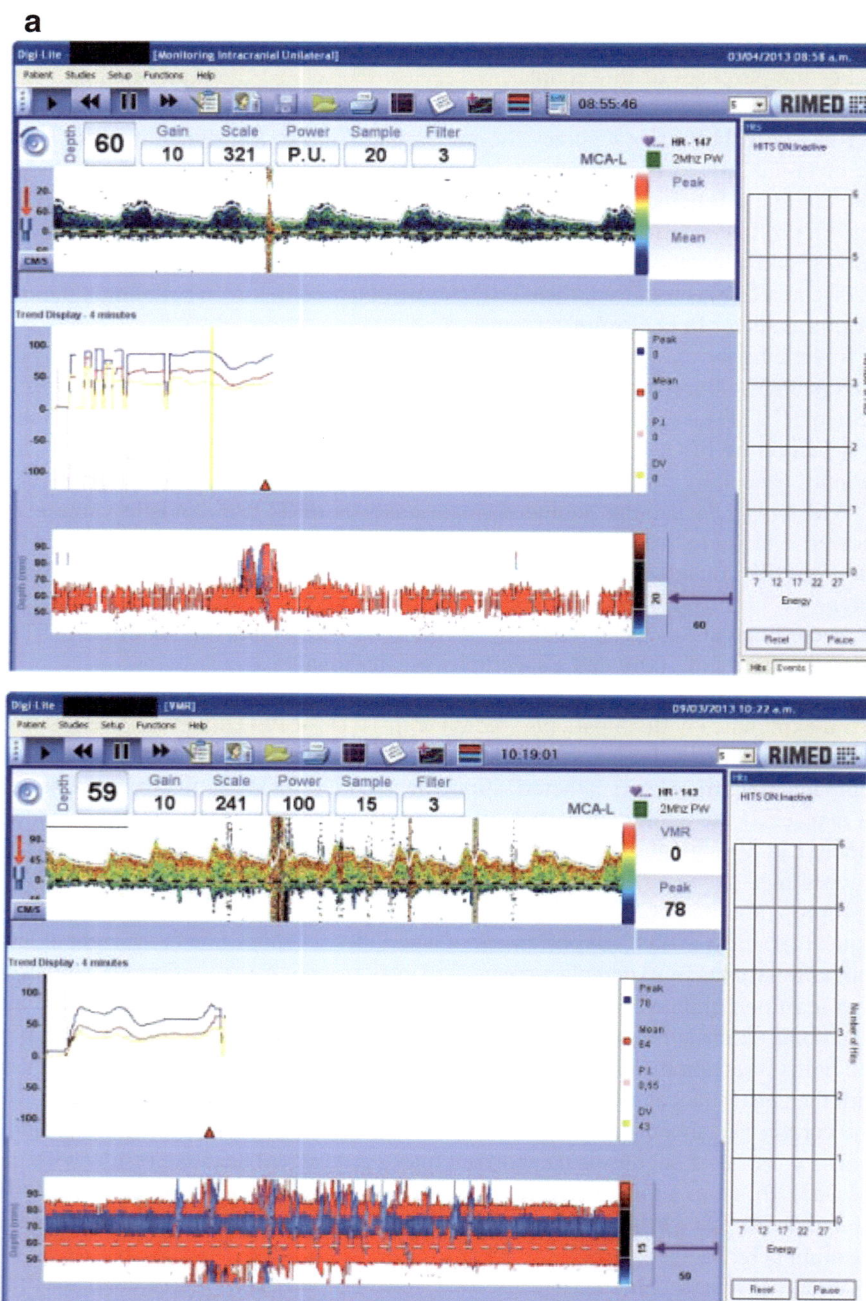

Fig. 18.1 TCD with stirred saline injection. Passage of "bubbles" is observed both in the spectral view and in M mode: (**a**) "drop" passage of a single bubble (less than 10 bubbles), (**b**) "rain" passage of more than 10 bubbles, (**c**) "curtain", bubbles can't be counted

b

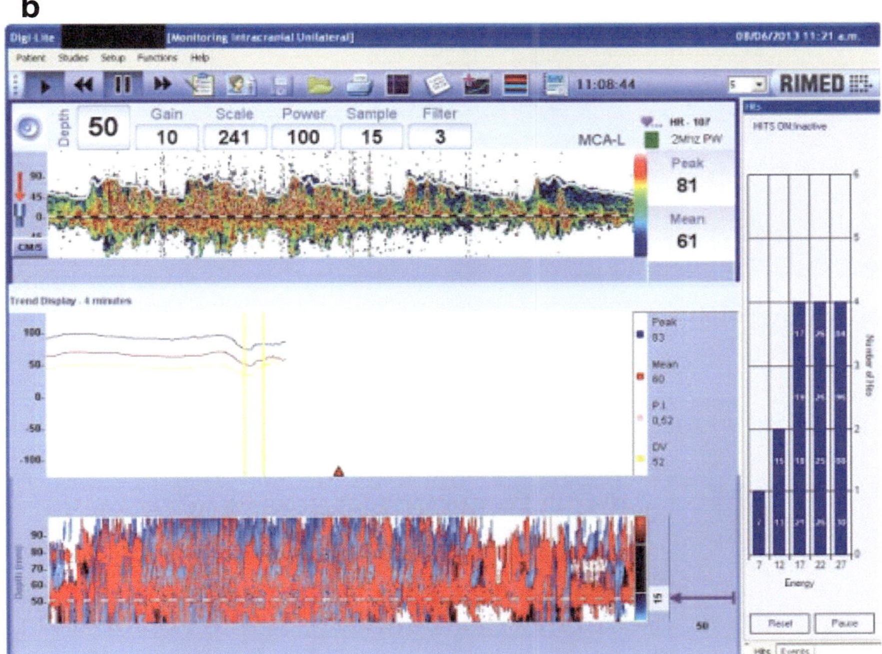

Fig. 18.1 (continued)

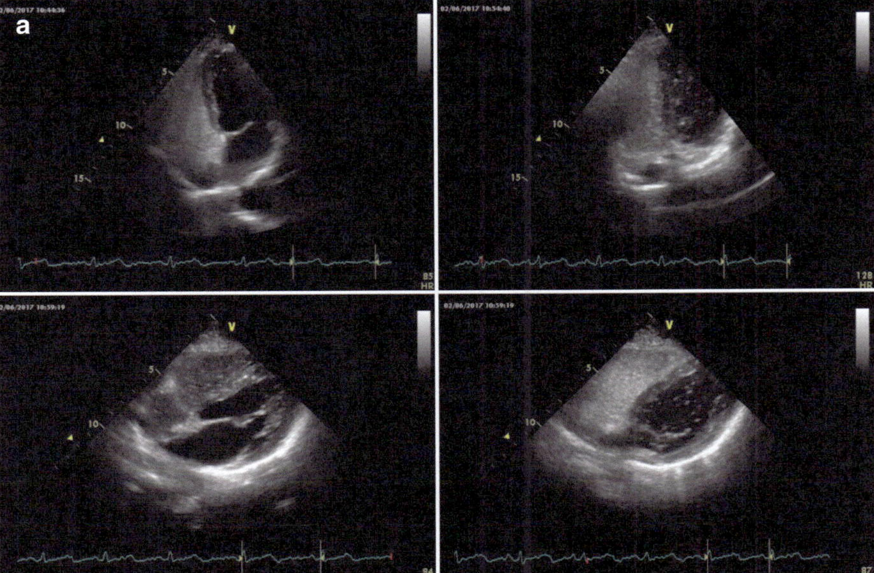

Fig. 18.2 Transthoracic echocardiography with stirred saline injection. Passage of "bubbles" is observed: (**a**) passage of more than 5 and less than10 bubbles, (**b**) passage of more than 10 bubbles, (**c**) passage of bubbles can't be counted

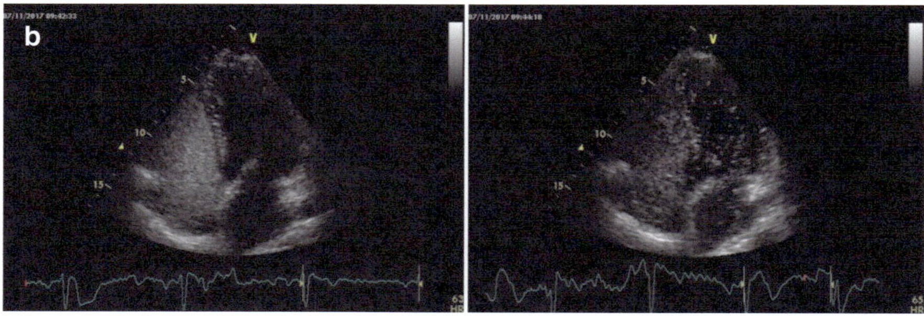

Fig. 18.2 continued

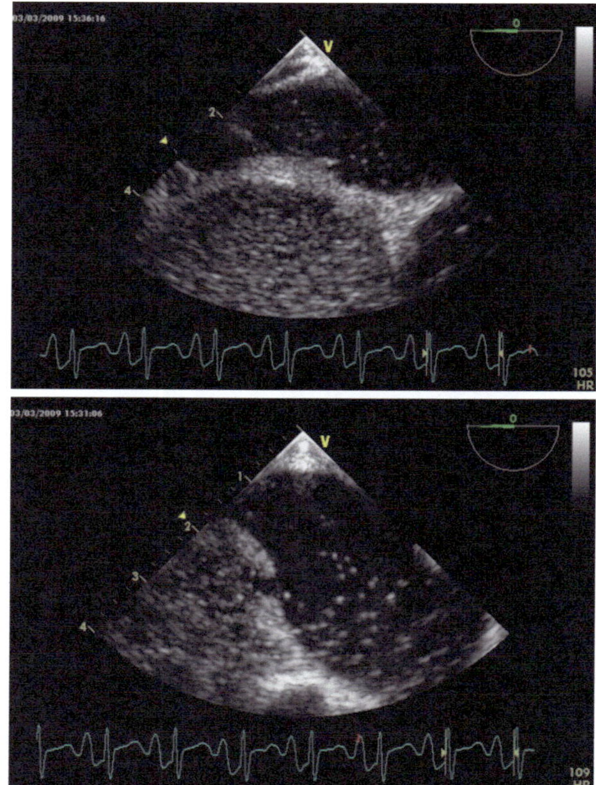

Fig. 18.3 Transesophagicechocardiography with stirred saline injection. Passage of "bubbles" is observed: (**a**) passage of more than 5 and less than 10 bubbles, (**b**) passage of more than 10 bubbles

In our experience TCD is the most reliable examination for PFO diagnosis, if it is negative no further exams are requested. If it is positive TTE is the elective test for confirmation, leaving TEE for complex cases in which PFO anatomy is important for clinical decisions.

Is any Indication for PFO Screening or Closure in Divers or Heigh Altitude Climbers?

PFO closure is a matter of debate. The 2021 Guideline for the Prevention of Stroke in Patients With Stroke and Transient Ischemic Attack [22] recommendations are as follows:

(a) In patients with a nonlacunar ischemic stroke of undetermined cause and a PFO, recommendations for PFO closure versus medical management should be made jointly by the patient, a cardiologist, and a neurologist, taking into account the probability of a causal role for the PFO (strong recommendation, expert opinion).
(b) In patients 18–60 years of age with a nonlacunar ischemic stroke of undetermined cause despite a thorough evaluation and a PFO with high-risk anatomic features, it is reasonable to choose closure with a transcatheter device and long-term antiplatelet therapy over antiplatelet therapy alone for preventing recurrent stroke (moderate recommendation, moderate evidence from randomized control trials (RTC)).
(c) In patients 18 to 60 years of age with a nonlacunar ischemic stroke of undetermined cause despite a thorough evaluation and a PFO without high-risk anatomic features, the benefit of closure with a transcatheter device and long-term antiplatelet therapy over antiplatelet therapy alone for preventing recurrent stroke is not well established (weak recommendation, limited evidence).
(d) In patients 18 to 60 years of age with a nonlacunar ischemic stroke of undetermined cause despite a thorough evaluation and a PFO, the comparative benefit of closure with a transcatheter device versus warfarin is unknown (weak recommendation, limited evidence).

A recent review article about PFO closure indications [23] included diving and high altitude pilots in them. Another review article [24] focused in PFO and hypoxemia highlights the condition relevance in high altitude pulmonary edema and decompression sickness, and hypothesized that some patients may have relief of symptoms and hypoxemia by eliminating the right-to-left shunt. An expert opinion editorial also agree with the above mention papers [25].

Last but not least there are three prospectives studies that demonstrate PFO closure benefit in professional and amateur divers [26–28].

The Controversial Aspects of Management, What we Are Calling the "Evidence Contour"

After reviewing most of the published literature on the subject there are some conclusions to be shared.

- First of all PFO presence worsened decompression sickness and high altitude pulmonary edema, as well as hypoxemia and sleep disorders in high altitude natural borned people.
- Second PFO size and anatomic conditions are closely related to clinical manifestations, the larger and complex PFO the worsen clinical condition.
- Third, PFO screaning should be indicated in professional climbers or divers with, at least, one clinical event. Although I didn't find a reference, according to this review, PFO searching should be bear in mind in high altitude non native workers (for example mine workers) with mild symptoms.
- Fourth PFO closure could be indicated according size and anatomic conditions assuming the similarity with cryptogenic stroke.

References

1. Powers WJ, Rabinstein AA, Ackerson T, et al. Guidelines for the early management of patients with acute ischemic stroke: 2019 update to the 2018 guidelines for the early management of acute ischemic stroke: a guideline for healthcare professionals from the American Heart Association/American Stroke Association. Stroke. 2019;50:e344–418.
2. Bornstein NM, Guekht A, Vester J, et al. Safety and efficacy of Cerebrolysin in early post-stroke recovery: a meta-analysis of nine randomized clinical trials. Neurol Sci. 2018;39:629–40.
3. Beghi E, Binder H, Birle C, et al. European Academy of Neurology and European Federation of Neurorehabilitation Societies guideline on pharmacological support in early motor rehabilitation after acute ischaemic stroke. Eur J Neurol. 2021;28:2831–45.
4. Telman G, Yalonetsky S, Kouperberg E, Sprecher E, Lorber A, Yarnitsky D. Size of PFO and amount of microembolic signals in patients with ischaemic stroke or TIA. Eur J Neurol. 2008;15:969–72.
5. Cho H, Kim T, Song IU, Chung SW. The prevalence of microembolic signals in transcranial doppler sonography with bubble test in acute ischemic stroke. J Ultrasound Med. 2021; https://doi.org/10.1002/jum.15724. Epub ahead of print
6. Saver JL, Carroll JD, Thaler DE, et al. RESPECT Investigators. Long-term outcomes of patent foramen ovale closure or medical therapy after stroke. N Engl J Med. 2017;377:1022–32.
7. Wardlaw JM, Valdés Hernández MC, Muñoz-Maniega S. What are white matter hyperintensities made of? Relevance to vascular cognitive impairment. J Am Heart Assoc. 2015;4:00114.
8. Lechat P, Mas J, Lascault G, Loron P, Theard M, Klimczac M, et al. Prevalence of patent foramen ovale in patients with stroke. N Engl J Med. 1988;318:1148–52.
9. Webster MW, Chancellor A, Smith HJ, Swift D, Sharpe D, Bass N, et al. Patent foramen ovale in young stroke patients. Lancet. 1988;2:11–2.
10. https://www.uptodate.com/contents/patent-foramen-ovale. Accessed May 2021.
11. Hackett PH, Rennie D, Levine HD. The incidence, importance, and prophylaxis of acute mountain sickness. Lancet. 1976;2:1149–55.

12. West BH, Fleming RG, Al Hemyari B, et al. Relation of patent foramen ovale to acute mountain sickness. Am J Cardiol. 2019;123(12):2022–5.
13. Allemann Y, Hutter D, Lipp E, et al. Patent foramen ovale and high-altitude pulmonary edema. JAMA. 2006;296:2954–8.
14. Lovering AT, Elliott JE, Davis JT. Physiological impact of patent foramen ovale on pulmonary gas exchange, ventilatory acclimatization, and thermoregulation. J Appl Physiol. 2016;121:512–7.
15. Brenner R, Pratali L, Rimoldi SF, et al. Exaggerated pulmonary hypertension and right ventricular dysfunction in high-altitude dwellers with patent foramen ovale. Chest. 2015;147(4):1072–9.
16. González-Alujas T, Evangelista A, Santamarina E, et al. Diagnosis and quantification of patent foramen ovale. Which is the reference technique? Simultaneous study with transcranial Doppler, transthoracic and transesophageal echocardiography. Rev Esp Cardiol. 2011;64:133–9.
17. Mojadidi MK, Roberts SC, Winoker JS, et al. Accuracy of transcranial Doppler for the diagnosis of intracardiac right-to-left shunt: a bivariate meta-analysis of prospective studies. JACC Cardiovasc Imaging. 2014;7(3):236–50.
18. Ren P, Li K, Lu X, Xie M. Diagnostic value of transthoracic echocardiography for patent foramen ovale: a meta-analysis. Ultrasound Med Biol. 2013;39:1743–50.
19. Mojadidi MK, Bogush N, Caceres JD, Msaouel P, Tobis JM. Diagnostic accuracy of transesophageal echocardiogram for the detection of patent foramen ovale: a meta-analysis. Echocardiography. 2014;31:752–8.
20. Sloan MA, Alexandrov AV, Tegeler CH, et al. Assessment: transcranial Doppler ultrasonography: report of the Therapeutics and Technology Assessment Subcommittee of the American Academy of Neurology. Neurology. 2004;62:1468–81.
21. Jauss M, Zanette E for the Consensus Conference. Detection of right-to-left shunt with ultrasound contrast agent and transcranial Doppler sonography. Cerebrovasc Dis. 2000;10:490–6.
22. AHA/ASA GUIDELINE. Guideline for the prevention of stroke in patients with stroke and transient ischemic attack. Stroke. 2021;2021(52):e364–467.
23. Giblett JP, Williams LK, Kyranis S, Shapiro LM, Calvert PA. Patent foramen ovale closure: state of the art. Interv Cardiol. 2020;15:e15.
24. Mojadidi MK, Ruiz JC, Chertoff J, et al. Patent foramen ovale and hypoxemia. Cardiol Rev. 2019;27:34–40.
25. Meier B. Offenes Foramen ovale: gute Gründe, es zu verschließen [Patent foramen ovele, good reasons to close it]. Dtsch Med Wochenschr. 2018;143(5):354–6.
26. Billinger M, Zbiden MR, Mordasini R, et al. Patent foramen ovale closure in recreational divers: effect on decompression illness and ischaemic brain lesions during long-term follow-up. Heart. 2011;97:1932–7.
27. Henzel J, Rudziński PN, Kłopotowski M, Konka M, Dzielińska Z, Demkow M. Transcatheter closure of patent foramen ovale for the secondary prevention of decompression illness in professional divers: a single-centre experience with long-term follow-up. Kardiol Pol. 2018;76(1):153–7.
28. Anderson G, Ebersole D, Covington D, Denoble PJ. The effectiveness of risk mitigation interventions in divers with persistent (patent) foramen ovale. Diving Hyperb Med. 2019;49(2):80–7.

Chapter 19
Preexisting Condition and Travel to High Altitude

Ranajit Chatterjee(Chattopadhyay) and Lalit Gupta

Case Discussion

A 55 year old male had arrived for tracking of around 4000 m and climbed an altitude of around 2500 m in a single day to a base camp. On night of arrival at this attitude he complained of sudden onset of chest pain, dyspnea, tiredness and exhaustion. After few hours, patient started irrelevant talking with improper behavior like refusal to feed and poorly responding to verbal commands. He was immediately managed at campsite healthcare facility with Oxygen and I/V fluids but his condition deteriorated at the very next day and he was shifted to the base camp hospital. There he had an episode of seizures which was immediately relieved with no focal deficit. On examining, the patient had GCS of 12/15 with pulse of 110 /min, BP 130/80 mmHg and respiratory rate of 35. Her oral temperature was around 101 °F, SpO_2 88% on room air. The rest of the systemic examination was unremarkable. His lab reports were: Hb of 13.6 g/dl with TLC of 24,000, platelets count 80,000, B.Urea 34 mg/dl, Creatinine 0.95 mg/dl, sodium 150 mEq/L, potassium 4.2 mEq/l, blood glucose 320 mg/dl. ABG values were suggestive of pH: 7.18, PaO2: 80 mmHg, PaCO2: 50 mm hg, HCO3: 14 mmol/l. ECG showed sinus tachycardia with RBBB and X- ray chest imperative of diffuse fine infiltrates with left lower zone opacity and prominent bronchopleural margins (Fig. 19.1). NCCT head was normal with CSF analysis also within normal limit. Baseline cultures were sent.

R. Chatterjee(Chattopadhyay) (✉)
Dept. of Anaesthesiology and Critical Care, Swami Dayanand Hospital, New Delhi, India

L. Gupta
Department of Anaesthesiology and Intensive care, Maulana Azad Medical college and Lok Nayak Hospital, New Delhi, India

J. Hidalgo et al. (eds.), *High Altitude Medicine*,
https://doi.org/10.1007/978-3-031-35092-4_19

211

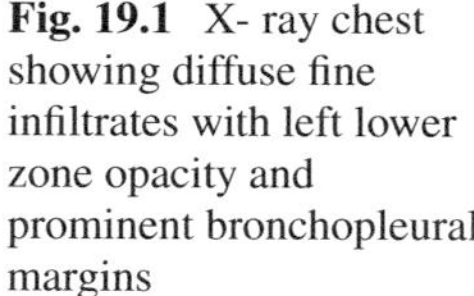

Fig. 19.1 X- ray chest showing diffuse fine infiltrates with left lower zone opacity and prominent bronchopleural margins

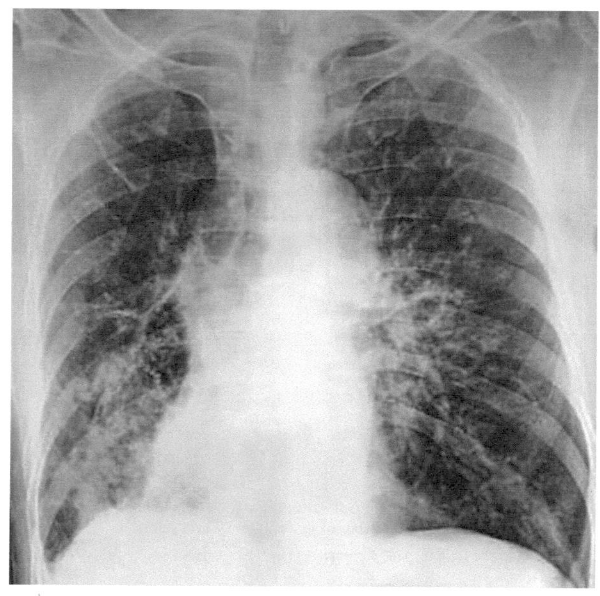

On careful examination and history taking it was found, patient was a known case of hypertension and diabetes mellitus irregular on treatment and was also regular smoker. The diagnosis of high altitude sickness with High altitude cerebral edema and High altitude pulmonary edema (HACE & HAPE) was made with diabetic ketoacidosis keeping in mind differential diagnosis of pneumonia with impending sepsis. Patient was immediately started on insulin infusion and broad spectrum antibiotics with CVP line and arterial line were placed for better monitoring. On second day of admission, GCS deteriorated to 7/15 and hypoxemia also increased. Patient was in respiratory distress; he was intubated, paralyzed and put on controlled mandatory ventilation. The blood sugars were still high around 250 mg/dl on average. During course of admission; ABG, hypoxemia and sugar improved, serial chest radiograph showed clearance of infiltrate and improved GCS. Patient was on ventilator for around 72 h, weaned off on fourth day and discharged to the ward after seventh day of admission.

Question 1 What is the probable diagnosis?

The diagnosis is high altitude cerebral edema with pulmonary edema and diabetic ketoacidosis.

Question 2 What approach should guide this patient's ventilator management?

This patient is having acute pulmonary edema secondary to the high altitude and all such patients should be managed by protective lung ventilation strategy in order to avoid ventilator associated lung injury. The patient is already having high grade fever and X ray changes suggestive of pneumonia, so all efforts should be made to save the patient further from ventilator associated pneumonia. This patient was started on controlled mechanical ventilation with a tidal volume of around 400 ml with FiO_2 of 100% with PEEP around 8 cmH_2O to start with and gradually increased to 12–15 cmH_2O over the time and later on decreased to 5 cmH_2O with FiO_2 of 40%. During this period, due to the pulmonary edema, the plateau airway pressure raised between 28 to 32 cmH_2O.

The broad spectrum antibiotics including tazobactum and meropenum were started immediately keeping in mind the possibility of developing sepsis. Initially the plan of low dose corticosteroid to start with was suggested but withhold in view of raised blood sugar. The patient had already been on insulin drip and it was difficult due to the stress induced hyperglycemia to maintain the blood sugar level less than 180 mg/dl. But as the stress controlled and hypoxia improved, the blood sugar level also came to the normal and remained satisfactory controlled on day fourth onwards. The patient was shifted to mannitol along with sliding scale insulin and transferred to the ward next day.

Question 3 What is high altitude cerebral edema?

High altitude cerebral edema also called HACE is a rare manifestation of high altitude acute mountain sickness. The patient feels lethargic, drowsy and confused like alcoholic intoxication and sometimes require immediate descend due to progressing hypoxemia. This condition is often associated with high altitude pulmonary edema (HAPE) manifested by severe breathlessness at rest, weakness, cough and hypoxemia. HAPE can be even more fatal than HACE [1, 2].

Question 4 What are the pre-existing medical problems which are often seen in patients going for high altitudes?

Travelers with medical conditions like heart failure, obstructive sleeve apnea, pre-existing hypoxemia due to elements of asthma or COPD are often advised to have a full medical checkup before undertaking high altitude travel [1, 3]. Patient with well controlled medical problems generally do not decompensate at high elevations. However, the patients with obstructive sleep apnea, if possible should carry there CPAP devices along with them with supplemental oxygen devices. Patients with hypertension should take their medicines regularly and should not do heavy activity at high altitude and should not forget to take their medicines on regular time.

While patients with diabetes can travel safely to high altitude, their blood glucose should be monitored regularly because high altitude illness can trigger diabetic ketoacidosis as in our case and it may be more difficult to treat in those patients who are taking acetazolamide for acclimatization at high altitude. Moreover, glucose meters do not read accurately at high divisions.

Apart from that, patients with pre-existing vision disorders like radial keratomy procedures may develop acute farsightedness (hyperopia) and cannot take proper care of themselves, so they should keep their glasses along with them [3]. Other disorders where patient should go at higher altitude carefully with pre-existing medical conditions are sickle cell anemia, pre-existing pulmonary hypertension, pre-existing decompensated heart failure or unstable angina, history of recent myocardial infection in last 90 days and previously space occupying lesions in brain. Patients with sickle cell disease are at high risk of painful crisis at high altitude due to hypoxemia, cold and dehydration. They are always needed to keep supplemental oxygen during high altitude travel.

Question 5 What are the various medications that should be used in patients with pre-existing medical disease going to high-altitude?

Most commonly used drug is acetazolamide (which prevent acute mountain sickness when taken before ascent as well as helps in speedy recovery). If the high altitude symptoms develop, it helps in reducing the respiratory alkalosis usually seen with high elevations while maintaining the arterial oxygenation. The second drug is dexamethasone, this drug is very useful in preventing HACE/HAPE. This drug should be taken very carefully in patients with pre-existing diabetes otherwise complications related to diabetic ketoacidosis may increase thus reserving this drug for patients particularly susceptible to high altitude pulmonary edema like the patients of pre-existing pulmonary hypertension and COPD.

Other medications that are of quite importance are nifidepine and phosphodiesterase 5 inhibitors (sildenafil, tadalafil), they will decrease the pulmonary hypertension and are reserved drugs for patents susceptible for HAPE. NSAIDS like ibuprofen also seems to be beneficial in preventing the signs of acute mountain sickness. Common medication dosing and uses to prevent and treat altitude illnesses is as per Table 19.1 [4].

Table 19.1 Medications to treat high altitude illness in patients with preexisting medical conditions

Medication	Use	Dose	Contraindications/Cautions
Acetazolamide	Prophylaxis: Acute mountain sickness (AMS) HACE prevention	Oral: 2.5 mg/kg in 2 divided doses	Hepatic and renal disorders, Metabolic acidosis, Diabetics, Pregnancy
Nifidepine	HAPE prevention and treatment	Oral: 30 mg/12 hrly, sustained release tablets	Hepatic insufficiency, concomitant use with other antihypertensive drugs, GI ulcers
Dexamethsone	Prophylaxis and prevention of AMS and HACE	Oral/ IV: 2 mg/6 hrly; 4 mg/12 hrly	Diabetic, Peptic/GI ulcers
Sildenafil	HAPE prophylaxis and prevention	Oral:50 mg/8 hrly	Concomitant use with nitrates or alpha blockers, Hepatic disorders
Tadalafil	HAPE prophylaxis and prevention	Oral:10 mg/12 hrly	Concomitant use with nitrates or alpha blockers, Hepatic disorders
Salmeterol	HAPE prophylaxis	Inhalation: 125 μg of salmeterol/12 hrly	CAD, concomitant use with beta blockers and tricyclic antidepressant

Question 6 What makes different peoples more or less susceptible to high altitude mountains sickness?

The spectrum of attitude sickness ranges from acute mountain sickness to high altitude pulmonary and cerebral edema with wide spectrum of manifestations in different people (25–85%) [5]. It has been found in some observational studies that women have a slightly higher risk than men. Moreover from the various studies it has also been seen that individuals between a 60 to 80 years. Age group have only 16% of incidence rate which is lower than younger peoples who had incidence of around 45%, this is related to higher exercise intensity in youngers and hence more respiratory complications [5].

External forces (e.g., medicine, nutrition, exercise, etc.) and longitudinal effects (e.g., changes in behavior, age, etc.) can modify the severity and/or presentation of many traits. As the altitude increases, the individual's ability to exercise decrease drastically. The oxygen saturation in blood is no longer maintained due to less oxygen level at high altitude and those with pre-existing lung disease suffers more than those who have a good pulmonary functions due to their good exercise tolerance. People with previous experience of high altitude even with coexisting medical disorders while going again to such areas may benefit from last travel and the premedication they learnt from last journey may also decrease the morbidity significantly.

Question 7 What are the various cardiovascular disorders associated with high altitude?

The most common disorder at high altitude of significant importance is hypertension. It has been seen the exaggerated effect of hypertension at attitudes is not seen till 3000 meters; however some patients have preexisting pathological reactions which result in sudden surge of hypertension [6]. The extent of pressure fluctuation depends on their exercise tolerance, genetics, degree of hypoxic stress, ambient temperature and medications they are compliant with. Always remember that hypertension is an independent risk factor for sudden cardiac death during tracking in patients with poorly controlled blood pressure. They should measure their blood pressure at regular intervals at high altitude end reserve medication should be kept as per their physicians advise. If hypertension is not controlled alpha adrenergic blockers are the drugs of choice at high attitude. Patients taking diuretics should think of substituting with another class of antihypertensive as diuretics may cause dehydration and electrolyte depletion. Furthermore, beta blockers should be taken with caution as they limit the heart rate response with increase physical activity at high altitude and may interfere with body's thermoregulatory mechanism of maintaining heat or cold.

Apart from hypertension, acute coronary artery disease is another cause of death at high altitude [7]. Acute hypoxia, dehydration, old environment leading to vasoconstriction and variability in heart rate with raised blood pressure may cause unstable angina or sometimes cardiac arrhythmias in high risk individuals at high altitude. Oxygenation in stenotic arteries significantly reduces at high altitude directly leading to further worsening of coronary artery disease. It is recommended that physical activities should be limited for duration of 3–5 days of acclimation. Persons with symptomatic heart failure or previous history of decompensated heart disease should give proper attention to the food balance and should monitor closely for signs of fluid retention while avoiding dehydration too. If there is impending chance of heart failure, the dose of acetazolamide may be adjusted in advance along with diuretics.

Sometimes at high altitude, ECG may show the changes of pulmonary hypertension which resolve with descend to the lower attitude [8]. Various types of arrhythmias related to increased heart rate may be evident during high altitude. Patients with left or right bundle branch block should be very cautious while going to the high altitude. Similarly for patients with congenital heart disease specifically associated with pulmonary hypertension, high altitude exposure is contraindicated. However if travel is necessary, symptomatic patients with congenital heart disease should take proper precautions for developing high altitude pulmonary edema and must take the nifedipine prophylactically to reduce their risk. Nifedipine reduce chest tightness and make breathing easier. It's also often part of an expedition's medical supplies.

Question 8 What are the various respiratory disorders associated with high altitude?

It should always be remembered that patients with COPD or allergic to cold atmosphere or previously hypoxemic from any respiratory illness sometimes develop high altitude pulmonary edema even at the lower elevations than younger people [9]. The decreased ventilatory response is usually the by result of decreased carotid body response due to chronic hypercapnia in such patients. Warm environment also result in pulmonary vasoconstriction and increased mean artery pressure, the smokers may have elevated levels of carboxy-hemoglobin and all these when associated together may cause performed hypoxemia, pulmonary hypertension, sleep disorder, laboured breathing and high altitude pulmonary edema. If there is an emergency and some patient has to go with such type of disorder to high altitude, he must undergo risk assessment test with proper prior pulmonary function tests and should ascend with caution to minimize the risk of adverse effects.

Patients of respiratory disorders should avoid exercise at high altitude and should learn self-respiratory physiotherapy. They should start spirometry and should halt smoking as long as possible before going for high altitude. Maintenance of hydration is very important to avoid problems associated with thickened mucus secretions [10]. Similarly there are increased chances of bronchial asthma due to bronchial hyper responsiveness because of cold and hypoxic air at high altitudes with decreased humidity. Bronchoconstriction at high altitude secondary to low barometric pressure may sometimes exaggerate hypoxemia leading to hypoxic pulmonary edema. The highest risk patients are those who are on inhaled bronchodilators and therefore should not be forgotten to take their bronchodilators along with supplementary oxygen when going to high altitudes. Any type of exertion should be avoided and they should not do excessive hyperventilation.

Similarly patients with obstructive sleep apnea and interstitial disease are at high risk of developing respiratory failure at high altitude patients [11]. Those who are using positive airway pressure methods at sea level may need to adjust their pressure settings to accommodate for decrease in barometric pressure at high altitude. If a patient of obstructive sleep apnea chooses for high altitude, it is reasonable to adjust to adjust the pressure setting of positive airway pressure device to accommodate for the decrease in barometric pressure at altitude [12].

Question 9 What are the various endocrine disorders that should be taken care at high altitude?

Diabetes is an independent risk factor for sudden cardiac death associated with high altitude mountain hiking [13]. While it has been seen that type-1 diabetes acclimatize well, there is little evidence to suggest that they are relative immune to attitude illness [14]. Always remember attitude exposure, moderate exercise with good glycemic control is all needed for such patients. There is high chances of deranged blood sugar at high altitude because of decrease in metabolic control as evident by elevation of HbA_1C and Insulin requirements. There is reduced insulin sensitivity with altered carbohydrate intakes and irregular exercise leading to development of poor blood sugar maintenance. Strenuous physical activity, decreased ambient temperature, nausea vomiting like GI symptoms of acute mountain sickness predispose diabetic Mountaineers to hypoglycemia requiring adjustment in insulin dose [15]. If a patient at high altitude develops pulmonary edema, it acts as another independent trigger for diabetic ketoacidosis in previously undiagnosed diabetic or well controlled diabetic patient. Also remember that inappropriate insulin dose, decreased calories, altered metabolism and exercises along with acetazolamide prophylaxis are independent factors for ketoacidosis. If patient takes dexamethasone like steroids, it may further aggravate the risk of glycemic irregularities at high altitude.

Precise energy intake and expenditure with frequent blood glucose monitoring should be done and flexible insulin dosing as imperative must be employed. Insulin vials may be sensitive to heat and cold and thus should be stored carefully to prevent it from freezing. All diabetic patients should be carefully screened for complications at sea level that could increase the risk associated with exercise or exposure to high altitude. Obesity along with diabetes is another risk factor at high altitude and may lead to obesity hypoventilation syndrome leading to further aggravation of metabolic disorders. Diabetic Retinopathy is a relative contraindication for such high altitude journey for risk of retinal hemorrhage at height more than 5500 m [16].

Question 10 What are the various neurological disorders to be taken care at high altitude?

The most important complications at high altitude are altitude related seizures that are believed to be the result of respiratory alkalosis, hypoxemia, sleep deprivation, and drugs lowering the seizure threshold like fluoroquinolones [17]. The risk of stroke at high altitude may be increased sometimes because of hyper viscosity syndrome of high altitude secondary to dehydration, cold atmosphere, inactivity and polycythemia. Always remember that travel to high altitude is contraindicated

Table 19.2 Checklist of recommendations for safe travel to high altitude

1.	(a) Medical advice before starting the trip. (b) Avoid travel in acute illness or with recently diagnosed new illness
2.	Ensure optimal fitness/ exercise tolerance/preemptive spirometry
3.	(a) Check interactions of currently using drugs with medications commonly used to treat altitude-related illness. (b) Avoid sedatives and opioid based cough suppressants. (c) Calibrate BP apparatus and glucometers
4.	Keep your positive airway pressure device and oxygen supplement if previously using them.
5.	Keep extra doses of regular medicine and separate doses of emergency medicines.
6.	If possible, travel in a group or with a partner
7.	Inform and educate travel companions about relevant medical conditions with written/oral instructions for emergency situation
8.	Maintain healthy nutrition and adequate hydration
9.	1. Do not ascend very fast and give time for acclimatization. 2. Do not overexert yourself. Only mild exercises for the first 48 hours.
10.	Call for help or descend to lower altitude immediately with the onset of symptoms.

for a 90 day period of post ischemic attack and if there is deemed necessary to travel to high altitude, all clinical situation and full physician estimation of stroke risk should be taken [18]. In some case, high altitude people also complained of migraine (with altered frequency, severity, and character) along with fever which sometimes confuse the diagnosis of high altitude meningitis [19].

Question 11 What is essential checklist for people traveling to high altitude with preexisting medical conditions?

Many people with preexisting medical conditions with proper planning and precautions, can safely take travel to high altitude [20] (Table 19.2).

Conclusion

Travelling to destinations at high altitude can be exciting, challenging, rewarding and sometimes life threatening too. All persons traveling to high altitude should be familiar with standard ascent and acclimatization protocols. They should have a physician checkup for identifying the possible risk of developing symptoms of high altitude illness. If they have the pre-existing medical conditions of cardiovascular system or respiratory system or related to their seizures activity they should adjust their drug doses with proper planning and precautions. Physician and patient must work together in coherence to plan a rational and informed approach for a safe and happy high altitude journey.

References

1. Bartsch P, Swenson ER. Acute high-altitude illnesses. N Engl J Med. 2013;369(17):1666–7.
2. Hackett PH, Roach RC. High altitude cerebral edema. High Alt Med Biol. 2004;5(2):136–46.
3. Pollard AJ, Murdoch DR. The high altitude medicine handbook. 3rd ed. Abingdon, UK: Radcliffe Medical Press; 2003.
4. Luks AM, Swenson ER. Medication and dosage considerations in the prophylaxis and treatment of high-altitude illness. Chest. 2008;133:744–55.
5. https://www.news-medical.net/health/What-Makes-Different-People-More-or-Less-Susceptible-to-Altitude-Sickness.aspx.
6. Luks AM. Should travellers with hypertension adjust their medications when travelling to high altitude? High Alt Med Biol. 2009;10:11–5.
7. Hultgren HN. Effects of altitude upon cardiovascular diseases [review]. J Wilderness Med. 1992;3:301–8.
8. Woods DR, Allen S, Betts TR, et al. High altitude arrhythmias. Cardiology. 2008;111:239–46.
9. Hackett PH, Roach RC. High-altitude medicine. In: Auerbach PS, editor. Wilderness medicine. 5th ed. Philadelphia: Mosby, Elsevier; 2007. p. 2–36.
10. Cogo A, Fischer R, Schoene R. Respiratory diseases and high altitude [review]. High Alt Med Biol. 2004;5:435–44.
11. Luks AM, Swenson ER. Travel to high altitude with pre-existing lung disease [review]. Eur Respir J. 2007;29:770–92.
12. Bloch KE, Latshang TD, Ulrich S. Patients with obstructive sleep Apnea at altitude. High Alt Med Biol. 2015;16(2):110–6.
13. Burtscher M, Pachinger O, Schocke MF, Ulmer H. Risk factor profile for sudden cardiac death during mountain hiking. Int J Sports Med. 2007;28:621–4.
14. Moore K, Thompson CJ. Diabetes and extreme altitude mountaineering. Br J Sports Med. 2001;35:83.
15. Leal C. Going high with type 1 diabetes [review]. High Alt Med Biol. 2005;6:14–21.
16. Mader TH, Tabin G. Going to high altitude with pre-existing ocular conditions [review]. High Alt Med Biol. 2003;4:419–31.
17. West JB, Schoene RB, Milledge JS. Pre-existing medical conditions at altitude. High altitude medicine and physiology. 4th ed. London: Hodder Arnold; 2000. p. 337–48.
18. Baumgartner RW, Siegel AM, Hackett PH. Going high with preexisting neurological conditions [review]. High Alt Med Biol. 2007;8:108–16.
19. Bartsch P, Swenson ER. Acute high-altitude illnesses. N Engl J Med. 2013;368:2294–302.
20. Luks AM, Auerbach PS, Freer L, et al. Wilderness medical society clinical practice guidelines for the prevention and treatment of acute altitude illness: 2019 update. Wilderness Environ Med. 2019;30:S3.

Chapter 20
Working at High Altitude

Kanwalpreet Sodhi, Ruchira Khasne, and Atul Phillips

Case Presentation

A 52-year-old male with hypertension on vacation in Leh-Ladakh (3500–6000 m height above sea-level) in India, had a road traffic accident and suffered a fracture to the right tibia-fibula. He is posted for open reduction internal fixation.

How Should this Patient Be Managed?

Major challenges in management of this patient are related to high altitude (HA) related physiological issues in the body and the equipment related issues that are to be used during surgical intervention for fracture fixation. Poor physiological reserve and low tolerance to compensate for blood loss during perioperative period places this patient at a high risk. After initial resuscitation, regional anesthesia should be provided for the surgery. While on one hand, a high risk of perioperative bleeding and poor tolerance to blood loss is present, on the other, polycythemia poses a high risk of perioperative thrombotic events.

K. Sodhi (✉)
Critical Care, Deep Hospital, Ludhiana, India

R. Khasne
SMBT Institute of Medical Sciences and Research Center,
Igatpuri, Nashik, Maharashtra, India

A. Phillips
Critical Care Medicine, St Stephens Hospital, Tis Hazari, Delhi, India

© The Author(s), under exclusive license to Springer Nature
Switzerland AG 2023
J. Hidalgo et al. (eds.), *High Altitude Medicine*,
https://doi.org/10.1007/978-3-031-35092-4_20

Standard Approach and Concerns of Management

What Are the Challenges in Health Care worker's (HCW's) Health while Working at High Altitude?

Working at HA is a challenging task for HCWs where the body is subjected to an essentially isolated hypoxic challenge. Low barometric pressures and decreased oxygen tension have their physiological effect on both acclimatized and un-acclimatized HCWs. At HA, a linear fall in atmospheric PO_2 leads to decrease in alveolar (PAO_2) and arterial (PaO_2) partial pressures of oxygen respectively, resulting in a reduction of oxygen delivery (DO2) [1]. If the body is gradually exposed to increasing altitude, it can adapt to these changes which is called "acclimatization". Acclimatization refers to an array of beneficial changes that occur in the body in response to hypoxia at HA, wherein one can function normally and restore DO2 as well.

What Is Acute Mountain Illness (AMS)?

The rate of ascent and the level of altitude determines altitude-related illnesses, which vary from mild AMS to potentially lethal high-altitude pulmonary oedema (HAPE). AMS is a benign form of altitude illness with self- limiting symptoms, developing after 6–12 h of ascent and improving within 2–3 days. Headache is the most common presenting symptom. Lake Louise AMS scoring system is used to assess the severity of AMS [2].

Lake Louise AMS scoring
- Recent ascent within last 4 days (>2500 m)
- Headache
- Presence of more than one symptom and each symptom is scored from 0–3 based on severity (none = 0, mild 1, moderate 2, severe 3): headache, gastrointestinal disturbance, insomnia, fatigue or weakness, dizziness or light-headedness

- (Mild AMS: Score of 3–5; Severe AMS: Score of >6)

HAPE is a type of non-cardiogenic pulmonary oedema occurring after rapid ascent due to exaggerated hypoxic pulmonary vasoconstriction (HPV) and elevated pulmonary artery pressure. It is characterized initially by dry cough, dyspnea, tachycardia, tachypnoea and crepitations. In later stages, hemoptysis, orthopnea and mental confusion can occur. Electrocardiography may reveal right ventricular strain or hypertrophy. When symptoms of AMS rapidly worsen developing encephalopathy characterized by ataxia and altered consciousness with diffuse cerebral involvement but generally without focal neurologic deficits then it is known as high-altitude cerebral oedema (HACE). It may be associated with papilledema and retinal hemorrhages [3].

Though pharmacologic prophylaxis may reduce symptoms of AMS but "controlled ascent" is the most effective preventive strategy. Drug of choice for AMS prevention is acetazolamide which is to be taken 1 day before ascent and to be continued for 2 or 3 days. It acts by carbonic anhydrase enzyme inhibition in the renal tubules causing a bicarbonate diuresis, and metabolic acidosis which stimulates ventilation and hastens respiratory acclimatization. However, it is contraindicated in people with sulfa allergy.

The mainstays of the treatment of AMS are descent from HA and oxygen supplementation. Patents with milder symptoms of AMS ((Lake Louise score < 4) do not need to be removed from HA. With adequate rest, hydration and symptomatic treatment, most symptoms of AMS resolve as acclimatization takes place. However, for symptoms which are moderate to severe (Lake Louise score >5) modest descent (>500 m), aided by combination of therapies with acetazolamide (higher doses may be required for HACE and HAPE), dexamethasone, analgesics and supplemental oxygen maybe required. Dexamethasone exerts an anti-inflammatory effect by reducing the production of reactive oxygen species and attenuation of hypoxic pulmonary vasoconstriction.

If AMS is severe and immediate descent is not possible, hyperbaric chambers (Gamow bags) as simulation of descent is used. Pulmonary vasodilators such as nifedipine or sildenafil can reduce pulmonary hypertension which helps to prevent and reduce symptoms in AMS [4].

What Physiological Changes Might Affect the Management of the Patient?

The physiological changes that the human body can adapt to and endure the changes in pressure due to HA has baffled physiologists and has remained an interesting area of research for many. Hyperventilation is most common physiological response to acclimatization. Acclimatization is achieved by body's physiological changes in cerebral vasculature, cardio-pulmonary system, fluid and electrolytes, hematological and temperature regulation. (**As per** Table 20.1) [5–14].

What Are the Challenges in the Intra and Postoperative Management of Patient?

The working environment in HA becomes challenging when acclimatization is not optimal. Following are the intra and post-operative challenges:

- Concerns for altered physical characteristics of respiratory gases and inhaled anaesthetic agents and calibration of equipment.
- Choice of anesthesia: The choice between administering general or regional anesthesia is dictated by the clinical scenario. General anesthesia is more

Table 20.1 Pathophysiological changes at high altitude

	System involved	Pathophysiological response
1	**Central Nervous System**	• Increase in cerebral blood flow • Raised intracranial pressure (ICP) • Altered behaviour, drowsiness • Incoordination and lack of judgment • Sleep–speech disturbances • Unconsciousness • Seizures
2	**Cardiovascular system**	• Tachycardia and hypertension due to increased sympathetic nervous activity • Increased blood volume by 30% • Increased erythropoiesis • Hematocrit increases from 40 to 65% • Local vasodilation due to tissue hypoxia • High altitude Pulmonary HTN (HAPH) due to hypoxic pulmonary vasoconstriction, pulmonary vessel remodeling, right ventricle hypertrophy • ECG changes: Arrhythmias, AV block • Hypotension • Negative inotropism
3	**Respiratory System**	• Reduced PiO_2 (partial pressure of oxygen in inspired gas) • Reduced ambient pressure • Reduced gas density • Hyperventilation and increased minute ventilation (hypoxic ventilatory response): With sudden exposure to hypobaric pressure, the decreased alveolar PO_2 stimulates the peripheral chemoreceptors in the carotid and aortic bodies • Increased diffusion capacity (normal 2.1 ml/mmHg/min) • Reduced oxygen gradient leading to ventilation perfusion mismatch • Hypoxia induced hyperpnea: Leftward shift of oxygen dissociation curve facilitating the release of oxygen to the tissues • Pulmonary edema: Most commonly neurogenic pulmonary edema due to increased hydrostatic pressure, increased pulmonary vascular permeability, coagulation defect, increased oxygen free radicals and increased autonomic activity
4	**Renal system**	• Rise in erythropoietin • Increase in the hematocrit and blood viscosity • Reduction in renal blood flow & GFR
5	**Hematological changes**	• Increased Fibrinogen, platelet factor V and VIII and platelet factor 3 are high • Increased risk of venous and arterial thrombosis • Platelet levels decrease, increased platelet aggregation and increased soluble platelet (sP) selectin levels by approximately 250%
6	**Temperature regulation**	• Risk of exposure to ultraviolet radiation • Exposure of extremes in temperature causing thermal injuries or hypothermia and cold injury such as frostbite.

challenging but even regional anesthesia is not free from its perils. Higher incidence of post-dural puncture headache after spinal anesthesia has been reported due to higher CSF pressure, decrease in alveolar ventilation, hypoxia and dehydration leading to inadequate decompensation for CSF leak [15].

- Drugs: Local anesthetics have shorter duration of action. Opioids suppress pulmonary hyperventilation which is an important compensatory mechanism for low oxygen tension and have an exaggerated respiratory depressant effect with higher chances of hypoxia and cyanosis. Therefore, supplemental oxygen is mandatory in case of any heavy sedation with hypnotics, narcotics, or other drugs [15].
- Intravenous (IV) fluids or blood products: All blood products and IV fluids should be warmed to body temperature before transfusion to avoid hypothermia. There is a risk of developing pulmonary edema, so IV fluids should be used judiciously to avoid fluid overload.
- According to Boyle's law, the volume of gases can change with changes in pressure, other additional concerns in certain situations such as during ascent a simple pneumothorax may expand to become tension pneumothorax, intestinal gas may expand to rupture a hollow viscus and an additional risk of gas embolism.
- Higher chances of oozing from wounds even with lower arterial pressure: related to polycythemia and coagulation abnormalities. Higher blood volume, increased venous pressure, vasodilation, increase in number of capillaries and capillary fragility have been noted in natives of HA.
- If the need arises to provide cardiopulmonary resuscitation, due consideration to scene safety, safety of rescuer, and hypothermia as a cause of arrest should be given.
- HA can cause postoperative cognitive and psychomotor dysfunction.
- Hypoxia can worsen patient's anxiety and pain which may mandate the need of continuous oxygen supply

What Are the Issues with the Medical Equipment while Working at High Altitudes?

Following are the major issues with the operating efficiency of medical equipment at HA:

- **Vaporizers**: Volatile agents vaporize more rapidly at HA due to decrease in the boiling point and delivers approximately 10% more. Variable-bypass vaporizers automatically compensate for changes due to HA because they put out a partial pressure that is determined by the position of the dial but it is not applicable to (Tec-9) desflurane vaporizers. At HA, the partial pressure of desflurane will be lower at a given vaporizer setting (volume percent) than at sea level, leading to under dosing of the anesthetic and to prevent this, a higher concentration of the dial is set to attain the same clinical effect as at sea level with desflurane (Tec-9) vaporizer. The following equation can be used to account for HA:

  [Required vaporizer setting = (Desired vaporizer setting at sea level × 760 mmHg)/(barometric pressure in mmHg)] [16]

- **Gas flowmeters**: The oxygen and other flowmeters are calibrated at sea level but the actual flow of gases through standard rotameters is higher than indicated at HA due to reduced gas density. The estimated error is @ 1% for every 1000m accent [17].

- **Ventilator performance**: Clinicians should be aware about the ventilator performance and its limitations to provide safe and effective ventilation especially during air transport. Certain ventilators compensate ventilator output to deliver the desired tidal volume regardless of changes in altitude and barometric pressure but others do not compensate for changes in altitude resulting in delivery of increasing tidal volumes with falling barometric pressure [18]. Most of the commercial ventilators failed at HA, delivering tidal volumes with up to 40% error from the set volume [19]. Altitude compensation is an active software algorithm incorporated into high-end ventilators.

- **Syringe infusion pumps**: Hypobaric conditions cause unpredictable, unintended higher drug delivery in pumps by bubble formation and expansion of existing bubbles. Insulin infusion therapy may thereby lead to unexpected hypoglycemia. This holds true for low-weight syringe infusion pumps also which deliver discontinuous flow. More prudence is required when drugs with a narrow safety margin such as vasoactive agents are being used where slight changes in administered volumes may lead to substantial hemodynamic changes [20, 21].

- **Capnograph**: Capnographs may show erroneous readings due to errors in calibration or sample line disconnections (due to development of air leaks). Regular recalibration and re-programming of the electronic equipment is needed with changes in altitude. Monitors designed for routine clinical use may be unsuitable for use at HA [22].

- **Pulse oximeters**: The pulse oximeters may show a decrease in saturation values below 70% to 75% which may be due to device errors or as a result of low baseline oxygen saturation in healthy individuals at HA [23]

- **BP monitors**: HA do not affect the accuracy of oscillometric noninvasive blood pressure monitors or manual sphygmomanometers.

- **Pressure transducers**: Pressure transducers are a form of electronic strain gauge which is vented with one side of the diaphragm and exposed to atmospheric pressure on one side and exposed to the patient's blood pressure/central venous pressure by a column of fluid. When zeroing the transducer, we are simply exposing both sides of the transducer to the same pressure, thus while zeroing, the altitude is irrelevant.

- Medical equipment that have an enclosed air space is affected due to the impact of Boyle's Law e.g. endotracheal tube cuffs and intravenous lines with flow driven by air-filled pressure bags.

- Power recovery and gas pressurization system of high-altitude diesel engines: At higher altitude, as air is not as good an insulator as it is at sea level, the creepage and clearance of the power supply has to take this into account.

Evidence Contour

Although there is not much literature available on the working of medical equipment at HA, following are the tips for acclimatization and medication dosing to prevent and treat altitude illness as per CDC and Wilderness Medical Society consensus guidelines [24, 25].

Tips for acclimatization
- Ascend gradually, avoiding rapid climbs (not more than 2750 m/day) without steep elevation. Once above 2750 m, more elevation no higher than 500 m/day.
- Consider using acetazolamide to speed acclimatization if abrupt ascent is unavoidable.
- Avoid alcohol for the first 48 h; continue caffeine if a regular user.
- Participate in only mild exercise for the first 48 hours.
- Having a high-elevation exposure (greater than 2750 m) for 2 nights or more, within 30 days before the trip, is useful, but closer to the trip departure is better.

Recommended medication dosing to prevent and treat altitude illness: [26]

• AMS prevention	Acetazolamide: 125 mg twice a day; 250 mg twice a day if >100 kg. Paediatrics: 2.5 mg/kg every 12 h
• AMS treatment	Acetazolamide: 250 mg twice a day Paediatrics: 2.5 mg/kg every 12 h
• AMS, HACE prevention	Dexamethasone: 2 mg every 6 h or 4 mg every 12 h Pediatrics: Should not be used for prophylaxis
• AMS, HACE treatment	AMS: Dexamethasone 4 mg every 6 h HACE: Dexamethasone 8 mg once, then 4 mg every 6 h Pediatrics: Dexamethasone 0.15 mg/kg/dose every 6 h up to 4 mg
• HAPE prevention and treatment	Nifedipine 30 mg SR version every 12 h
• HAPE prevention	Tadalafil 10 mg twice a day Sildenafil 50 mg every 8 h

References

1. Guyton and Hall. Text book of medical physiology. 12th ed. Philadelphia: Elsevier. p. 527–34. chapter 43
2. Luks AM. Physiology in medicine: a physiologic approach to prevention and treatment of acute high-altitude illnesses. J Appl Physiol. 2015;118:509–19.
3. Lumb A. Nunn's applied respiratory physiology. 9th ed. Elsevier; 2010. chapter 16. p. 205–17.
4. McGraw-Hill Education. Harrison's principles of internal medicine, vol. 2. 20th ed. McGraw-Hill Education; 2018. chapter 453. p. 3333–46.

5. Wolfel EE, Levine BD. The cardiovascular system at high altitude. In: Hornbein TF, Schoene RB, editors. High altitude: an exploration of human adaptation. New York: Marcel Dekker; 2001.
6. Naeje R. Physiological adaptation of the cardiovascular system to high altitude. Prog Cardiovasc Dis. 2010;52:456–66.
7. Zhu L, Fan M. Impact of plateau environment hypoxia on human cognitive function and intervention measures. Chin J Pharmacol Toxicol. 2017;31:87–92.
8. Pugh LGCE. Blood volume and haemoglobin concentration at altitudes above 18,000 ft. (5500 m). J Physiol. 1964;170:344–54.
9. Wagner PD. A theoretical analysis of factors determining VO2 Max at sea level and altitude. Respir Physiol. 1996;106:329–43.
10. Singh MV, Salhan AK, Rawal SB, Tyagi AK, Kumar N, Verma SS, et al. Blood gases, hematology, and renal blood flow during prolonged mountain sojourns at 3500 and 5800m. Aviat Space Environ Med. 2009;74:533–6.
11. Palubiski LM, O'Halloran KD, O'Neill J. Renal physiological adaptation to high altitude: a systematic review. Front Physiol. 2020;11:756. https://doi.org/10.3389/fphys.2020.00756.
12. Vij A. Effect of prolonged stay at high altitude on platelet aggregation and fibrinogen levels. Platelets. 2009;20:421–7.
13. Lehmann T, Mairbaurl H, Pleisch B, Maggiorni M, Bartsch P, Reinhart WH. Platelet count and function at high altitude and in high-altitude pulmonary edema. J Appl Physiol. 2006;100(2):690–4.
14. Anand A, Jha S, Saha A, Sharma V, Adya C. Thrombosis as a complication of extended stay at high altitude. Natl Med J India. 2001;14:197–201.
15. Wani Z, Sharma M. Anesthesia considerations: high altitude and anesthesia. J Card Crit Care. 2017;1:30–3.
16. Miller RD. Md Ms, Md MPBasics of Anesthesia, vol. 83. 6th ed. Philadelphia, PA: Saunders; 2011. p. 202–3.
17. Safar P, Tenecila R. High altitude physiology in relation to anesthesia and inhalational therapy. Anesthesiology. 1964;35:515–31.
18. Rodriquez D Jr, Branson RD, Dorlac W, Dorlac G, Barnes SA, Johannigman JA. Effects of simulated altitude on ventilator performance. J Trauma. 2009;66:S172-7. https://doi.org/10.1097/TA.0b013e31819cdbd1.
19. Blakeman T, Britton T, Rodriquez D, Branson R. Performance of portable ventilators at altitude. J Trauma Acute Care Surg. 2014;77:S151-5. https://doi.org/10.1097/TA.0000000000000379.
20. Blancher M, Repellin M, Maignan M, Clapé C, Perrin A, Labarère J, et al. Accuracy of low-weight versus standard syringe infusion pump devices depending on altitude. Scand J Trauma Resusc Emerg Med. 2019;27:65. https://doi.org/10.1186/s13049-019-0643-1.
21. King BR, Goss PW, Paterson MA, Crock PA, Anderson DG. Changes in altitude cause unintended insulin delivery from insulin pumps: mechanisms and implications. Diabetes Care. 2011;34:1932–3. https://doi.org/10.2337/dc11-0139.
22. Myers KS, Gardner-Thorpe C. Problems with capnography at high altitude. Anesthesia. 2004;59:69–72. https://doi.org/10.1111/j.1365-2044.2004.03447.
23. Luks M, Swenson ER. Pulse oximetry at high altitude Andrew. High Alt Med Biol. 2011;12:109–19.
24. Luks AM, McIntosh SE, Grissom CK, Auerbach PS, Rodway GW, Schoene RB, et al. Wilderness medical society consensus guidelines for the prevention and treatment of acute altitude illness. Wilderness Environ Med. 2010;21:146–55.
25. Hackett PH, Shlim DR. High-altitude travel & altitude illness. In: Brunette GW, Nemhauser JB, editors. Disease control and prevention. CDC yellow book 2020: health information for international travel. New York: Oxford University Press; 2017.
26. Butterworth JF. Morgan & Mikhail's clinical anesthesiology, vol. 63. 5th ed. McGraw-Hill; 2013. p. 170.

Chapter 21
High Altitude Sickness Not a Challenge but a Risk

Souvik Mukherjee

Being hit by acute mountain sickness made me realize that it can happen to anyone.

I was leading a trek to Kalindi Khal. The day before going to the Kalindi Khal we were on acclimatization hold at Vasuki Taal. My SpO2 (Oxygen Saturation) level was 99%. My pulse rate was 67.

With Gods grace weather cleared up quite a bit on the pass crossing day. It was extremely sunny, and the entire trail was covered with 2–3 feet of snow.

We started the pass crossing climb at 6:08 a.m. towards Khar Pathar at 17,000 Ft.

While Progressing ahead, realized that around 3 trekkers were too slow and were lagging behind.

So, to check on them I quickly went 1 km up towards the pass. It was a 15 minutes' walk up again.

After a while I got a throbbing headache and I started feeling pukish. The headache soon turned severe. It was a 9 on a scale of 1 to 10. I was extremely fatigued, dehydrated, and hungry at that time.

I immediately took Paracetamol 650 and Pan-D started munching some chocolates. Because of my condition I took the call of reshuffling the team. I went ahead with the lead guide descending as quickly as possible. My SpO2 level was around 90% at the altitude of 16,250 ft.

As I reached back at Meru Glacier campsite, I ate some more snacks, and hydrated self and rested for 1 h. By then the headache had subsided considerably. I was still feeling fatigued.

My SpO2 level came up to 95% at 14,000 ft. By night time my headache and all other symptoms had subsided.

An incident like this makes me realize how AMS can hit anyone. I have been in a high-altitude region for quite some time. I had even done a recce of the Kalindi Khal acclimatization trail up to 16,000 ft. on previous day and day before.

S. Mukherjee (✉)
Center of Exellence, Ghaziabad, India

J. Hidalgo et al. (eds.), *High Altitude Medicine*,
https://doi.org/10.1007/978-3-031-35092-4_21

What went wrong was not eating enough breakfast and lunch on the glacier crossing day. I also drank very little water till I reached the 17,000 Ft.

When you have varicose veins, your mind is consistently searching for answers. You may find yourself looking for clues about what helps you to feel more comfortable, and about what causes discomfort to increase. We often look at factors such as weight and how long we sit or stand, but did you know that there may also be a correlation with the presentation of venous insufficiency and where you are located at any given moment?

Things Are Heating up

It is common for people to look at the ways that cold weather affects the body. Joints seem to get a little more creeky and cranky when the temperature drops. When it comes to veins, though, pay attention to how you feel when things heat up. Some studies indicate increased symptoms and complications with varicose veins in warmer temperatures. These include not only that sense of pressure, but also cramping in the leg muscles, swelling, and itching.

Knowing your Risks and Acting Accordingly

So, if varicose veins become more symptomatic in hot weather, the next step is to take appropriate action. This does not mean staying indoors in the nice, cool, air-conditioning. Physical activity is integral to managing vein health. To offset the effects of heat, experts recommend taking extra care to hydrate. When we drink plenty of water, we have more water and salt running through the body; its muscles and tissues, and even the blood. Hot weather makes us sweat, which decreases salt-levels, which causes the body to retain fluids. Fluid retention equals swelling. Swelling means pooling blood. You see the pattern.

Going to New Heights

We're relatively safe from exorbitant heat now that summer is behind us, but many people may be planning a winter vacation that will take them to new heights. Heading up to the top of a mountain, or traveling by plane to see loved-ones, may feel unnerving if you've heard that altitude will affect the presentation of varicose veins. Fortunately, this is more myth than fact. Yes, flying could cause varicose veins to feel more "pent-up" or swollen. However, experts believe that he may have much more to do with the lack of movement than altitude. If you plan to fly, take time to walk during layovers, or before and after flights. Also, when possible, get up and move around the cabin to prevent stagnation in the lower extremities.

A Beginner's Guide to Acute Mountain Sickness

Picture this, you're enjoying a beautiful trek through a Snow line above 12,000 Ft when suddenly your partner complains of a headache and feels a little dizzy. You get to your Camp site and he doesn't feel like eating anything. Sound familiar? He might be suffering from Acute Mountain Sickness or AMS. AMS is one of the most common risks that trekkers face while trekking at high altitudes. This usually occurs at altitudes above 2500 m and is the degradation of health due to the gain in altitude (Pictures 21.1, 21.2, 21.3, 21.4, 21.5, 21.6 and 21.7).

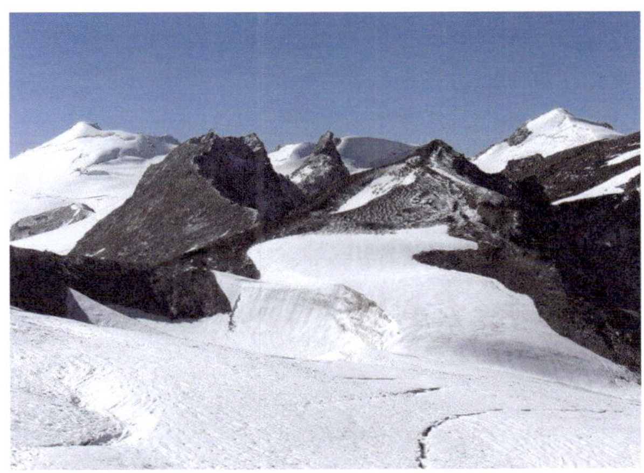

Picture 21.1 Himalayan Glacier, Picture courtesy of: **Souvik Mukherjee**

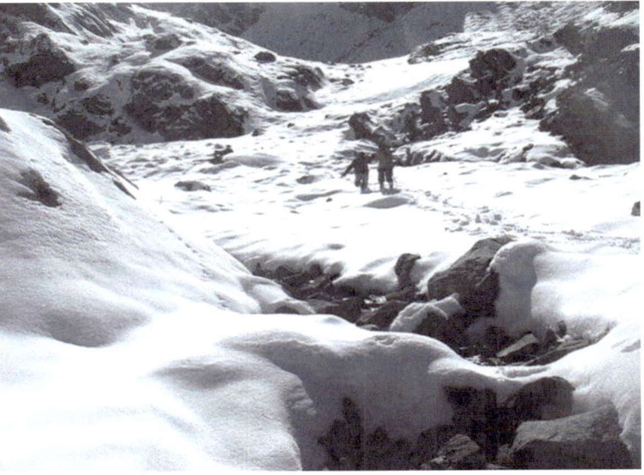

Picture 21.2 Himalayan Glacier, Picture courtesy of: **Souvik Mukherjee**

Picture 21.3 The peak as in heaven, Picture courtesy of: **Souvik Mukherjee**

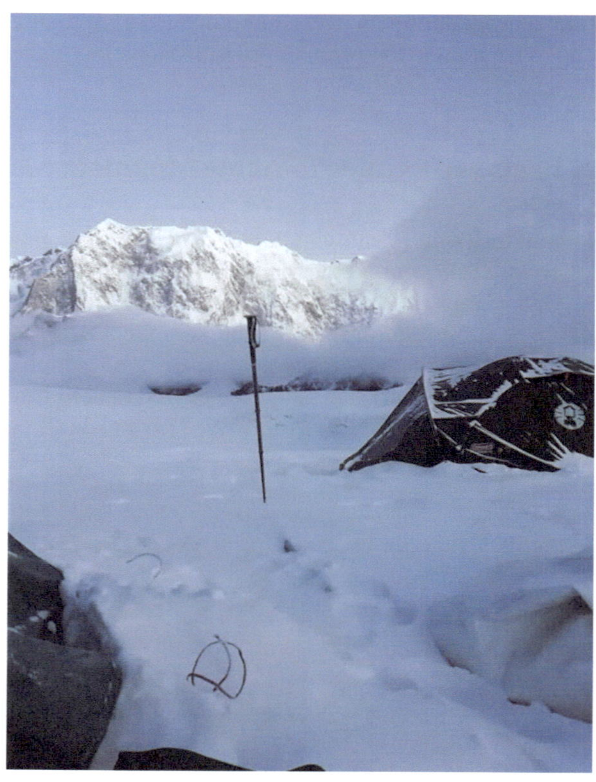

Picture 21.4 The trail, Picture courtesy of: **Souvik Mukherjee**

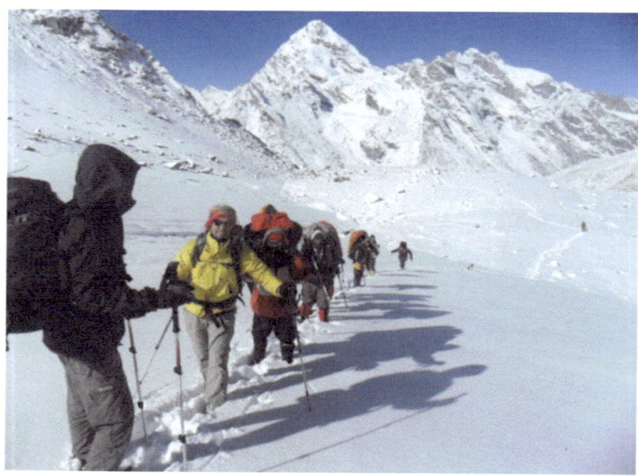

Why does it happen? When one gains altitude, the density of air reduces correspondingly reducing the amount of oxygen absorbed by the lungs with each breath. AMS occurs as the body does not have time to adjust to this reduction of oxygen. Mild AMS is a common phenomenon, and the symptoms are usually easy to identify.

Picture 21.5 The Trail, Picture courtesy of: **Souvik Mukherjee**

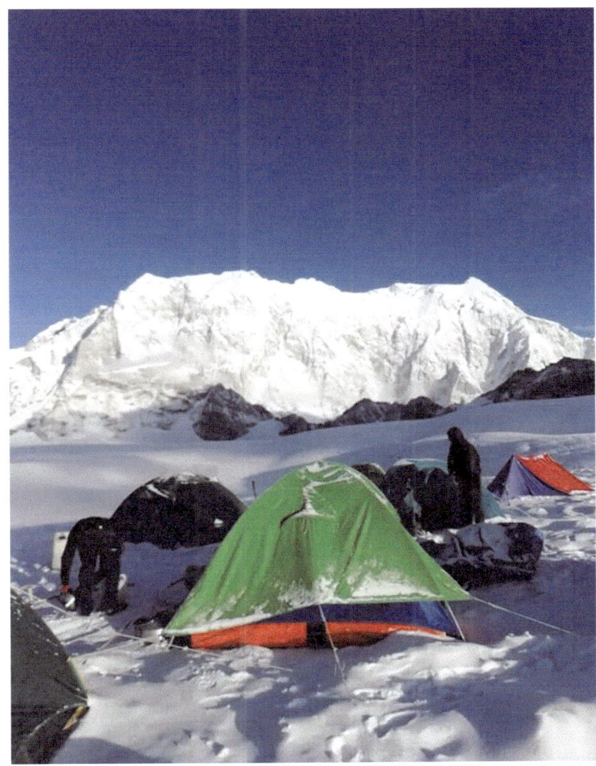

Picture 21.6 The tent, Picture courtesy of: **Souvik Mukherjee**

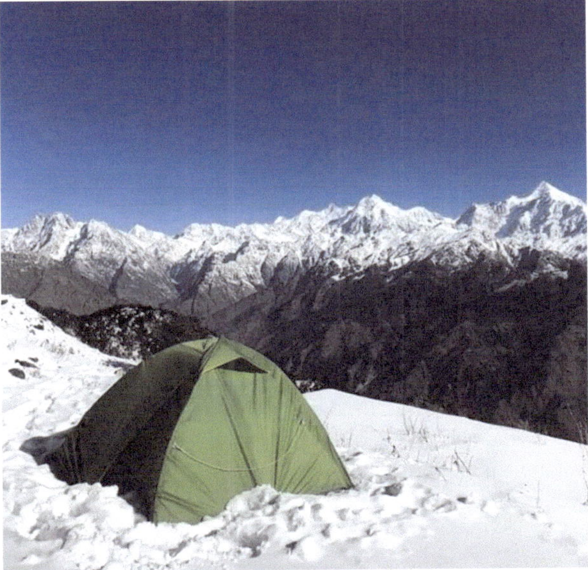

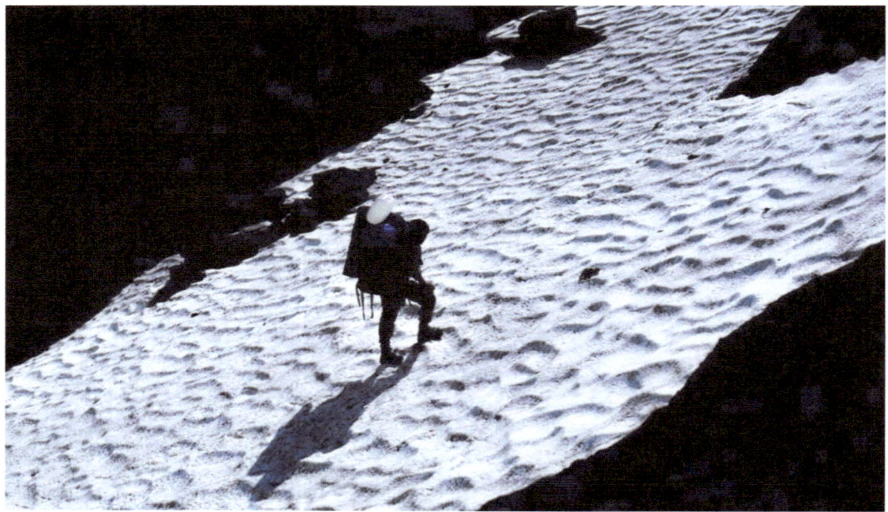

Picture 21.7 The tireless climber, Picture courtesy of: **Souvik Mukherjee**

By far the best method to prevent AMS is through a process known as acclimatization however, Drugs such as Diamox are effective at reducing the symptoms.

Acclimatization is the process in which an individual adjusts to a change in its altitude, allowing it to maintain performance across a range of environmental conditions. Some basic principles for acclimatization are:

Don't gain altitude too fast i.e. maintain a slow pace while trekking at high altitudes

- Avoid exerting yourself for the first 24 h at a high altitude
- Take one acclimatization or rest day for roughly every 900 ft. gain in altitude
- "Climb High and sleep low." You can climb more than 1000 feet (305 m) in a day as long as you come back down and sleep at a lower altitude.
- Stay properly hydrated. Acclimatization is often accompanied by fluid loss, so you need to drink lots of fluids to remain properly hydrated (at least 3–4 L/day). Urine output should be copious and clear.
- Avoid gaining altitude if you have some symptoms of AMS.
- Keep in mind that different people will acclimatize at different rates and the group must ensure that everyone is properly adjusted to the altitude before moving higher.

There are more to it from the Medical point of view. Above are from my experience as an High Altitude trekker for 20 plus years. Have been affected by AMS and have witnessed and rescued few seasoned trekkers as well. High Altitude Sickness should not be taken lightly, Every trekker or Mountaineer must know the symptoms to prevent further deuteration.

A Lone Ranger
Souvik Mukherjee
I am Project Management Professional in the field of Risk & Compliance with HCL Tech. Been a Mountaineer and Search & Rescue Specialist have served Indian Armed Forces.

Index

J. Hidalgo et al. (eds.), *High Altitude Medicine*,
https://doi.org/10.1007/978-3-031-35092-4

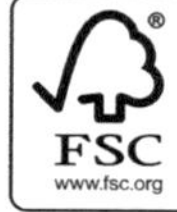